1 CD-ROM

Occupational Therapy and Dementia Care

Occupational Therapy and Dementia Care

THE HOME ENVIRONMENTAL SKILL-BUILDING PROGRAM FOR INDIVIDUALS AND FAMILIES

Laura N. Gitlin, PhD, and
Mary A. Corcoran, PhD, OTR/L, FAOTA

With Contributions by
Yeon Kyung Chee, PhD; Pamalyn Kearney, MS, OTR/L;
Rosalyn S. Lipsitt, MHL, OTR/L; Geri Shaw, OTR/L;
Susan Toth-Cohen, PhD, OTR/L; and Tracey Vause Earland, MS, OTR/L

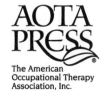

AOTA PRESS
The American
Occupational Therapy
Association, Inc.

Vision Statement

AOTA advances occupational therapy as the preeminent profession in promoting the health, productivity, and quality of life of individuals and society through the therapeutic application of occupation.

Mission Statement

The American Occupational Therapy Association advances the quality, availability, use, and support of occupational therapy through standard-setting, advocacy, education, and research on behalf of its members and the public.

AOTA Staff

Frederick P. Somers, Executive Director
Christopher M. Bluhm, Chief Operating Officer
Audrey Rothstein, Director, Marketing and Communications

Chris Davis, Managing Editor, AOTA Press
Barbara Dickson, Production Editor

Robert A. Sacheli, Manager, Creative Services
Sarah E. Ely, Book Production Coordinator

Marge Wasson, Marketing Manager
Elizabeth Sarcia, Marketing Specialist

American Occupational Therapy Association, Inc.
4720 Montgomery Lane
Bethesda, MD 20814
Phone: 301-652-AOTA (2682)
TDD: 800-377-8555
Fax: 301-652-7711
www.aota.org
To order: 1-877-404-AOTA (2682)

Disclaimers

This publication is designed to provide accurate and authoritative information in regard to the subject matter covered. It is sold or distributed with the understanding that the publisher is not engaged in rendering legal, accounting, or other professional service. If legal advice or other expert assistance is required, the services of a competent professional person should be sought.
— *From the Declaration of Principles jointly adopted by the American Bar Association*
  and a Committee of Publishers and Associations

It is the objective of the American Occupational Therapy Association to be a forum for free expression and interchange of ideas. The opinions expressed by the contributors to this work are their own and not necessarily those of the American Occupational Therapy Association.

ISBN: 1-56900-203-7

Library of Congress Control Number: 2005923702

Design by Sarah E. Ely
Composition by Electronic Quill, Silver Spring, MD
Printed by Boyd Printing, Albany, NY

Contents

PART III: Fundamentals of the Intervention

PART IV: Practicalities of Implementing the Home Environmental Skill-Building Program

APPENDIXES

List of Tables, Figures, Exhibits, Models, and Case Examples

Preface

Dementia is a devastating, progressive, terminal disease that currently affects more than 4 million adults in the United States. This number is expected to increase exponentially to 13 million people in the near future as the Baby Boom generation reaches retirement age.

The vast majority of people with dementia lives in the community at large and eventually is assisted by family members who become the "hidden" patients along the pathway of the disease. Families face many challenges—adjusting to and coping with the diagnosis; learning how to strike the right balance between doing for the person with dementia and providing oversight yet autonomy; safe-proofing the home; ensuring appropriate hydration and nutrition; assisting with toileting, bathing, and grooming; and creating meaning, life quality, and dignity, all while managing their own stress, fatigue, and profound sadness and loss.

Families become involved in the care of people with dementia in a progressive fashion, such that, as the disease advances, more hands-on assistance and oversight are increasingly required, leading many to live what is often referred to as the "36-hour" day.[1] Thus, the impact of dementia on family members is typically profound, placing families at significant financial, emotional, and physical health risk, including mortality.

Supporting people with dementia and their family members in managing the disease process and maximizing their life quality is complex, necessitating a multidisciplinary and team approach among health and human services professionals. Although new understandings of the etiology of dementia are emerging with hope for treatment on the horizon, we remain now and into the near future in desperate need of approaches for helping people with dementia and families in their daily heroic efforts.

---

[1]Mace, N. L., & Rabins, P. V. (1981). *The 36-hour day: A family guide to caring for persons with Alzheimer's disease, related dementing illnesses, and memory loss in later life.* Baltimore, MD: Johns Hopkins University Press.

Our research has been in the forefront of creating the evidence to show that occupational therapy should and must be a primary player—a critical member of the multidisciplinary management team in dementia care. This book, based on more than 15 years of systematic research on the role of occupational therapy in helping families manage dementia care at home, presents an evidence-based intervention that can be implemented by therapists in home care or in a variety of settings such as assisted living and in consultation with other health and human services professionals. The research evidence indisputably shows that occupational therapy, long neglected in the clinical care of this dyad, has a critical role in maintaining the ability of families to provide care at home.

We have been on a long journey—we have been in and out of the homes and lives of many families and individuals with dementia—we have been gripped by the devastation of the disease, as well as by the strength, spirit, creativity, innovation, grace, and dignity of families. Our research goal, as reflected in the chapters that follow, is to bridge academic and clinical acumen to advance the quality of life of families and individuals with dementia. Our intent is to provide the empirical support and foundation by which occupational therapy and other health professionals can make a real-world difference in dementia care.

—Laura N. Gitlin, PhD

Acknowledgments

The intervention that we present here, the Home Environmental Skill-Building Program (ESP), began with a pilot study initially supported in part by funds from the American Occupational Therapy Foundation. This initial pilot study provided the basis for refining the intervention and testing it using randomized clinical trial methodology. These randomized trials and other related studies to evaluate different components of the intervention have been supported in part by funds from the National Institute on Aging (5-U01-AG13265, RO1-AG10947, and R03-AG15517-01). More recently, building on the knowledge gained from these studies, we are currently experimenting with different approaches to target troublesome behaviors associated with dementia (National Institute on Aging and National Institute on Nursing Research, R01-AG22254) and with strategies for enhancing the quality of life of individuals with dementia living at home (National Institute on Mental Health, 1-R21-MH069425). We gratefully acknowledge and thank our funding sources for continued support, without which this research effort could not have been undertaken.

We also acknowledge our gratitude to the occupational therapists who worked with us in pilot testing and then formally testing and refining the approach reported here. Their creativity, impressive clinical reasoning, and commitment significantly contributed to the success of this project.

Finally, it is the families and the individuals with this terrible disease for whom we must ultimately thank for opening up their homes and revealing their lives to us. We hope, in turn, to have made at least a small positive difference in their daily struggles.

Introduction

The Home Environmental Skill-Building Program (ESP)

Laura N. Gitlin, PhD
Mary A. Corcoran, PhD, OTR/L, FAOTA
Susan Toth-Cohen, PhD, OTR/L

In this book, we present an intervention, the Home Environmental Skill-Building Program (ESP), which has been rigorously tested over the past 15 years using randomized, controlled-trial methodology by the Center for Applied Research on Aging and Health in collaboration with the Department of Occupational Therapy, Jefferson College of Health Professions at Thomas Jefferson University in Philadelphia. We present the background information, theoretical frameworks, and essential elements of ESP, an important non-pharmacological approach to improving the quality of life of families and individuals dealing with this disease.

ESP is an intervention that is best delivered by occupational therapists; nevertheless, the principles of ESP and the vision that it embraces about the critical role of the physical and social environment in managing day-to-day care should be of interest and adapted for use by other health and human services professionals.

ABOUT THE INTERVENTION

The intervention presented here originally was designed for use with caregivers who live at home and provide care to a person with dementia. Although occupational therapists have an important intervening role across the trajectory of decline associated with dementia, the ESP primarily targets families of people who are at the mild–moderate to moderate–severe stages of the disease process, stages in which caregivers become increasingly involved in day-to-day dementia care.

Essentially, the ESP helps family caregivers understand the effects of physical and social environmental factors on people with reduced cognitive abilities, including the physical set-up of the home and caregiver communication style. Further, ESP is designed to help caregivers learn how to problem-solve and devise solutions involving modifications of different dimensions of home life, including

- The physical environment (how objects are used),
- The task environment (how daily routines and activities are carried out), and
- The social environment (how other family members and informal and formal supports can be organized and involved in daily care).

Specifically, ESP engages caregivers in building important skills such as problem-solving, communication, and environmental simplification and provides technical support for implementing specific solutions to targeted care challenges. Caregivers are empowered to engage their family members in work and leisure activities, support their participation in daily self-care, minimize or control troublesome behaviors (e.g., resistance to care, wandering, mobility difficulties), and manage their own issues of fatigue and stress. The problem areas that are addressed in ESP reflect concerns identified by caregivers themselves. The strategies that are introduced to address each concern or problem area are customized to the particular physical and social caregiving context and environment of the home. The strategies are designed to minimize disparities between external or environmental demands and the capabilities of people with dementia, referred to here as care recipients, as well as enable caregivers to enhance predictability and control within their life space.

With regard to the procedural aspects or delivery characteristics, ESP consists of up to five or six 1 ½-hour home visits and one 20- to 30-minute telephone contact that occur over a 6-month period and is referred to as the *active phase.* Sessions during this phase are spaced according to caregiver availability and need as well as the occupational therapist's clinical reasoning as to the best pacing of visits to enable skills to be adapted, practiced, and integrated by families. The active phase can be followed by additional telephone and in-home contact if necessary, referred to in our research as the *maintenance phase.* In our research (see Chapter 2), the maintenance phase consisted of three telephone contacts and one home visit over an additional 6-month period to help caregivers maintain their newly learned skills and generalize strategies to emerging difficulties. However, our research shows that, for some caregivers, more hands-on opportunities (e.g., additional in-home visits) might be necessary and more effective than telephone check-ins.

ESP is designed as a stand-alone intervention. However, families caring for people with dementia have many different needs and thus can benefit from a wide range of services. As such, ESP can and should be combined or integrated with other intervention approaches, including psychoeducational counseling, information and referral, or other supportive services. The essential characteristics of ESP are presented in Exhibit I.1.

ESP AS A PRACTICE FRAMEWORK

ESP is similar in approach to other programs of public health import that involve skill-building, behavioral change, and behavioral management principles for

EXHIBIT I.1. Essential Characteristics of the ESP Intervention

- Is theory based
- Is replicable
- Has standard components
- Has strategies tailored to specific family concerns
- Offers hands-on skill training in
  - Problem-solving
  - Communication
  - Task simplification
  - Stress management
  - Modification of physical and social environmental factors.

Note. ESP = Home Environmental Skill-Building Program.

managing chronic and progressive diseases. In these types of health and behavioral change programs (e.g., exercise, smoking cessation, medication management), the essential principles for intervention, as in ESP, include the assessment and specification of a particular problem or target behavior, collaborative goal setting and identification of barriers and motivating factors, provision of personalized skills as needed, and follow-up support (Glasgow et al., 1999).

ESP follows these essential elements and thus is consistent with other behavioral change strategies. Nevertheless, to understand ESP as an evidence-based therapeutic approach within occupational therapy, we draw on the *Occupational Therapy Practice Framework: Domain and Process* and its associated diagram (American Occupational Therapy Association, 2002) and adopt it to the specific context of intervening with family caregivers and people with dementia living at home (Figure I.1).

The overall goal of ESP, as shown in the box at the top center of the diagram shown in Figure I.1, is to address the quality of life and occupational performance of both the family caregiver and individual with dementia (referred to here as caregiver–care recipient, or CG–CR, dyad). Moving clockwise from the top box to the outer right box is the implementation of ESP, which involves the basic steps of problem identification, implementation of strategies, and strategy refinement. The next outer box moving clockwise and to the left indicates that success of ESP is based on initial and ongoing analysis of the occupational profiles and independent and interactive performance of both caregiver and care recipient. The *Framework* and the arrows connecting the three outer

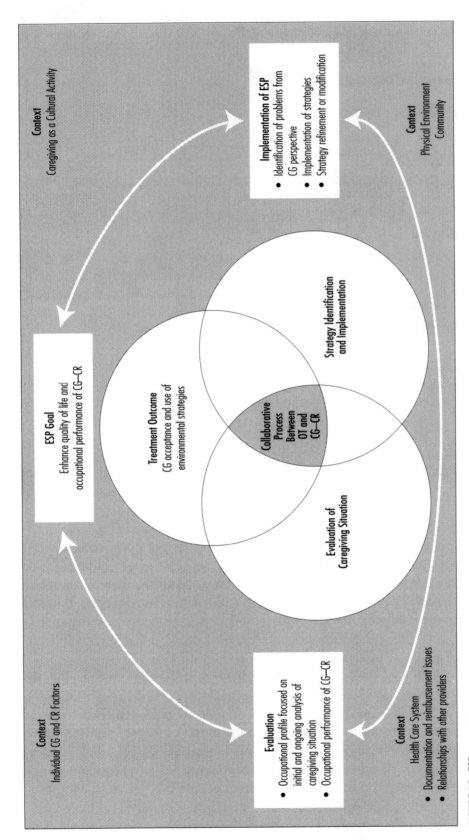

FIGURE I.1. ESP processes.

Note. ESP = Home Environmental Skill-Building Program; CG = caregiver; CR = care recipient (person with dementia).

Adapted from American Occupational Therapy Association. (2002). Occupational therapy practice framework: Domain and process. *American Journal of Occupational Therapy, 56,* 609–639.

Text within figure:

Context
Caregiving as a Cultural Activity

Implementation of ESP
• Identification of problems from CG perspective
• Implementation of strategies
• Strategy refinement or modification

Context
Physical Environment
Community

Context
Individual CG and CR Factors

ESP Goal
Enhance quality of life and occupational performance of CG–CR

Strategy Identification and Implementation

Treatment Outcome
CG acceptance and use of environmental strategies

Collaborative Process Between OT and CG–CR

Evaluation of Caregiving Situation

Evaluation
• Occupational profile focused on initial and ongoing analysis of caregiving situation
• Occupational performance of CG–CR

Context
Health Care System
• Documentation and reimbursement issues
• Relationships with other providers

boxes indicate the interactive and nonlinear nature of the ESP and the influence of one component on the other.

The three inner-connected circles (evaluation, strategy implementation, and treatment outcome) suggest that the intervention is an iterative process. At the heart of ESP is the therapeutic relationship or collaborative process that evolves between therapist and families.

THE ESP PROCESS

As the model suggests, evaluation, implementation, and ongoing reassessment are fluid, dynamic processes similar to traditional occupational therapy models. Let's examine each component of the model more carefully.

Evaluation of the Caregiving Situation

As in the *Occupational Therapy Practice Framework*, the ESP process begins with a two-step evaluation that sets the stage for that which follows (AOTA, 2002, p. 615). This process is intended to develop a holistic understanding of the overall caregiving situation on which to base the ESP for a particular CG–CR situation.

The first step is an assessment of the occupational profile of the caregiver and care recipient. An understanding of CG–CR concerns, problems, and risks is critical to the success of the intervention process. Specifically, this initial step provides an understanding of the CG–CR occupational history, patterns of daily living, interests, values, needs, and daily concerns. The occupational profile also involves obtaining specific information about the way in which caregivers define dementia, view their role, and define their own personal goals for caring. The specific areas of concern about caregiving are identified, and initial priorities for treatment are determined.

The second step is to analyze the occupational performance of CG–CR and to determine target areas for skill development. Actual performance of the caregiver during specific caregiving tasks is observed in context to identify factors that support and hinder performance of both caregiver and care recipient. Performance skills, performance patterns, context or contexts, activity demands, and CG–CR factors are all considered, but only selected aspects may be specifically assessed based on the caregiver's self-identified concerns (Chapters 7 and 8 provide a description of assessment approaches).

Implementation of ESP

The next aspect of the ESP process involves developing a treatment plan to guide treatment actions. This is developed in collaboration with the caregiver (and care recipient, if possible). Implementation strategies are rooted in three theoretical frameworks, including personal control, competence–environmental–press, and stress–health process (see Chapter 5). For each targeted problem area, a specific treatment outcome is identified, discussed, confirmed, and agreed on with the caregiver (e.g., reduction of number of incontinence incidents, more time for self each week). Based on the identified treatment outcomes, specific strategies are developed, implemented, and refined to improve CG–CR performance. CG–CR responses are monitored, and strategies are added, refined, modified, or removed based on continual review (refer to Chapters 8 and 9).

Caregiver Acceptance and Use of Environmental Strategies

Occupational therapists continue to observe and monitor CG–CR responses to treatment strategies and outcomes relative to treatment goals. Initial responses (e.g., rejection, acceptance, modification of strategies) determine next treatment steps (e.g., refinement of strategies, reinforcement and continued practice, new strategies introduced, new problem area targeted). The acceptance and use of strategies by caregivers, referred to as the "enactment" of treatment (Burgio et al., 2001), is an important step in the intervention process that is necessary to achieve a positive improvement in occupational performance.

Context

Finally, it is important to note that consistent with the *Occupational Therapy Practice Framework* (AOTA, 2002), the ESP service delivery process takes place within multiple contexts. We view context as an overarching, underlying, and embedded influence on the process of service implementation. The context reflects the characteristics of families (e.g., education, religiosity) and the illness (e.g., cognitive status, impairment, preserved capabilities), micro-level cultural activity (e.g., familial and home life, the physical environment, community), and macro-level factors such as health care system features (e.g., availability of respite, reimbursement for needed services, long-term-care policy, community-based programs and supports). Context influences the service delivery process as well as the caregiver's specific engagement and performance patterns.

Each component of the ESP practice framework is discussed in more detail in the chapters that follow.

TRANSITIONS: FROM "BENCH TO BED" TO HOME

Moving an intervention from bench to bed to home so to speak, or from a controlled research environment to real-world practice, requires adjustments to a "research protocol." Nevertheless, to make adjustments to the intervention to fit practice and the restrictions that may be imposed by third-party insurers, occupational therapists must not change several critical elements or intervention principles of ESP. These immutable principles, shown in Exhibit I.2, represent the essential or fundamental elements of ESP without which we do not believe intervention efforts will be effective. We view these principles as core to what

EXHIBIT I.2. Immutable ESP Intervention Principles

- Assessment and treatment of the dyad (CG and CR)
- Use of a collaborative framework in which CGs are viewed as partners in the process (e.g., lay practitioners)
- Minimum of 2 treatment sessions with a recommendation of at least 3–6 sessions to allow for assessment, introduction of strategies, and then their modification or refinement
- Use of problem-solving that actively involves CGs (and CRs, if possible)
- Introduction of linguistically and culturally appropriate customized strategies to address CG-identified target problem areas
- Active engagement of CGs in skill-training through use of modeling, demonstration, and role-play.

Note. ESP = Home Environmental Skill-Building Program; CG = caregiver; CR = care recipient (person with dementia).

may be referred to as the mechanism of action, or why and how the intervention may work.

Although ESP is designed as a home-based approach, its essential elements are easily transferable to other care contexts such as outpatient rehabilitation or consultative contexts in adult day centers or assisted-living facilities especially designed for people with dementia.

THERAPEUTIC STANCE

The trajectory of dementia and hence caregiving is complex and ultimately reflects the confluence of many factors. Of utmost importance is the context, including a family's underlying culture; financial, social, and emotional resources; and also the unique manifestations of the disease. On entering the home or life space of the CG–CR dyad, one is immediately confronted by the fluidity and magnitude of the day-to-day challenges of living with dementia. Thus, ESP requires reflective practitioners who are willing and capable of being non-prescriptive, who relish the challenge of discovery and putting together bits of information to derive a meaningful set of tailored strategies that has the potential of making a difference in a complex context. To this end, we recommend that health professionals who use the ESP seek colleagues to share cases and problem solve to share strategies and derive a more in-depth understanding as to what might work best and for whom. We found the debriefing process very important, and sharing clinical stories has been shown to enhance the ability of therapists to be reflective, a critical stance of therapists who want to implement ESP (Mattingly & Fleming, 1994; Parham, 1987; Slater & Cohn, 1991). Moreover, case sharing assists in developing individualized approaches for treating clients (Mattingly & Gillette, 1991).

HOW TO USE THIS BOOK

Each section and chapter moves readers through the essential elements of the ESP Practice Framework as discussed briefly above and shown in Figure I.1. As such, the book is organized into four major sections. Part I provides an overview of the research evidence in support of the approach that is subsequently presented and provides the justifications for implementing ESP; Part II provides an important and basic overview of the main characteristics of dementia as a disease process and its impact on caregiving; Part III represents the core or heart of the matter, a detailed description of the intervention (the "how-to" piece); and Part IV concludes the book with considerations about the practicalities of implementing the ESP in real-world contexts.

The appendices are particularly useful—they contain the essential assessment tools and resources necessary for implementing the intervention as well as related reference material for readers who wish to further their understanding of environmental principles of care.

Each chapter incrementally builds on the other in a logical sequence. Each chapter also can stand alone to maximize its utility and adaptability for use in training, educational, and continuing education programming.

WHO SHOULD USE THIS BOOK

This book is designed principally for use by occupational therapists and, in particular, practitioners at the intermediate and advanced levels. Nevertheless, graduate students in occupational therapy as well as other health and human services professionals also may find this book a useful guide for understanding the role and impact of the physical and social environment in dementia care, strategies that can minimize environmental stressors in the home, and the unique role of occupational therapists in the management of the disease process and concomitant caregiver concerns.

REFERENCES

American Occupational Therapy Association. (2002). Occupational therapy practice framework: Domain and process. *American Journal of Occupational Therapy, 56*, 609–639.

Burgio, L., Corcoran, M., Lichstein, K. L., Nichols, L., Czaja, S., Gallagher- Thompson, D., et al. (2001). Judging outcomes in psychosocial interventions for dementia caregivers: The problem of treatment implementation. *The Gerontologist, 41*, 481–489.

Glasgow, R. E., Wagner, E., Kaplan, R., Vinicor, F., Smith, L., & Norman, J. (1999). If diabetes is a public health problem, why not treat it as one? A population-based approach to chronic illness. *Annals of Behavioral Medicine, 21*, 159–170.

Mattingly, C., & Fleming, M. F. (1994). *Clinical reasoning: Forms of inquiry in a therapeutic practice.* Philadelphia: F. A. Davis.

Mattingly, C., & Gillette, N. (1991). Anthroplogy, occupational therapy, and action research. *American Journal of Occupational Therapy, 45,* 972–978.

Parham, D. (1987). Toward professionalism: The reflective therapist. *American Journal of Occupational Therapy, 41,* 555–561.

Slater, D. Y., & Cohn, E. S. (1991). Staff development through analysis of practice. *American Journal of Occupational Therapy, 45,* 1038–1044.

The Research Evidence

Why Dementia?
Why Caregiving?
Why Occupational Therapy?

Laura N. Gitlin, PhD
Mary A. Corcoran, PhD, OTR/L, FAOTA

The occupational therapist really advised me. That's why it was so wonderful. Because like I said, the therapy at [the facility] was 50% my wife and 50% me. . . . They talked to me as they improved her therapy. Like, they showed me.

—Caregiving Styles Study (Corcoran) NIA R29-A613019 30501#1:142–150

In its 2003 *Progress Report on Alzheimer's Disease*, the U.S. Department of Health and Human Services highlighted the following facts:

- Four and a half million people in the United States have dementia.
- It is anticipated that 13 million people will have dementia in 2013.
- Thirty-four million people have dementia worldwide.
- One in 10 people has dementia after age 65.
- Half of people older than 85 have dementia.
- The average duration of dementia from diagnosis to death is 8 years, with a range of 4 to 20 years.
- One in four people can expect to be a caregiver for a family member with dementia.
- Dementia will touch all families in the United States by 2020.
- To date, there is no cure for dementia.

These painful facts speak to the grave public health concern and the societal and personal costs of dementia in the United States and worldwide. Dementia is a progressive, devastating, terminal disease that robs people of memory, cognition, intellectual functioning, and physical capacity. The trajectory of decline is so dramatic that dementia takes a heavy toll not only on the person with the disease but also on all who care about and for the person, and in particular the person who is primary caregiver during the 4 to 20 years, or more, that the disease persists. This chapter examines the essential characteristics of the disease process from which to highlight the specific and critical role of occupational therapists in the long-term care of this population.

DEMENTIA AS A PUBLIC HEALTH CONCERN

Several characteristics of dementia highlight why dementia has become a major public health concern and, in turn, support the added value of occupational therapy in dementia care. These include

- The unpredictable course of the disease,
- Its long duration,
- The characteristic behavioral disturbances,
- The need for around-the-clock care,
- The costs of the disease to society, and
- Varying prevalence rates across groups.

Unpredictability

Dementia does not follow a uniform or single predictable course. Although *dementia* is an umbrella term for an array of conditions or syndromes (see Chapter 3), even within a specified type of dementia (e.g., Alzheimer's disease, vascular dementia), the disease trajectory can be highly variable. Although there are general patterns and particular behavioral manifestations typical of specific and identifiable disease stages, care recipients may experience weekly or even daily fluctuations in abilities, memory, and behavioral disturbances within a spiral downward. Caregivers frequently report that "this week is a good week," or "yesterday was good, but today he can't dress himself," or "you should visit in the morning because that is when she is at her best."

For the individual with dementia, fluctuations in basic memory, judgment, and performance can be frightening, particularly in the early stage of the disease when some insight and self-awareness persist. For family members as well, the unpredictability and oscillations in performance can be very upsetting, and this aspect of the disease can be difficult to manage. The unpredictability adds to the challenges caregivers encounter in planning day-to-day life, understanding the capabilities of the affected person, and ensuring his or her safety and overall well-being.

Unpredictability also characterizes the transitions of the affected person from one stage of the disease to the next. For example, the caregiver must continually evaluate at what point it becomes unsafe for the affected family member to participate in cherished and long-standing activities such as driving, going to the corner store alone, swimming at the local health club, or riding the bus independently. Sometimes it is only after an incident that compromises the family member's safety, such as becoming lost in the neighborhood or being involved in a car accident, that the caregiver and family recognize that their loved one has reached a new stage in which the current level of autonomy is no longer viable. Family members experience great stress as they adjust to the disease's course and as they seek to exert some level of control over the immediate environment to keep things "normal" and to maximize quality of life for both their loved one and themselves.

Prolongation: The Long Goodbye

Another challenging characteristic of dementia is that it is prolonged. Families must undergo an extensive and grueling grieving process in which they become firsthand eyewitnesses to the slow deterioration of a loved one's mind and body. The disease process does not offer any respite; as it progresses, hands-on assistance and constant oversight to ensure safety and well-being become increasingly necessary. The prolonged course of the disease results in an immense financial, emotional, and social drain on families that increases psychosocial and health risks for all who provide care (Schulz & Beach, 1999).

A particular irony of dementia caregiving is that, as the disease progresses, the social networks of families typically shrink as the need for help grows. Chief among the reasons is that it customarily becomes increasingly difficult to involve others in the household because of the daily complexities associated with dementia care. For example, some individuals with dementia become paranoid or extremely agitated with "strangers" in the home, and their caregivers may avoid having visitors as a consequence.

Behavioral Disturbances

The families of people with dementia must contend with a wide range of behavioral disturbances that are considered a secondary but devastating consequence of the disease. Behaviors such as agitation, repetitive questioning, shadowing, resistance to care, and verbal or physical aggressiveness are disruptive and troubling to families and pose a safety risk to both the person affected and the caregiver. Behavioral disturbances provoke concern on other levels as well. Caregivers speak not only of the physical and emotional distress of caregiving but also, and equally important, of the ethical dilemmas that plague them at each progressive stage of the disease as they seek to preserve the dignity and personhood of the care recipient (Hasselkus, 1988). Additionally, research evidence suggests that the need to manage behaviors triggers the most financially burdensome aspect of dementia caregiving: the need for a caregiver to terminate employment, provide constant oversight, and seek additional formal or paid assistance in the home. Some behaviors, such as elopement (wandering away from the home) and incontinence, may trigger nursing home placement (Ballard, Lowery, Powell, O'Brien, & James, 2000; Boucher, 1999).

The "24/7" Caregiver

The variations and decline inherent in the disease process eventually entail what Mace and Rabins (1981) referred to as "the 36-hour day." Families find that they are "on" 24 hours a day, 7 days a week. Such intensive caregiving requires that the caregiver continually adjust his or her personal goals and daily routines, reevaluate the feasibility of continued employment and the financial implications of leaving the workforce, cope with the profound personal loss of a loved one, and recognize and adapt to what the loved one can no longer do.

A critical consequence of the continuous, never-ending quality of caregiving for a person with dementia is that family caregivers often become hidden patients who experience a range of health-related difficulties, yet another reason why the disease is a public health concern. These difficulties have been well documented in the research literature and include emotional distress, clinical depression, poor health, fatigue, and a higher rate of mortality compared with noncaregivers (Ory, Hoffman, Yee, Tennstedt, & Schulz, 1999; Schulz & Beach, 1999; Schulz, O'Brien, Bookwala, & Fleissner, 1995). Moreover, prolonged exposure to chronic stress such as that experienced in caregiving has been shown to compromise the immune system, leading to heightened risk for a wide range of diseases and to reduced reserve and capacity for recovery (Kiecolt-Glaser, Glaser, Gravenstein, Malarkey, & Sheridan, 1996; Kiecolt-Glaser, Marucha, Malarkey, Mercado, & Glaser, 1995).

Societal Costs

Dementia is a public health concern because of its cost to society in terms of both the value of caring for someone with dementia and the decreased productivity of employees who assume caregiving responsibilities. The value of services that caregivers provide has been estimated to be $197 billion per year, and the aggregate costs of caregiving in lost productivity to U.S. business is conservatively estimated to be $11.4 billion annually (1997 dollars; Metropolitan Life Insurance Company [MetLife], 1997). The economic value and impact of caregiving is thus considerable and is often not apparent (Gitlin & Schulz, 2003).

Disparities in Prevalence Across Groups

Although dementia affects all racial and ethnic groups, epidemiological studies suggest a higher prevalence in Black people than in White people, with the expectation that the number of Black people ages 65 years and older who have dementia will double to 6.9 million by 2030. Furthermore, compared with White people in the same age category, Black elderly people are more likely to be diagnosed later in the disease process and thus to miss opportunities for medical and psychosocial interventions that may benefit both the patient and the family. In view of these trends, the national Alzheimer's Association has put forth a call to action and has made numerous recommendations that are aimed at reducing health risks among Black patients with dementia and their family members, as well as patients and families with low incomes (Alzheimer's Association, 2004). One of their recommendations is for further development, testing, and implementation of in-home interventions that provide skills training to families and effective approaches for working with individuals from diverse cultural and socioeconomic groups. The collaborative and client-driven frameworks within occupational therapy in general and ESP in particular are ideal for addressing the Alzheimer's Association's recommendations and, in particular, for providing culturally sensitive and linguistically appropriate interventions to enable caregivers to manage caregiving at home.

SERVICE DELIVERY IN THE HOME

Dementia and caregiving have become a public health concern because of the number of people afflicted; the financial, emotional, social, and health affects on the person afflicted and his or her family; the societal costs; and disparities in prevalence across groups. A keen focus has emerged on finding a cure, developing effective services, and helping families manage the disease at home to not only postpone nursing home placement but also to enhance the life quality of households affected by dementia. Given that most scientists estimate a cure to be at least 20 years away, strategies for helping families effectively cope are a high priority.

The vast majority of people with dementia are cared for at home by one or more family members for the duration of the disease (Haley & Bailey, 1999), a fact that is often overlooked. Caregivers experience a wide range of service needs that change and evolve over time as their caregiving responsibilities increase, and the home, as the natural life space and context of caregiving, is an ideal setting in which to provide services to families that are designed to support their efforts to enable aging in place. Although services delivered in the home have become a routine component of long-term care for elderly patients, families rarely receive in-home formal services that address their specific needs as caregivers.

Why offer services to families in their homes? National health care trends suggest that homes and communities will increasingly serve as the primary care setting for the delivery of a vast array of health and human services to people with dementia and their family caregivers (Spitzer, 1998; Wahl & Gitlin, 2003). There are distinct advantages to providing support in the home. For example, because caregivers do not have to leave their home, it may be easier to receive help in that setting and to learn different skills for caregiving; they can learn and practice new techniques in the context in which it will be used, and they do not have to worry about care arrangements during training. Although offering help in the home of families may be beneficial, there are also unique challenges in providing services in this setting. First, such services are labor intensive; they constitute one-on-one intervention requiring the time and expertise of a health or human services professional. Second, caregivers may find it difficult to dedicate the time or to focus when a health professional is in the home while they are also attending to other family members and responsibilities. Additionally, having a stranger in the home may increase the confusion, fear, and agitation of a patient with dementia, and managing the aftermath of an in-home training session can result in additional burden for the caregiver.

Nevertheless, unexpected interruptions and behavioral difficulties that manifest during a home intervention session can serve as a critical teaching moment, enabling the occupational therapist to model a particular communication approach or to make recommendations that the caregiver can try out and receive feedback on immediately. Consequently, the advantages of an in-home session far outweigh the potential negatives, and most caregivers welcome health professionals into their homes. Caregivers rarely encounter professionals who focus on them and the issues they personally experience. Thus, caregivers tend to view a visit from an occupational therapist who is willing to listen and help in the areas that caregivers themselves identify as important as a great opportunity.

SKILLS-TRAINING OF CAREGIVERS

Most services and tested interventions for family caregivers that have been developed are derived from the perspectives of psychology that emphasize the cognitive management of the stressful situation. Research in this area has typically involved testing the effects of different psycho-educational counseling (either group or individual) involving a combination of counseling, education, stress management, and problem-solving skill development.

Recent reviews of existing caregiver interventions have concluded that a broad range of intervention strategies to address the multiple needs of caregivers at each stage of the illness trajectory remain important to test (Bourgeois, Schulz, & Burgio, 1996). Training caregivers in specific skills such as problem solving, communicating effectively, and care coordination has been identified as an important need and one that occupational therapists are uniquely qualified to address (Corcoran, 2000; Miller & Butin, 2000; Hinrichsen & Niederehe, 1994; Biegel & Schulz, 1999).

WHY OCCUPATIONAL THERAPY?

Unique Expertise

Families are the hidden patients affected by dementia, and many need help in managing their distress and a wide range of daily shifting challenges. Occupational therapists are uniquely qualified to assist families not only with the skill building they need but also in evaluating the patient with dementia to help families understand what the person is unable to do and what he or she is still capable of doing. Thus, occupational therapists are in a unique position to help families understand the disease process, set up predictable and simplified daily routines, help caregivers effectively involve and coordinate others in daily caregiving tasks, and support the preserved capabilities of people with dementia.

Occupational therapists bring important professional skills and expertise to families. They provide knowledge about the disease, help families access services, and train caregivers to use positive and productive coping strategies in adjusting to each disease stage. They are also able to teach skills in managing progressively complex behaviors and functional dependency.

Current perspectives on understanding dementia-related behaviors suggest that these behaviors are a consequence of the confluence of person-based, caregiver-centered, and environmental factors that conspire and exacerbate the underlying cognitive deficits. The Home Environmental Skill-Building Program (ESP) uses occupational therapists' unique skill set to assess these three influences and intervene with each to derive the best fit between person and home as a way to control, minimize, or manage difficult behaviors. Of importance is the therapist's knowledge of the influence of the environment on behavior and environmental strategies to compensate for declines in a person's competency.

An Emerging Area of Practice

Medicare, Medicaid, private health insurers, special education programs, vocational programs, community health and social programs, mental health systems, and other service providers recognize occupational therapy as a health and rehabilitation profession. Occupational therapists provide services to individuals in a range of health and community settings, including nursing homes, hospitals, day programs, patients' homes, hospices, and many other types of facilities and programs. This wide experience gives occupational therapy the potential to make a critical contribution to the care of people at all stages of the disease process.

The specific nature of the intervention depends on the stage of illness and the manner in which cognitive impairment is manifested in activities of daily living. Traditionally, occupational therapists have worked directly with people with cognitive impairments and have consulted with other health care providers about treatment approaches and environmental modifications. Occupational therapists help family members typically by providing education and training in specific rehabilitative approaches for their loved one.

Working directly with families who care for individuals with dementia represents a relatively new practice arena for occupational therapists. There are several reasons for the delay in entering this arena, foremost of which has been the restrictions imposed by third-party reimbursement. In the past, this has severely limited an occupational therapist's engagement with families who are not eligible to receive direct services unless they focus on functional improvement or maintenance goals for the patient with dementia. Although this remains true today, ESP, which is described in this book, involves providing training to a family that is designed to help sustain functionality of the person with dementia, thus heightening its reimbursable potential.

Another reason that occupational therapists have not traditionally worked with dementia caregivers is that they have lacked an appropriate framework and an evidence-based approach, which ESP now offers. ESP provides a dynamic approach the occupational therapist can use in evaluating the person with dementia, the caregiver, and the home environment and developing specific modifications to address caregiving challenges in collaboration with the caregiver. The occupational therapist introduces the caregiver to a problem-solving approach that involves targeting a particular behavior or problem area, understanding the impact of the environment on dementia and the targeted area, and identifying ways to simplify tasks, communication, objects, and daily routines to match a person's capabilities. As shown in Table 1.1, occupational therapists can implement a vast array of environmental strategies to benefit both the caregiver and the patient with dementia, or care recipient.

CONCLUSION

For people with dementia and their families, the home is the natural life space and context in which caregiving occurs over a prolonged time. It is an ideal setting in which to provide services to families that are designed to support their

TABLE 1.1. Examples of Environmental Strategies and Potential Benefits for Areas
of Caregiver and Care Recipient Functioning

Targeted Area of Functioning	Examples of Environmental Strategy	Potential Benefits to Person With Dementia	Potential Benefits to Caregiver
Safety of care recipient	Remove dangerous items (medications, cleaning fluids, sharp objects) Remove objects in pathways	Decreased risk of falls or ingestion of dangerous fluids	Decreased need for constant vigilance
Orientation and awareness of care recipient	Label objects Use bold solid-color placemat to contrast with white plate Use large calendars, clocks	Increased recognition of common household objects Orientation to time and day Decreased agitation	Decreased level of assistance required
Self-care of care recipient	Label and set out objects for grooming Install grab bars, tub chair Use tactile cueing to initiate activity and help with sequencing	Support for participation in daily activities of living Decreased agitation	Decreased level and type of assistance required Reduced caregiver upset
Engagement in meaningful activities of care recipient	Introduce an activity board and simplified or enlarged games Introduce activities requiring repetitive motion (e.g., bead sorting, window washing, folding clothes)	Support for engagement in meaningful activity Increased attention span Decreased agitation	Decreased need for constant vigilance Respite opportunities Decreased caregiver upset
Comfort of care recipient	Place meaningful objects to touch or look at Set up photos Set up a control center with meaningful objects to manipulate and use (e.g., glass of water, newspaper, television controls)	Decreased agitation Enhanced sustained engagement Enhanced sense of control, personhood, and comfort	Decreased need for constant vigilance Respite opportunities Decreased caregiver upset
Caregiver concerns (e.g., fatigue, guilt, inability to care for self)	Help caregiver coordinate social network to provide care Introduce routines to enable respites and to increase predictability Validate caregiver skills	Decrease agitation, facilitate ability to remain at home	Increase caregiver mastery and use of effective strategies

efforts to maintain the well-being and functionality of the family member with dementia. Helping families modify the home environment to effectively manage complex behaviors and functional dependency is an important strategy that occupational therapists are uniquely qualified to implement.

REFERENCES

Alzheimer's Association. (2004). *African-Americans and Alzheimer's disease: The silent epidemic.* Retrieved November 12, 2004, from www.alz.org/Resources/Diversity/downloads/AA_EDU-SilentEpidemic.pdf.

Ballard, C., Lowery, K., Powell, I., O'Brien, J., & James, I. (2000). Impact of behavioral and psychological symptoms of dementia on caregivers. *International Psychogeriatrics, 12*(1), 93–105.

Biegel, D. E., & Schulz, R. (1999). Caregiving and caregiver interventions in aging and mental illness. *Family Relations, 48,* 345–354.

Boucher, L. A. (1999). Disruptive behaviors in individuals with Alzheimer's disease: A behavioral approach. *American Journal of Alzheimer's Disease, 14,* 351–356.

Bourgeois, M. S., Schulz, R., & Burgio, L. (1996). Interventions for caregivers of patients with Alzheimer's disease: A review and analysis of content, process, and outcomes. *International Journal of Aging and Human Development, 43,* 35–91.

Corcoran, M. A. (2000). Enhancing the health of family caregivers: Implications for health care providers. In F. Burke & J. Laramie (Eds.), *Primary care for the older adult: A multidisciplinary approach* (pp. 578–588). St. Louis, MO: Mosby.

Gitlin, L. N., & Schulz, R. (2003, Winter). Current data, future directions: Researchers look at caregivers and caregiving. *Healthcare and Aging, 10*(4), 5–8.

Haley, W. E., & Bailey, S. (1999). Research on family caregiving in Alzheimer's disease: Implications for practice and policy. In B. Vellas & J. L. Fitten (Eds.), *Research and practice in Alzheimer's disease* (Vol. 2, pp. 321–332). Paris: Serdi Publisher.

Hasselkus, B. R. (1988). Meaning in family caregiving: Perspectives on caregiver/professional relationships. *The Gerontologist, 28,* 686–691.

Hinrichsen, G. A., & Niederehe, G. (1994). Dementia management strategies and adjustments of family members of older patients. *The Gerontologist 34,* 95–102.

Kiecolt-Glaser, J., Glaser, R., Gravenstein, S., Malarkey, W., & Sheridan, J. (1996). Chronic stress alters the immune response to influenza virus vaccine in older adults. *Proceedings of the National Academy of Sciences, USA, 93,* 3043–3047.

Kiecolt-Glaser, J. K., Marucha, P. T., Malarkey, W. B., Mercado, A. M., & Glaser, R. (1995). Slowing of wound healing by psychological stress. *Lancet, 346,* 1194–1196.

Mace, N. L., & Rabins, P. V. (1981). *The 36-hour day: A family guide to caring for persons with Alzheimer's disease, related dementing illnesses, and memory loss in later life.* Baltimore: Johns Hopkins University Press.

Metropolitan Life Insurance Company [MetLife]. (1997, June). *The MetLife study of employer costs for working caregivers.* Westport, CT: MetLife Mature Market Institute.

Miller, P. A., & Butin, D. (2000). The role of occupational therapy in dementia—C.O.P.E. (Caregiver Options for Practical Experiences). *International Journal of Geriatric Psychiatry, 15*(1), 86–89.

Ory, M. G., Hoffman, R. R., Yee, J. L., Tennstedt, S., & Schulz, R. (1999). Prevalence and impact of caregiving: A detailed comparison between dementia and nondementia caregivers. *The Gerontologist, 39,* 177–185.

Schulz, R., & Beach, S. (1999). Caregiving as a risk factor for mortality: The caregiver health effects study. *Journal of the American Medical Association, 282,* 2215–2219.

Schulz, R., O'Brien, A. T., Bookwala, J., & Fleissner, K. (1995). Psychiatric and physical morbidity effects of dementia caregiving: Prevalence, correlates, and causes. *Gerontologist, 35,* 771–791.

Spitzer, A. (1998). Nursing in the health care system of the postmodern world: Crossroads, paradoxes and complexity. *Journal of Advanced Nursing, 28*(1), 164–171.

U.S. Department of Health and Human Services. (2003). *2003 Progress report on Alzheimer's disease*. Retrieved November 12, 2004 from http://www.alzheimers.org/pr03/2003_Progress_Report_on_AD.pdf.

Wahl, H.-W., & Gitlin, L. N. (2003). Future developments in living environments for older people in the U.S. and Germany: Potential and constraints. In K. W. Schaie, H.-W. Wahl, H. Mollenkopf, & F. Oswald (Eds.), *Aging independently: Living arrangements and mobility* (pp. 281–301). New York: Springer.

2

Evidence in Support of the Home Environmental Skill-Building Program

Laura N. Gitlin, PhD
Mary A. Corcoran, PhD, OTR/L, FAOTA

I think I also take a lot of strength in the realization that I am doing some good for him. Not just everything I can but that I can do quite a bit for him. And that is a source of satisfaction, which is extremely important. It is extremely important that you consider yourself a good caregiver. . . . It would be nice every once in a while if he showed some kind of recognition of it. I don't see it at all.

—Corcoran, Styles of Caregiving, Interview #10013#2:243–254

This chapter identifies the evidence that supports the use of the Home Environmental Skill-Building Program (ESP) as a practice approach for family caregivers and people with dementia living at home. We developed the intervention we present in this book over the course of 15 years and 8 funded research studies (Table 2.1). Each study incrementally and logically built on the other and, taken as a whole, they have provided an evolving understanding of the treatment effects, who benefits most, delivery characteristics, and specific guidelines for implementing an environmental skill-building intervention for managing dementia care.

PREVIOUS CAREGIVER STUDIES

The past 20 years have witnessed a proliferation of caregiver intervention studies designed to support families in their efforts to care for people with dementia at home. Most tested interventions are based on a stress process model (see

TABLE 2.1. Main Research Studies on the ESP Approach

Study Title	Funding Source	Focus of Study
Field-Based Training Approach for Occupational Therapists Working With Demented Elderly and Caregivers	Tirlawyn (1988–1989)	Approaches to training occupational therapists in collaborative care
Environmental Adaptation for Chronically Disabled Community Elderly	American Occupational Therapy Foundation (1987–1989)	Feasibility and acceptability of adaptive equipment Identification of collaborative strategies in working with elderly patients in the home
Improving Role Competency of Spouses Caring for the Elderly With Dementia	American Occupational Therapy Foundation; Thomas Jefferson University Stipend (1988–1990)	Feasibility and acceptability of environmental strategies with spousal caregivers
Dementia Management: Home Intervention for Caregivers	National Institute on Aging (1992–1995)	Randomized controlled trial to test 3-month environmental-based intervention
Research Minority Supplement	National Institute on Aging (1992–1995)	Black caregiver needs and resources
A Tool to Measure Home Environments of Persons With Dementia	National Institute on Aging (1998–2000)	Evaluation of observational tool (Home Environmental Assessment Protocol) to assess supportive environmental features
Home Environmental Skill-Building Program for Caregivers	National Institute on Aging (1996–2002)	Randomized controlled trial to test 6-month environmental-based intervention
Research Minority Supplement	National Institute on Aging (1992–1995)	Predictors of treatment adherence Delivery characteristics of the intervention

Chapter 5) and psychoeducational approaches. Typically, these interventions involve a combination of individual or group counseling, education, stress management, and problem-solving skill development and tend to be delivered primarily by social workers, care managers, or educational counselors. Despite the multitude of caregiver intervention studies (see Bourgeois, Schulz, & Burgio, 1996; Kennet, Burgio, & Schulz, 2000; Schulz et al., 2003), few have tested in-home skill-building approaches (for an exception, see Burgio, Stevens, Guy, Roth, & Haley, 2003), and fewer still have evaluated a home modification approach for managing daily challenges in caring for people with Alzheimer's disease and related disorders (ADRD).

Thus, an important public health priority, and one that ESP addresses, is to develop and test new approaches that teach families specific skills in providing quality home care and that, in turn, decrease caregiver burden and enhance well-being. This priority is supported as well by recent reviews of caregiver studies concluding that, although some psychoeducational interventions are effective in reducing caregiver distress and postponing nursing home placement (see Mittelman, Roth, Coon, & Haley, 2004), it remains important to develop and test a broader range of intervention strategies that address the multiple needs of caregivers at each stage of the illness trajectory (Bourgeois et al., 1996). These studies also suggest the need for interventions to be tailored to specific characteristics of caregivers (Biegel & Schulz, 1999; Gitlin, Belle, et al., 2003) and to combine information and referral-type services with hands-on skills training.

ESP differs from previously tested psychosocial and educational caregiver interventions with respect to its theoretical base and goals and the specific caregiver concerns that it targets for intervention. The intervention is based on a competence–environmental press framework (Lawton & Nahemow, 1973) and personal control theory (Schulz & Heckhausen, 1999). As described in more detail in Chapter 5, its goal is to lower the press (demands) of the social and physical environment for the caregiver and person with dementia and to provide the caregiver with primary strategies to maintain personal control through effective management of complex daily care problems. An environmental approach emphasizes the objective stressors or conditions in the caregiving situation (e.g., care recipient behaviors, home condition, and social network) that can be modified to ease caregiver burden and reduce or manage the dependence and behavioral manifestations of a patient with dementia.

PREVIOUS RESEARCH ON ENVIRONMENTAL INTERVENTIONS FOR FAMILY CAREGIVERS

Although home safety recommendations have traditionally been a part of hospital and home care with patients with dementia (Alzheimer's Association, 1997), only recently have approaches involving environmental modification been evaluated systematically. Early exploratory and descriptive studies on home environments showed that family caregivers modified their homes and perceived these modifications as helpful. These studies also showed that families tended to implement environmental strategies to cope with safety concerns and that they needed professional guidance to apply strategies to other behavioral problems. Nevertheless, this first wave of studies with family caregivers used primarily single-case or panel designs, and outcomes were limited to utilization rates of environmental strategies and self-reported benefits (Olsen, Ehrenkrantz, & Hutchings, 1993; Pynoos & Ohta, 1991).

Although few researchers have studied environmental modification with family caregivers, studies in other settings and with physically frail older adults provide empirical justification for the use of this approach in the households of people with dementia. For example, the severity of delirium in hospitalized older people was associated with modifiable environmental risk factors (McCusker et al., 2001), and interventions involving environmental modifications to prevent delirium in the hospital were shown to be effective (Inouye, Bogardus, Baker, Leo-Summers, & Cooney, 2000). A randomized controlled study testing an assistive device and home modification intervention found lowered long-term-care costs and postponement of relocation among the physically frail older people in the treatment group (Mann, Ottenbacher, Fraas, Tomita, & Granger, 1999).

STUDY FINDINGS IN SUPPORT OF THE HOME ENVIRONMENTAL SKILL-BUILDING PROGRAM

Each of the studies listed in Table 2.1 contributed incrementally to the evidence that supports ESP approach. Table 2.2 summarizes the specific treatment effects found from studies using randomized controlled trial methodology.

In one randomized controlled study with 202 caregivers for people with dementia, we found that a 3-month intervention involving hands-on problem solving and environmental recommendations resulted in improvements for both caregivers and care recipients (Gitlin, Corcoran, Winter, Boyce, & Hauck, 2001). Specifically, caregivers who received the intervention, compared with caregivers in usual care, reported fewer declines in instrumental activities of daily living (IADL), a trend toward fewer declines in self-care, and fewer behavior problems at the 3-month posttest. Additionally, spouses who received the intervention reported less upset with behavioral manifestations, female caregivers reported enhanced self-efficacy in managing troublesome behaviors, and female and Black caregivers reported enhanced self-efficacy in managing functional dependency compared with their counterparts in the control group.

Another randomized controlled trial with 272 families (the REACH I study) was part of the National Institutes of Health REACH (Resources for Enhancing Alzheimer's Caregiver Health) initiative (Wisniewski, et al., 2003). We found that ESP reduced stress in targeted areas of objective and subjective burden and

TABLE 2.2. Summary of Key Treatment Effects of the ESP Approach Based on Randomized Controlled Studies

Factor	Treatment Outcomes	Study
Care Recipient Quality of Life		
ADL dependence	Intervention female CGs reported less decline in CR ADLs compared with control female CGs.	Dementia Management study (Gitlin et al., 2001)
IADL dependence	Intervention CGs reported less decline in CR IADLs compared with control CGs.	Dementia Management study (Gitlin et al., 2001)
Behaviors	Intervention CGs reported fewer occurrences of behavior problems related to memory loss compared with control CGs.	REACH I long-term effects (Gitlin et al., in press)
Caregiver Quality of Life		
Efficacy	Intervention female CGs reported enhanced self-efficacy in managing IADLs compared with control female CGs. Intervention non-White CGs reported enhanced self-efficacy in managing IADLs compared with control non-White CGs. Intervention female CGs report enhanced self-efficacy in managing behaviors compared to control female CGs.	Dementia Management study (Gitlin et al., 2001)
Emotional well-being (upset, positive affect)	Intervention CGs and spouse CGs in particular reported less upset with behaviors compared with control spouse CGs. Intervention CGs reported improved affect compared with control CGs.	Dementia Management study (Gitlin et al., 2001) REACH I study (Gitlin, Winter, Corcoran, Dennis, Schonfeld, & Hauck, 2003)
Mastery and skill	Intervention female CGs reported greater overall CG mastery. Intervention CGs reported greater use of task simplification strategies compared with control CGs.	REACH I study (Gitlin et al., 2003)
Need for help	Intervention CGs reported less need for outside assistance than control CGs.	REACH I study (Gitlin et al., 2003)

Note. ADL = activities of daily living; CG = caregiver; CR = care recipient; IADL = instrumental activities of daily living.

enhanced selected aspects of caregiver well-being. Furthermore, the findings confirmed our previous research that an environmental approach reduces upset with behaviors for spouses but does not appear to be as effective for nonspouses and that women gain more from this approach than men. However, in contrast to the findings from our previous study, we did not find treatment effects for the person with dementia. One explanation for this discrepancy in findings is that our REACH sample was much more impaired cognitively and functionally than our previous samples. Thus, it may be that intervention at the mild to moderate stage of the disease process, as opposed to moderate to severe, would be important to make a difference in life quality. Finally, as we had anticipated, we did not find any differential treatment effects for white and non-White caregivers. However, non-White caregivers were more likely to remain in the study than White caregivers, an indication of the utility and social validity of the intervention for this group, which is typically underserved.

More specifically, the REACH I study showed that caregivers who received ESP improved over 6 months in three areas: (a) objective burden, as measured by the amount of help received from family and friends for activities of daily living (ADL) assistance; (b) subjective burden, as measured by the level of upset with memory-related behaviors; and (c) perceived change in affective well-being. In contrast, control group participants showed declines in all of these areas over 6 months. Caregivers did not show statistically significant improvements in other outcome variables as we had initially hypothesized. We expected but did not find less burden with managing ADL and IADL care. We also did not find a decline in time spent overseeing IADL performance or a slower rate of decline in functional dependence among care recipients, nor did we find that caregivers reported fewer disruptive behaviors. The lack of statistically significant change in burden levels may be due to a floor effect, in that caregivers reported very little burden at baseline with ADL and IADL dependence. Consequently, there may have been little room for improvement in this area. Another explanation may be a mismatch between the intervention and the outcome measures; outcome measures may not have been specific or sensitive enough to detect the environment-related impact of ESP.

Differential Effects for Caregiver Subgroups

Caregivers represent a highly diverse population with widely differing needs, cultural beliefs and values, and caregiving preferences. Consequently, a given intervention approach may not be suitable for all caregivers. The few studies that have examined caregiver characteristics in relationship to service use and treatment outcomes suggest differential effects along a number of dimensions. For example, Cox (1998) found that Black caregivers benefited more than White caregivers from a psychosocial intervention, and Zarit, Stephens, Townsend, Greene, and Leitsch (1999) showed that spouse caregivers used adult day services for briefer periods than nonspouse caregivers. Thus, to understand the impact of an intervention on caregivers with varying characteristics, it is very important to examine who may or may not benefit (Biegel & Schulz, 1999).

ESP requires caregivers to actively problem solve, change lifelong daily routines, use new care strategies, and adjust or remove material aspects of the environment that may have personal meaning. This is a behaviorally demanding intervention. ESP involves helping families change ineffective management approaches that may represent lifelong patterns. Hence, this intervention may not be right for all people; some caregivers may respond more favorably than others to ESP.

We have examined whether caregivers respond differently to ESP based on their gender, race, and relationship to the care recipient. Previous research has shown that these characteristics account for significant differences in caregiver functioning, coping, and responses to caregiving demands. For example, research shows that female caregivers reported more psychiatric symptoms and provided more hands-on involvement in caregiving (e.g., level of responsibility, number of tasks, and hours spent in hands-on care) than male caregivers (see Yee & Schulz, 2000, for a comprehensive review). In contrast, male caregivers tended to seek more assistance from family members and other informal services than female caregivers and expressed more objective than subjective burden (Neal, Ingersoll-Dayton, & Starrels, 1997; Schulz, O'Brien, Bookwala, & Fleissner, 1995). Additionally, although a sense of control is an expressed need for both genders, being assertive or exerting control may be accompanied by strain for women who may not be used to assuming authority or who may not have the skills to assume it effectively (Miller, 1987). As discussed previously, females seem to benefit from ESP more than males.

Research has also consistently shown that spouse caregivers have higher rates of upset and depression than nonspouse caregivers (Pruchno & Resch, 1989; Schulz et al., 1995). Little is known about how such differences affect participation in treatment and outcomes, however. Zarit and colleagues (1999) showed differences in adult day center use such that spousal caregivers tended to be briefer users than nonspouse caregivers. Our research consistently has shown that spouses who receive the ESP intervention report less upset than nonspouses over disruptive behaviors.

Whereas much research has shown racial differences in how caregiving is appraised, with Black people showing lower levels of upset or depression, little is known about whether intervention outcomes vary by race or ethnicity (see Haley et al., 2004). A few studies suggest differential effects for psychosocial interventions. Cox (1998) found that Black caregivers benefited more than White caregivers from a psychosocial intervention. Burgio et al. (2003) also found that Black caregivers gained more from participation in an in-home skills program, whereas White caregivers benefited more from telephone contact. However, our research (Gitlin, et al., 2001; Gitlin, Winter, et al., 2003) shows that, for an environmental intervention, Black caregivers demonstrated greater gains in only one caregiving domain—self-efficacy in managing functional dependence—relative to controls. Additionally, Black caregivers were more likely than White caregivers to stay in treatment. It is still unclear why these differences occur and whether socioeconomic status or educational level accounts for differential effects.

Thus, some groups of caregivers benefit more than others from ESP intervention. Women, for example, are more likely than men to comply with a home environmental intervention (Gitlin, Corcoran, Winter, Boyce, & Marcus, 1999) and report many more-important benefits from participation, including greater emotional gains and enhanced mastery and skill (Gitlin, et al., 2001). Additionally, spouses are more likely to show reduced upset than are nonspouses, and there are few differences in treatment effects for Black and White caregivers.

The stance toward culture embedded in ESP (see Chapter 4) is that the occupational therapists must view and understand each household as a microcultural unit from which to develop appropriate strategies that will be appropriate for that context. In evaluating the cultural dynamics of the care context, the occupational therapist interventionist must consider numerous aspects, including the physical and social environment, and the characteristics of the caregiver, including age, gender, education level, ethnic and religious orientation, preferred style of care, and understanding of dementia. Thus, the particular strategies that the professional introduces and the way he or she introduces them (e.g., by emphasizing verbal over written information) must be appropriate to the specific cultural context.

We believe that this stance toward culture optimizes the social relevance and validity of ESP and should minimize differences in treatment benefits across cultural or ethnic groups. Nevertheless, it is striking that women consistently benefit more than men do from the ESP approach. This may be a consequence of gender differences in basic approaches to providing care in general, with women favoring more hands-on, direct forms of assistance and men tending to prefer delegation and coordination of care providers. Given that the central thrust of ESP is building skills in providing hands-on management of dementia, it appears to favor women's preferred approaches and to better support their concerns and efforts.

Treatment Adherence

Adherence to treatment is important. One must participate in a treatment process to realize a clinically meaningful outcome. The ability to sustain engagement in an intervention and to integrate environmental strategies into daily routines is also an indicator of the feasibility, social acceptability, and validity of the intervention. Thus, examining adherence is an important aspect of verifying the efficaciousness of the intervention.

Table 2.3 summarizes the dose intensity features of the REACH I study. Caregivers received an average of nearly six visits and fell well within the protocol with regard to minutes spent in treatment and number of problems addressed. Caregivers reported or interventionists observed that the caregivers actively used and integrated into daily routines 54% of the strategies that were introduced during intervention sessions (Chee, Gitlin, Dennis, & Hauck, 2004).

TABLE 2.3. Treatment Characteristics for the REACH I Study Group (*N* = 116)

Component	Mean (SD)	Actual Range	Range by Protocol
Number of contacts	5.8 (1.6)	1–10	6
Time in intervention (minutes)	477.2 (145.1)	55–855	480
Number of problem areas addressed	4.36 (1.7)	1–12	3–5
Percentage of strategies integrated	54.0 (26.4)	0–100	0–100

The integration of strategies is somewhat lower than our previous research, which showed that caregivers actively used up to 84% of strategies by the completion of the intervention (Corcoran & Gitlin, 2001). This difference may reflect the more severe impairment of the REACH study sample compared to earlier samples (Corcoran & Gitlin, 2001). The findings of the REACH I study show that, overall, caregivers find the treatment approach acceptable, are able to sustain engagement over the six active sessions, and are selective in which strategies they accept and ultimately use.

Additionally, we consistently have found that caregivers who are either female or Black have higher retention rates (e.g., participate in more intervention sessions and spend more time with interventionists) than either male or White caregivers as a whole. Furthermore, caregivers who start the intervention with high readiness for change (i.e., willingness to learn new strategies and change caregiving approaches) use the intervention strategies more than caregivers with low readiness for change. Finally, it is important to note that the active involvement of caregivers in the therapeutic process—for example, by engaging families in role play, demonstration, and practice opportunities to learn intervention strategies—yields a higher level of adherence to the intervention than using a strictly didactic approach or providing written information alone (Belle et al., 2003; Chee et al., 2004).

Evidence for the Home as the Context for Intervention

The home is the primary care setting for more than 4 million Americans who have been diagnosed with ADRD (Haley & Bailey, 1999). National health care trends suggest that homes and communities will increasingly serve as the primary setting for delivering a vast array of health and human services to patients and their family caregivers. Future population projections suggest that families will continue to be the principal source of support for patients with dementia and that the home will remain the predominant setting for dementia care (Czaja, Eisdorfer, & Schulz, 2000; Wahl & Gitlin, 2003).

Thus, there is ample evidence that the home is an important context in which dementia care occurs. It is important to understand the evidence in support of providing an occupational therapy–based program in the home. Presently, there is no empirical evidence to suggest that providing intervention to families in their own homes is more effective or beneficial than providing the same intervention in a formal care setting (Wallace et al., 1998). That is, we do not know if the home setting affords greater benefit than a formal care setting for a person to receive a particular intervention. Nevertheless, there is evidence that home visits by health professionals yield more knowledge of care difficulties and result in greater compliance with care recommendations and that patients improve more quickly in their own homes (Ramsdell, Swart, Jackson, & Renvall, 1989). Additionally, recent research has shown that home visits enable professionals to identify more critical home safety and caregiver issues than a clinic-based interview (Ramsdell, Jackson, Guy, & Renvall, 2004). Adult learning theory also supports the practice of providing services to families in their own homes in that it suggests that adults learn most effectively when new skills are taught in the context in which they are actually used. Moreover, adult learners may benefit from repeated opportunities to practice new skills in real-life situations.

Evidence for Use of the Environment as a Treatment Modality

The use of environmental modifications is an important nonpharmacological approach to the management of behavioral manifestations of ADRD. Environmental interventions have been used in assisted living and nursing home facilities, as well as in hospital and home health care practices. Nevertheless, the full range of environmental strategies is not widely used across the continuum of care for people with ADRD, and no one has systematically developed clinical guidelines for implementing environmental strategies. The lack of systematic clinical guidelines is chiefly due to the lack of clear evidence about which environmental strategies afford positive outcomes, the range of benefits of any one strategy, and whether strategies used in one living context can be transferred to another.

Is the use of the physical and social environment as a treatment modality effective in managing troublesome behaviors associated with dementia such as agitation, wandering, or loss of function? There is some evidence to suggest that most environmental interventions do accomplish their intended purpose. In a recent review of 64 studies, Gitlin, Liebman, and Winter (2003) found that the vast majority of studies (90%) reported some level of success and that 10 of the 11 randomized clinical trials reviewed showed statistically significant improvements for experimental group participants in comparison to control group participants.

It is important to note that there does not appear to be one single environmental strategy that is more effective than others, suggesting that distinct environmental strategies may afford similar benefits for people with dementia.

For example, there are numerous environmental strategies to reduce agitation that appear to be effective. Strategies as diverse as Holmberg's (1997) social environment intervention involving group walking and Goddaer and Abraham's (1994) use of soothing music at mealtimes similarly resulted in reduced agitation among nursing home residents with dementia. Moreover, although the majority of studies in Gitlin, Liebman, et al.'s (2003) review evaluated the effect of an environmental modification on agitated behaviors, these studies also targeted a broad range of other outcomes and have reported improvements. For example, environmental strategies have been used to reduce exiting behavior, enhance nutritional intake, and improve affective well-being, activity engagement, attention, cognitive functioning, and medication use. This suggests the breadth of potential benefits derived from simple, low-cost environmental changes such as covering doorknobs with cloth, placing tape on floors, and using white noise. Furthermore, the outcomes these studies targeted are of high clinical relevance; that is, they have direct implications for well-being and daily quality of life.

Thus, studies conducted in institutional settings suggest that environmental adaptations may have multiple benefits for people with dementia (Gitlin, Liebman, et al., 2003). Environmental strategies have been shown to help manage such behaviors as wandering, agitation, and restlessness (Novak & Guest, 1989; Royall, Mahurin, & Gray, 1992; Steinfeld & Shea, 1993) and to enhance daily function and the performance of ADLs (Gitlin et al., 2001; Namazi & DiNatale Johnson, 1991; Novak & Guest, 1989).

CONCLUSION

Occupational therapists increasingly recognize evidence-based practice as a critical approach to improving patient care and quality of life. In using any therapeutic approach, it is important to evaluate the evidence regarding its benefits, its relevance to the target population, and the essential or immutable elements of the approach that must be implemented to derive treatment effects. The 15 years of research on environmental approaches in dementia care with caregivers at home provide critical evidence-based knowledge about

- The key benefits of the ESP approach,
- Which groups derive the biggest gains (female caregivers, spouse caregivers),
- The acceptability of strategies (54% to 84% of strategies are implemented),
- Which groups adhere to the intervention (e.g., Black caregivers, female caregivers, and caregivers who express a readiness to learn new techniques),
- Which groups have more difficulty with the treatment process (male caregivers and caregivers with depressive symptoms), and
- Which implementation techniques are most effective (e.g., use of therapeutic engagement and active involvement of caregivers in the treatment process).

REFERENCES

Alzheimer's Association. (1997, June). *Key elements of dementia care*. Chicago: Author.

Belle, S. H., Czaja, S. J., Schulz, R., Burgio, L. D., Gitlin, L. N., Jones, R., et al. (2003). Combining diverse interventions using a new taxonomy to combine the uncombinable: Integrating results across diverse caregiving interventions. *Psychology and Aging, 18*, 396–405.

Biegel, D. E., & Schulz, R. (1999). Caregiving and caregiver interventions in aging and mental illness. *Family Relations, 48*, 345–354.

Bourgeois, M. S., Schulz, R., & Burgio, L. (1996). Interventions for caregivers of patients with Alzheimer's disease: A review and analysis of content, process, and outcomes. *International Journal of Aging and Human Development, 43*, 35–91.

Burgio, L., Stevens, A., Guy, D., Roth, D. L., & Haley, W. E. (2003). Impact of two psychosocial interventions on White and African American family caregivers of individuals with dementia. *The Gerontologist, 43*, 568–579.

Chee, Y. K., Gitlin, L. N., Dennis, M. P., & Hauck, W. W. (2004, November 21). *Predictors of adherence to in-home caregiver interventions for managing dementia*. Paper presented at the meeting of the Gerontological Society.

Corcoran, M., & Gitlin, L. N. (2001). Family caregiver acceptance and use of environmental strategies in occupational therapy intervention. *Physical & Occupational Therapy in Geriatrics, 19*(1), 1–20.

Cox, C. (1998). The experience of respite: Meeting the needs of African American and White caregivers in a statewide program. *Journal of Gerontology: Social Work, 30*, 59–72.

Czaja, S., Eisdorfer, C., & Schulz, R. (2000). Future directions in caregiving: Implications for intervention research. In R. Schulz (Ed.), *Handbook on dementia caregiving: Evidence-based interventions for family caregivers* (pp. 283–320). New York: Springer.

Gitlin, L. N., Belle, S. H., Burgio, L., Czaja, S., Mahoney, D., Gallagher-Thompson, D., et al. (2003). Effect of multi-component interventions on caregiver burden and depression: The REACH multi-site initiative at six months follow-up. *Psychology and Aging, 18*(3), 361–374.

Gitlin, L. N., Corcoran, M. A., Winter, L., Boyce, A., & Hauck, W. W. (2001). A randomized, controlled trial of a home environmental intervention to enhance self-efficacy and reduce upset in family caregivers of persons with dementia. *The Gerontologist, 41*, 15–30.

Gitlin, L. N., Corcoran, M. A., Winter, L., Boyce, A., & Marcus, S. (1999). Predicting participation and adherence to a home environmental intervention among family caregivers of persons with dementia. *Family Relations, 48*, 363–372.

Gitlin, L. N., Hauck, W. W., Dennis, M. P. & Winter, L. (in press). Long-term effects of the Home Environmental Skill-building Program for families caring for persons with Alzheimer's disease and related disorders. *Journal of Gerontology: Medical Sciences*.

Gitlin, L. N., Liebman, J., & Winter, L. (2003). Are environmental interventions effective in the management of Alzheimer's disease and related disorders? A synthesis of the evidence. *Alzheimer Care Quarterly, 4*, 85–107.

Gitlin, L. N., Winter, L., Corcoran, M., Dennis, M., Schinfeld, S., & Hauck, W. (2003). Effects of the Home Environmental Skill-building Program on the caregiver-care recipient dyad: Six-month outcomes from the Philadelphia REACH initiative. *The Gerontologist, 43*, 532–546.

Goddaer, J., & Abraham, I. L. (1994). Effects of relaxing music on agitation during meals among nursing home residents with severe cognitive impairment. *Archives of Psychiatric Nursing, 3,* 150–158.

Haley, W. E., & Bailey, S. (1999). Research on family caregiving in Alzheimer's disease: Implications for practice and policy. In B. Vellas & J. L. Fitten (Eds.), *Research and practice in Alzheimer's disease* (Vol. 2, pp. 321–332). Paris: Serdi Publisher.

Haley, W. E., Gitlin, L. N., Wisniewski, S. R., Mahoney, D. F., Coon, D. W., Winter, L., et al. (2004). Well-being, appraisal, and coping in African-American and Caucasian dementia caregivers: Findings from the REACH study. *Aging and Mental Health, 8,* 316–329.

Holmberg, S. K. (1997). Evaluation of a clinical intervention for wanderers on a geriatric nursing unit. *Archives of Psychiatric Nursing, 11,* 21–28.

Inouye, S. K., Bogardus, S. T., Jr., Baker, D. I., Leo-Summers, L., & Cooney, L. M. (2000). Hospital Elder Life Program: A model of care to prevent cognitive and functional decline in older hospitalized patients. *Journal of the American Geriatrics Society, 48,* 697–706.

Kennet, J., Burgio, L., & Schulz, R. (2000). Interventions for in-home caregivers: A review of research 1990 to present. In R. Schulz (Ed.), *Handbook on dementia caregiving: Evidence-based interventions for family caregivers* (pp. 61–125). New York: Springer.

Lawton, M. P., & Nahemow, L. E. (1973). Ecology and the aging process. In C. Eisdorfer & M. P. Lawton (Eds.), *The psychology of adult development and aging* (pp. 619–674). Washington, DC: American Psychological Association.

Mann, W. C., Ottenbacher, K. J., Fraas, L., Tomita, M., & Granger, C. V. (1999). Effectiveness of assistive technology and environmental interventions in maintaining independence and reducing home care costs for the frail elderly. *Archives of Family Medicine, 8,* 210–217.

McCusker, J., Cole, M., Abrahamowicz, M., Han, L., Podoba, J. E., & Ramman-Haddad, L. (2001). Environmental risk factors for delirium in hospitalized older people. *Journal of the American Geriatrics Society, 49,* 1327–1334.

Miller, B. (1987). Gender and control among spouses of the cognitively impaired: A research note. *The Gerontologist, 27,* 447–453.

Mittelman, M. S., Roth, D. L., Coon, D. W., & Haley, W. E. (2004). Sustained benefit of supportive intervention for depressive symptoms in caregivers of patients with Alzheimer's disease. *American Journal of Psychiatry, 161,* 850–856.

Namazi, K. H., & DiNatale Johnson, B. (1991). Physical environmental cues to reduce the problems of incontinence in Alzheimer's disease units. *American Journal of Alzheimer's Care and Related Disorders & Research, 6*(6), 22–28.

Neal, M. B., Ingersoll-Dayton, B., & Starrels, M. E. (1997). Gender and relationship differences in caregiving patterns and consequences among employed caregivers. *The Gerontologist, 37,* 804–815.

Novak, M., & Guest, C. (1989). Application of a multidimensional caregiver burden inventory. *The Gerontologist, 29,* 798–803.

Olsen, R. V., Ehrenkrantz, E., & Hutchings, B. (1993). Creating supporting environments for people with dementia and their caregivers through home modifications. *Technology and Disability, 2,* 47–57.

Pruchno, R., & Resch, N. L. (1989). Aberrant behaviors of Alzheimer's disease: Mental health effects on spouse caregivers. *Journal of Gerontology, 44,* S177–S182.

Pynoos, J., & Ohta, R. J. (1991). In-home interventions for person's with Alzheimer's disease and their caregivers. *Occupational Therapy and Physical Therapy in Geriatrics, 9,* 83–92.

Ramsdell, J. W., Jackson, J. E., Guy, H. J. B., & Renvall, M. J. (2004). Comparison of clinic-based home assessment to a home visit in dementia elderly patients. *Alzheimer Disease and Associated Disorders, 18,* 145–153.

Ramsdell, J. W., Swart, J. A., Jackson, E., & Renvall, M. (1989). The yields of a home visit in the assessment of geriatric patients. *Journal of the American Geriatric Society, 37*(1), 17–24.

Royall, D. R., Mahurin, R. K., & Gray, K. F. (1992). Bedside assessment of executive cognitive impairment: The executive interview. *Journal of the American Geriatrics Society, 40,* 1221–1226.

Schulz, R., & Heckhausen, J. (1999). Aging, culture and control: Setting a new research agenda. *Journal of Gerontology: Psychological Sciences, 54B,* P139–P145.

Schulz, R., O'Brien, A. T., Bookwala, J., & Fleissner, K. (1995). Psychiatric and physical morbidity effects of dementia caregiving: Prevalence, correlates, and causes. *The Gerontologist, 35,* 771–791.

Schulz, R., O'Brien, A. T., Czaja, S., Norris, M. A., Martire, L., Belle, S., et al. (2003). Dementia caregiver intervention research: In search of clinical significance. *The Gerontologist, 42,* 589–602.

Steinfeld, E., & Shea, S. (1993). Enabling home environments: Identifying barriers to independence. *Technology and Disability, 2*(4), 69–79.

Wahl, H.-W., & Gitlin, L. N. (2003). Future developments in living environments in the U.S. and Germany: Potential and constraints. In K. W. Schaie, H.-W. Wahl, H. Mollenkopf, & F. Oswald (Eds.), *Aging in the community: Living arrangements and mobility* (pp. 281–301). New York: Springer.

Wallace, J. I., Buchner, D. M., Grothaus, L., Leveille, S., Tyll, L., LaCroix, A. Z., et al. (1998). Implementation and effectiveness of a community-based health promotion program for older adults. *Journal of Gerontology: Medical Sciences, 33A,* 301–306.

Wisniewski, S. R., Belle, S. H., Coon, D. W., Marcus, S. M., Ory, M. G., Burgio, L. D., et al. (2003). The Resources for Enhancing Alzheimer's Caregiver Health (REACH): Project design and baseline characteristics. *Psychology and Aging, 18,* 375–384.

Yee, J. L., & Schulz, R. (2000). Gender differences in psychiatric morbidity among family caregivers: A review and analysis. *Gerontologist, 40,* 147–164.

Zarit, S. H., Stephens, M. A. P., Townsend, A., Greene, R., & Leitsch, S. (1999). Patterns of adult day service use by family caregivers: A comparison of brief versus sustained use. *Family Relations, 48,* 355–361.

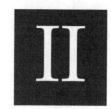

Essentials of Dementia and Caregiving

3

Trajectory of Dementia and Impact on Families

Pamalyn Kearney, MS, OTR/L
Geri Shaw, OTR/L
Laura N. Gitlin, PhD

He had a cup of coffee, and he set it down on one of my paintings, and five or six of my paintings had splashes of coffee on them. And I came in and saw it, and I just exploded. I exploded in anger and then tears. And I cried and cried and I cried all night. I found myself waking up in tears all night. And I said, hey, you are depressed. This is what they call depression.

—Caregiving Styles Study (Corcoran) NIA R29-AG13019 10061#1:740–747

*D*ementia is derived from the Latin roots *de,* which means *from* or *away,* and *mens,* which means *mind* (Merriam-Webster Online, 2004). Thus, a literal translation of dementia is *away from the mind.* Today, *dementia* is used to refer to a group of disorders that result in impaired cognition, decreased functional performance in routine activities, and declines in socially acceptable behavior. To be diagnosed with dementia, the individual must have an acquired memory impairment combined with one or more of the following—aphasia (disordered language), apraxia (disordered movement), agnosia (difficulty recognizing objects despite intact sensory function), or disordered executive functions (e.g., problem solving, abstract thinking, planning, organization)—resulting in significant decline in social and occupational performance (American Psychiatric Association, 2000). For an individual to be diagnosed with dementia, these deficits must be severe enough to interfere with work, relationships, and customary social activities; they must clearly represent a change in level of functioning; and they must not be attributable to delirium or any other psychiatric disease (Knopman, Boeve, & Petersen, 2003).

In 2000, an estimated 4 million Americans were living with Alzheimer's disease (AD), the most common cause of dementia for individuals ages 65 years and older (DeKosky, 2003; Herbert, Scherr, Bienias, Bennett, & Evans, 2003; Knopman et al., 2003; National Institute on Aging [NIA], 2003a; Prigerson, 2003; Sadik & Wilcock, 2003). Researchers expect the incidence and prevalence of AD to climb sharply over the next 50 years. The midrange estimate for 2050 is more than 13 million Americans, a 300% increase, with nearly 1.5 million new diagnoses yearly (Herbert et al., 2003; NIA, 2003a; Prigerson, 2003; Sadik & Wilcock, 2003). The reasons behind this growth in the number of Americans living with Alzheimer's disease and related disorders (ADRD) are an increase in the number of people living into old age, a projected decline in the death rate, and the extended life spans of people with dementia (Herbert et al., 2003).

The impact of dementia is pervasive. Dementia affects not only the affected individual and the health care system but also family members, who typically are responsible for the care of the person with dementia as the disease progresses until death. This caregiver role can be a lengthy one, potentially lasting up to 20 years or more (NIA, 2003a). Almost 70% of people with dementia live at home, with family and friends providing the majority of their care (Rymer et al., 2002). This chapter provides an overview of the known causes of dementia, its clinical stages and current treatments, and the impact of the disease process on the person with the condition and his or her informal support system.

NEUROPATHOLOGY

In the 19th century, scientists first recognized dementia as an actual illness with associated structural changes in the brain. Dr. Alois Alzheimer described these pathological changes as plaques and neurofibrillary tangles early in the 20th century (Schneck, Reisberg, & Ferris, 1982). Our understanding of neuropathology has progressed over the past century. We now know that plaques and tangles also exist in the brains of nonaffected individuals. A large quantity of these plaques and tangles, combined with brain atrophy, are the hallmark of the disease process of AD (DeKosky, 2003; NIA, 2003a, 2003b; Tariot & Federoff, 2003).

AD alone accounts for up to 60% of all cases of dementia; AD in combination with other types of dementia accounts for 80% of dementia cases (Knopman et al., 2003). Other common types of dementia include vascular dementia (VaD), Lewy body dementia (LBD), and frontotemporal dementia (FTD). These four types combine to account for 90% of individuals with dementia (Souder, Chastain, & Williams, 2002). Although AD, LBD, FTD, and VaD account for so many dementia cases, there are many other disorders, including Huntington's disease and Creutzfeldt–Jakob disease, that result in or present as dementia, some of which are reversible. Table 3.1 provides an overview of the more common disorders and their presentations.

The plaques that are so prevalent in the brains of individuals with AD are known technically as *beta-amyloid plaques*. For those individuals who develop AD in middle adulthood, the development of these plaques has been linked to one of three possible genetic mutations. The vast majority of people who develop AD do so in older adulthood; for these people the cause of plaque development is not known (NIA, 2004). These plaques are dense clusters of beta-amyloid proteins and other cellular materials. Neurofibrillary tangles result from a chemical change to a specific protein known as *tau*, which is a component of internal neuronal structure. This modified tau joins with other pieces of tau to create tangled clumps of protein (NIA, 2003b; Tariot & Federoff, 2003). The exact relationship of these changes to each other and to the development and progression of AD is not yet clear, although it appears that these processes work together to decrease synaptic connections between neurons and to cause neuronal death and brain atrophy (DeKosky, 2003; NIA, 2003b; Tariot & Federoff, 2003). Severity of AD seems to correlate more strongly with the degree of neurofibrillary tangles present than with the number of plaques. In addition, the person with AD typically experiences abnormalities with neurotransmitter systems, particularly with the cholinergic and glutamatergic systems (Sadik & Wilcock, 2003; Tariot & Federoff, 2003); current pharmacological interventions target these neurotransmitter systems.

Other types of dementia display different patterns of pathodynamics. VaD is the result of damage to brain structures caused by inadequate blood supply, which is in turn caused by cardiovascular or cerebrovascular disease; VaD may be found in combination with other etiologies such as AD (Fleming, Adams, & Petersen, 1995; National Institute of Neurological Disorders and Stroke [NINDS],

TABLE 3.1. Types of Dementia and Their Presentation

Type of Dementia	Presentation May Include	
Alzheimer's disease	Gradual, progressive onset	Changes in mood and personality
	Memory loss	Loss of initiative
	Difficulty performing familiar tasks	Visuospatial impairment
	Disorientation to time and place	Difficulty with daily activities
	Poor judgment	Incontinence
	Difficulty with language	
Vascular dementia— Includes multi-infarct dementia and Binswanger's disease	Onset can be sudden or a stepwise progression	Difficulty with daily activities
	Difficulty with language	Emotional outbursts
	Memory problems	Weakness in one or more extremities
Lewy body dementia	Progressive onset	Difficulty with language
	Memory loss	Hallucinations and paranoia
	Poor judgment	Parkinsonian symptoms
	Confusion	Day-to-day fluctuations in symptom severity
Frontotemporal dementia— Includes Pick's disease and primary progressive aphasia	Progressive onset	Language impairment
	Socially inappropriate behavior	Motor or balance impairment
	Distractibility	Memory loss, typically later in disease process
	Repetitive actions	
Huntington's disease	Degenerative hereditary disease	Personality change
	Involuntary movement of arms, legs, or face	Difficulty with memory
		Slurred speech
	Difficulty concentrating	Impaired judgment
Creutzfeldt–Jakob disease	Rare, rapidly progressive disease	Involuntary movements
	Behavioral changes	Social withdrawal
	Impaired coordination	Difficulty with speech
	Memory loss	

2004; Souder et al., 2002). Diagnosis of VaD requires either a new onset or a substantial worsening of cognitive decline within 3 months of a confirmed cerebrovascular accident or evidence of bilateral brain infarctions in cortical or subcortical gray matter on neuroimaging (Knopman et al., 2003). VaD is present in up to 20% of cases of dementia among elderly people (Martin, 2001; NINDS, 2004). The onset of VaD may be more abrupt than that of AD, often marked by a stepwise progression of symptoms rather than a gradual decline. In addition, dysfunction in VaD may appear to be more localized and focal than that of AD (NINDS, 2004).

LBD is a progressive, global dementia that appears to be caused by the development of abnormal structures (Lewy bodies) in the brain (McKeith et al., 1996; NINDS, 2004). Lewy bodies are also associated with Parkinson's disease and AD, but the exact relationship between LBD and these other diseases is unclear (NINDS, 2004). The literature suggests that LBD may be present in up to 25% of people with dementia (Martin, 2001; McKeith et al., 1996). Symptoms of LBD include fluctuations in cognitive functioning, visual and auditory hallucinations, delusions, bradykinesia (loss of spontaneous movement), muscle rigidity, and other motor impairments common in people with Parkinson's disease (McKeith et al., 1996; NINDS, 2004; Souder et al., 2002).

FTD is believed to account for up to 10% of dementia cases. FTD is associated with degeneration of nerve cells in the frontal and temporal lobes of the brain and with neurofibrillary tangles similar to those described for AD (NINDS, 2004). Because of the nature of frontal and temporal lobe function, people with FTD may experience changes in personality, impaired executive functions, difficulty with social interactions, and socially inappropriate behaviors. FTD can also result in impaired language, decreased balance, and ritualistic behaviors. In contrast to AD, memory is preserved until later stages of the disease (Knopman et al., 2003; Martin, 2001; NINDS, 2004).

Exhibit 3.1 lists conditions that can mimic the symptoms of dementia and that should be ruled out before a diagnosis of AD or any other dementia is made. Although we recognize that the different forms of dementia progress in different ways, the following sections provide an overview of the stages of dementia based on AD, which accounts for the largest percentage of people with dementia.

STAGES OF DEMENTIA

AD is typically a slow but relentlessly progressive disease that often presents at onset with subtle cognitive changes (Petersen, 2000; Reisberg, Ferris, DeLeon, & Crook, 1982). As the disease progresses, most individuals with dementia develop one or more of the following behavioral alterations: withdrawal, aggression,

EXHIBIT 3.1. Major Conditions That May Mimic Dementia

Metabolic abnormalities	Lead poisoning
Endocrine abnormalities	Brain tumor
Vitamin B1, B6, or B12 deficiency	Anoxia
Dehydration	Normal pressure hydrocephalus
Systemic infection	Depression
Subdural hematoma	Delirium

anxiety, sleep disturbances, wandering, hallucinations, or delusions (Bullock & Hammond, 2003; DeKosky, 2003; Holtzer et al., 2003; Sadik & Wilcock, 2003). Functional impairments also develop and progress, from difficulty with instrumental activities of daily living (IADL) such as work performance and bill paying to inability to perform basic activities of daily living (ADL) such as dressing and feeding (Reisberg, 1984; Reisberg et al., 1982; Sadik & Wilcock, 2003).

A variety of frameworks can be used to organize discussions related to stages of disease progression and functional impairment in individuals with AD. The following discussion is organized based on the progression of the disease from mild cognitive impairment to mild, moderate, and severe dementia, terminology consistent with the Alzheimer's Association's (2003) educational resources for individuals, families, and professionals and with the classifications of the Global Deterioration Scale (see Reisberg et al., 1982). Table 3.2 provides an overview of this framework for AD stage progression.

Mild Cognitive Impairment

Petersen (2000) characterized mild cognitive impairment (MCI) as a new onset of both subjective and objective memory impairment that is evident when the individual is compared with people of similar age and education. The individual with MCI demonstrates general cognitive functioning that is normal and has typical ADL and IADL performance, although one study identified a decline in some financial abilities such as bank statement management and bill payment compared with nonimpaired peers (Griffith et al., 2003). Memory deficits may not be apparent in casual interactions. Overall, memory is impaired beyond what is typically expected for the individual's age, but the impairment is not severe enough to fit the diagnostic criteria for dementia (DeKosky, 2003; NIA, 2003a; Petersen, 2000). Vogel et al. (2004) found that people with MCI ranged from full awareness to substantial loss of insight regarding their impairments.

Many researchers consider MCI to be either a transient state between normal aging and early probable dementia or a very early stage of dementia (DeKosky, 2003; NIA, 2003a; Petersen, 2000). Individuals with MCI develop diagnosable dementia at a rate of 10% to 15% yearly, compared with 1% to 2% of the general population (DeKosky, 2003). The NIA (2003a) has reported that up to 40% of individuals with MCI develop AD within 3 years of diagnosis.

Caregiving issues are generally not noteworthy for individuals with MCI, who are typically able to function quite well in all occupational roles. Families may begin to see mild changes and may have concerns about the long-term prognosis and adequacy of the current living situation, but hands-on care is typically not required. Caregiver involvement may be more intense at this stage, however, when neuropsychiatric symptoms are present. Lyketsos et al. (2002) evaluated 320 individuals with MCI who were part of a larger longitudinal Cardiovascular

TABLE 3.2. Stages of Dementia, Associated Changes, and Family Caregiver Needs

Stage	Memory and Cognitive Changes	Behavioral Changes	Functional Changes	Caregiving Demands and Caregiver Needs
Mild cognitive impairment	Subjective and objective memory loss	Possible anxiety Forgetfulness Some confusion	Isolated, if present, and limited to high-level IADL deficits	Caregiving demands: Mild anxiety Caregiving needs: Education
Mild dementia	Loss of new or recent memory Word-finding difficulties Decreased concentration Decreased problem-solving skills Lack of initiative	Mood and personality changes Emotional withdrawal Increased anxiety Depression	Difficulties with financial management Difficulty managing medication routine Tendency to become lost traveling to unfamiliar places Impaired work and social performance	Caregiving demands: Assistance with IADLs Caregiving needs: Education Behavior management strategies Skills for coping with disease process Financial planning Referral to community resources
Moderate dementia	Continued decline in memory Increased confusion Difficulty with personal information Disorientation to time and place Difficulty with new learning Incontinence	Paranoia Hallucinations Delusions Compulsive behavior Repetitive behavior Agitation Aggression Restlessness Wandering Withdrawal Apathy Anxiety Inappropriate behavior Depression	Difficulty with self-care, including clothing selection, dressing, bathing, and toileting Difficulty with communication Difficulty with mobility Inability to drive safely	Caregiving demands: Moderate assistance with ADL Total assistance with IADL Caregiving needs: Assistance with increased physical burden Assistance with behavior management Assistance reevaluating employment situation Stress reduction techniques
Severe dementia	Profound loss of function in all areas Increased amount of time spent sleeping Inability to recognize familiar faces Lost capacity for understanding speech Decreased ability to swallow Incontinence of bladder and bowel	Apathy Restlessness Increased amount of time sleeping	Profound loss of function in all areas Eventual loss of all mobility	Caregiving demands: Total assistance in IADL and most or all ADL Caregiving needs: All above

Health Study and found that 20% had symptoms of depression, 15% symptoms of apathy, and another 15% symptoms of irritability. Clearly, individuals diagnosed with or suspected to have MCI who demonstrate more profound memory or functional impairments should be evaluated for other possible psychiatric conditions so that appropriate treatment can be provided.

Mild Dementia

Mild dementia is characterized by the gradual development of memory or cognitive deficits (Bullock & Hammond, 2003) that are noteworthy enough for family, friends, and coworkers to notice. The person with mild dementia frequently has decreased knowledge of new or recent events and acquaintances. Memory of personal history begins to fade. The individual with mild dementia is oriented to self, time, familiar faces, and familiar locations (Alzheimer's Association, 2003; Reisberg, 1984; Reisberg et al., 1982). Word and name finding become mildly impaired, as do judgment and problem solving (Alzheimer's Association, 2003; NIA, 2003b; Knopman et al., 2003). Concentration abilities decrease, and the ability to plan, organize, and complete complex tasks gradually becomes compromised (Alzheimer's Association, 2003; Reisberg, 1984; Reisberg et al., 1982).

In the mild stage of dementia, behavioral concerns and depression may develop. The person may feel overwhelmed and may respond to this feeling with mood and personality changes such as denial, emotional withdrawal, flattened affect, or increased anxiety (NIA, 2003b; Reisberg, 1984; Reisberg et al., 1982). Holtzer et al.'s (2003) study of 236 individuals with mild AD found that 57% had issues with wandering and that 22% were physically aggressive. Clearly, behavioral impairments increase the demands on caregivers. Depression is also a concern for this population; Zubenko et al. (2003) found that one-third of their study participants with AD had developed a major depressive episode at or after the onset of cognitive impairment. It is vital that professionals address this depression, because treatment can often result in an overall improvement in cognitive functioning.

Individuals with mild dementia often experience difficulty with accurate and efficient completion of tasks. This contributes to IADL dysfunction in the areas of financial management, medication management, travel to unfamiliar places, and performance in work and social situations (Alzheimer's Association, 2003; Bullock & Hammond, 2003; NIA, 2003b; Knopman et al., 2003; Reisberg, 1984; Reisberg et al., 1982). Individuals with mild dementia may misplace or lose valuable items (Alzheimer's Association, 2003; Reisberg et al., 1982). In spite of these deficits, ADL performance remains independent, and individuals with mild dementia often are able to continue to live alone with support from family and friends (Bullock & Hammond, 2003).

Recent research suggests that individuals with mild dementia have the capacity for more new learning than was previously thought. Loewenstein, Acevedo, Czaja, and Duara (2004) found that people mildly impaired with AD who were also taking cholinesterase inhibitors had clinically and statistically significant improvements (after cognitive rehabilitation) in their ability to count change for a purchase (71% improvement) and recall faces and names (170% improvement). These findings are consistent with those of Lustig and Buckner (2004), who reported that individuals in the mild stage of AD retained their implicit memory (relatively unconscious and automatic recall). These two studies may support new strategies for introducing compensatory techniques in the early stages of dementia to improve functioning (Alzheimer's Disease Education and Referral Center [ADEAR], 2004b).

Moderate Dementia

Declines in performance and functioning are typically dramatic in the moderate stage of dementia. The individual experiences a continued decline in memory and may have difficulty recalling his or her address, telephone number, other personal information, or personal history (Alzheimer's Association, 2003; NIA, 2003b; Reisberg, 1984; Reisberg et al., 1982). The person with moderate dementia usually remembers his or her own name and the names of close relatives, such as his or her spouse or children, but he or she may forget names of grandchildren and friends (Alzheimer's Association, 2003; NIA, 2003b; Reisberg, 1984; Reisberg et al., 1982). These individuals are no longer oriented to time, place, or season. Attention span, organized and logical thinking, mental arithmetic abilities, and impulse control are decreased (Alzheimer's Association, 2003; NIA, 2003b).

The person with moderate dementia has difficulty with new learning and with managing unexpected situations (NIA, 2003b). Deficits at the moderate stage of dementia are variable, making these changes difficult and unpredictable for both the individual and the caregiver and resulting in "good days" and "bad days." For a person at the moderate stage, the world has become a frightening place to be (Reisberg, 1984).

Apraxia and disordered language can develop during this stage (Bullock & Hammond, 2003; NIA, 2003b) and can affect, to a great extent, functional performance and communication. In a study of 255 individuals with and without AD, Edwards, Deuel, Baum, and Morris (1991) found that 58% of individuals with AD had apraxic motor performance, compared with fewer than 1% of those without AD. Although this apraxia initially may occur during the mild dementia stage, there is a graded increase in dysfunction as the disease progresses. The degree of language impairment is variable for individuals with AD; typical areas of difficulty include name and word finding, language comprehension and fluency

(Hebert et al., 2000; Knopman et al., 2003) and can impact both verbal and written communication. Combined with the cognitive deficits identified above, these losses have a profound impact on ADL performance.

Additionally, important behavioral changes occur during the moderate stage of dementia. Assessment of more than 1,000 individuals with AD in the Consortium to Establish a Registry for Alzheimer's Disease (CERAD) database found that more than 50% were reported to have experienced some form of behavioral or personality change (Neumann et al., 2001). Behavioral changes typically increase as cognitive skills decline throughout the moderate stage. These changes are of considerable concern, because research indicates that management of behavioral issues is more difficult and stressful for families than management of ADL and IADL dysfunction, resulting in increased caregiver burden and prompting consideration of nursing home placement (Haley, Wadley, West, & Vetzel, 1994; Sadik & Wilcock, 2003). Common behavioral manifestations include suspiciousness, paranoia, hallucinations, delusions, compulsive or repetitive behaviors, agitation, violence, aggression, restlessness, and wandering (Alzheimer's Association, 2003; Bullock & Hammond, 2003; Holtzer et al., 2003; NIA, 2003b; Reisberg, 1984; Reisberg et al., 1982). Psychosocial and emotional changes include denial, anger, emotional lability, withdrawal, apathy, depression, and anxiety (Bullock & Hammond, 2003; NIA, 2003b; Reisberg, 1984; Reisberg et al., 1982). Disruptions in sleep–wake cycles are also common, frequently leading to disruptions in family sleep patterns (Alzheimer's Association, 2003; Bullock & Hammond, 2003).

Because of cognitive, motor, and behavioral impairments, the moderate stage of dementia is a time of considerable decline in most areas of occupational performance. Continued decline in memory and organized thinking exacerbate the deficits seen in the mild stage with work and social activities. Individuals at the moderate stage of AD can no longer manage in the community without support and may not be able to live alone (Bullock & Hammond, 2003; Reisberg, 1984). Although they become lost easily, they may still be able to manage travel in very familiar environments (Alzheimer's Association, 2003; NIA, 2003b; Reisberg et al., 1982). Individuals who continued to drive their cars through the mild stage are now more impaired (Reisberg, 1984) and may become lost while driving or have accidents, or both, because of difficulty with memory and cognitive processes.

At this stage, ADL become more difficult to complete. The individual requires assistance to choose clothing that is appropriate for the season or occasion and may require assistance with other aspects of dressing, such as sequencing (Alzheimer's Association, 2003; Reisberg, 1984; Reisberg et al., 1982). The individual with moderate impairment may require coaxing or even assistance for bathing (Bullock & Hammond, 2003; Reisberg, 1984; Reisberg et al., 1982). Many individuals remain independent with toileting during the early phases of this stage, but assistance to complete the steps involved in toileting and increasing incidences of incontinence characterize progression toward the severe stage (Alzheimer's Association, 2003; Reisberg, 1984; Reisberg et al., 1982).

Severe Dementia

Damage to and atrophy of brain structures is widespread in the severe stage of dementia (NIA, 2003b), with a profound loss of functioning in all areas. The individual has considerable cognitive disability and may sleep, or appear to be in a stupor or coma, much of the time (Haley et al., 1994; NIA, 2003b; Reisberg, 1984). He or she is unable to recognize family or loved ones and is unable to speak so that others can understand. The person with severe dementia may be able to sporadically utter a word or phrase, but most vocalizations are nonsensical (Alzheimer's Association, 2003; NIA, 2003b; Reisberg, 1984; Reisberg et al., 1982). It is difficult at this point to decipher the meaning of these vocalizations and determine if they are attempts to communicate or expressions of discomfort, leading to a risk of overmedication if these utterances are mistakenly attributed to discomfort (Reisberg, 1984). The individual with severe dementia typically becomes dysphagic (difficulty or inability to swallow) and is at risk for aspiration (Alzheimer's Association, 2003; Bullock & Hammond, 2003; NIA, 2003b; Reisberg, 1984).

Physical function is much more impaired than at earlier stages (Haley et al., 1994), with most people demonstrating apraxic motor performance (Edwards et al., 1991). People with severe dementia may be able to ambulate with assistance for a time but will eventually lose even this ability. Use of assistive devices for mobility is impractical at this stage because of the affected individual's inability to learn to use them (Alzheimer's Association, 2003; Reisberg, 1984). As motoric decline progresses, the individual becomes unable to sit upright without support and eventually to hold his or her head upright (Alzheimer's Association, 2003). Well-being may be further compromised by weight loss, seizures, and skin infections (NIA, 2003b).

The behavioral issues so prevalent in the moderate stage of the disease decrease for the most part during the severe stage. Although the individual may continue to appear apathetic, the substantial cognitive and physical impairments seem to limit the expression of problematic behaviors (Haley et al., 1994). Depression remains a concern, however. Zubenko et al. (2003) found that 50% of study participants with severe cognitive impairment also had major depression. All IADL and most ADL functions are lost in the severe stage. The individual may be able to feed himself or herself with assistance for a time but will eventually need total assistance (Alzheimer's Association, 2003; Bullock & Hammond, 2003; Reisberg et al., 1982). A similar process occurs with toileting, leading to complete incontinence of bowel and bladder (Alzheimer's Association, 2003; Reisberg et al., 1982).

PROGRESSION OF DEMENTIA

There are no clear indicators to guide prediction of rate of decline for people with dementia. The 2001–2002 *Alzheimer's Disease Progress Report* (NIA, 2003a) reported that the average life expectancy after diagnosis is 8 to 10 years, with some individuals living as long as 20 years or more after diagnosis. In contrast, Wolfson et al. (2001) reported results of the Canadian Study of Health and Aging indicating that the average survival after diagnosis is 3.33 years. Estimates may vary because of differences in when families seek diagnosis.

The likelihood of an individual transitioning from one stage of the disease to another within any given year seems to be independent of the length of time in the current stage (Neumann et al., 2001). The reasons for this are unclear. In their review of data from the CERAD database, Neumann et al. found that nearly 40% of individuals in the mild or moderate stages of AD progressed to a more severe stage or died in 1 year. Santillan, Fritsch, and Geldmacher (2003) explored this progression with 236 men and women who had mild AD. They found that the strongest predictor of decline within 1 year for their participants was a Mini-Mental State Examination score of less than 20 (out of 30 possible). Psychotic symptoms and impaired insight were predictors of faster decline, possibly because they indicated more advanced disease process. Higher levels of education were also associated with more rapid decline, although the authors acknowledged that this finding is controversial and inconsistent in the literature. Indeed, Wolfson et al. (2001) found no significant differences in progression relative to education level.

Disease progression in other types of dementia varies from that seen in AD. VaD generally progresses in a more stepwise pattern than the gradual decline seen in AD. The rate of progression is dependent on the level of success in treating underlying vascular disease (NINDS, 2004). In a review of people registered in the Mayo Clinic's Alzheimer's Disease Patient Registry, Knopman et al. (2003) found a median survival of 3 years for individuals who had a vascular component to their dementia. The same authors found that people with LBD tended to have a faster progression of their disease than did people with AD. The NINDS reported that those with LBD lived an average of 7 years after their symptoms began. FTD progresses rapidly, with noteworthy decline in only 2 to 4 years for some people, whereas others experienced a more gradual decline and appeared more stable over time. Average life expectancy was 5 to 10 years after diagnosis (Knopman et al., 2003; NINDS, 2004).

PHARMACOLOGICAL STRATEGIES FOR DEMENTIA

The most established pharmacological strategy to date is the use of cholinesterase inhibitors to facilitate improved cholinergic neurotransmission (Bullock & Hammond, 2003). At this time, approved cholinesterase inhibitors in the United States include tacrine (Cognex, First Horizon Pharmaceutical), donepezil (Aricept, Eisai Inc.), rivastigmine (Exelon, Novartis Pharmaceuticals Corporation), and galantamine (Reminyl, Janssen Pharmaceutica) (Hake, 2002; NIA, 2003b; Tariot & Federoff, 2003). Benefits of these drug interventions include improvement, stabilization, or slowing of decline in cognitive, behavioral, or functional performance for individuals with AD, VaD, and LBD in the mild to moderate stages (Bullock & Hammond, 2003; Doody et al., 2001; Hake, 2002; Knopman et al., 2003; Martin, 2001; NIA, 2003b; NINDS, 2004; Tariot & Federoff, 2003). In clinical trials with people with AD, researchers found that cholinesterase inhibitors effected marked improvement in cognition from baseline measures in 15% to 20% of participants and less dramatic improvement in another 30% of participants.

Overall, 80% of participants in clinical trials either improved or maintained cognitive performance over the duration of the clinical trial (Tariot & Federoff, 2003). In addition, cholinesterase inhibitors have been found to either delay the development or decrease the frequency of the problematic behaviors that are common in dementia (Doody et al., 2001; Hake, 2002; Tariot & Federoff, 2003). There is no evidence of the superiority of one drug over another (Tariot & Federoff, 2003). It is important to note, however, that cholinesterase inhibitors cannot prevent the eventual progression of dementia. Their benefit lies in their ability to delay decline and preserve function for longer than no intervention (Doody et al., 2001; Hake, 2002; Tariot & Federoff, 2003).

Researchers are beginning to explore the benefit of cholinesterase inhibitors for people with MCI. Recently, ADEAR (2004a) announced preliminary findings from a study linking donepezil with reduced risk of progressing to AD when taken by people with MCI. The duration of this risk reduction was limited to 18 months, but researchers continue to explore it as one potential to delay progression from MCI to AD.

Memantine (Namenda, Forest Pharmaceuticals) is the most recently approved pharmacological intervention for AD in the United States. Memantine was approved for use in late 2003 after several years of use in Europe ("FDA Approves," 2003). Apparently, memantine affects the glutamatergic system by regulating excess glutamate (NIA, 2003b). In clinical trials, memantine seems to slow the rate of cognitive and functional decline for individuals with moderate to severe AD (Tariot & Federoff, 2003). It is the only drug currently available that has a significant impact on this population.

Selegiline and vitamin E have both been shown to slow the progression of cognitive impairment, although neither results in improved cognition (Doody et al., 2001). Ginkgo biloba, a popular herbal therapy, has been found to be safe for people with dementia and has resulted in some improvement of cognition and ADL performance based on clinician assessment and cognitive testing (Doody et al., 2001; Ernst, 2002). Wong, Smith, and Boon (1998) reported that people with AD and VaD who have moderate to severe memory impairment may show improvements with ginkgo biloba use that are small but noticeable to caregivers. However, the use of ginkgo biloba with all types of dementia needs to be further researched (Doody et al., 2001).

Based on their review of the research literature, Doody et al. (2001) recommended that agitation and psychosis be treated first with modification of environmental triggers, and many researchers and clinicians agree. This perspective underlies the Home Environmental Skills-Building Program (ESP), described in this book. When environmental strategies are not completely successful, antipsychotic medications should then be tried. The exception is individuals with LBD, whose extrapyramidal symptoms can worsen with the use of antipsychotics (Martin, 2001). Antidepressants, selected with consideration of side effects, are also recommended for the treatment of depression (Doody et al., 2001).

Other pharmacological interventions for people with dementia are available for risk factors and symptom management. For example, pharmacological intervention for individuals with VaD should address underlying vascular disease and risk factors (Knopman et al., 2003). People with LBD should receive treatment appropriate for Parkinson's disease when gait and balance deficits are present (Knopman et al., 2003; Martin, 2001; NINDS, 2004). Currently, there is no pharmacological intervention to slow the progression of FTD, although symptom management via antipsychotics and antidepressants is recommended (Martin, 2001; NINDS, 2004).

IMPACT OF DISEASE PROGRESSION ON FAMILIES

The Family Caregiver Alliance (2001) reported that up to 5 million informal caregivers provide care for people with dementia in the United States. Caregiving exacts a substantial toll on family caregivers, causing emotional strain, distress, and physical exhaustion. When compared to noncaregivers, family caregivers are more likely to report their own health as fair to poor, more likely to use psychotropic drugs, more likely to use medical care, and less likely to engage in health-promoting behaviors (Clyburn, Stones, Hadjistavropoulus, & Tuokko, 2000). The experience of caregiving is influenced by a variety of issues, including the preexisting relationship with the person with dementia, competing roles and responsibilities, abilities and behaviors of the care recipient, abilities and experience of the caregiver, and the context in which the caregiving interactions occur.

Caregiving during the mild stage of dementia may consist primarily of supervision, setup, and support. As the person with dementia moves into the moderate stages of the disease, the demands on the caregiver increase considerably. The person with dementia typically requires extensive assistance with IADL and increasing help with ADL. Living arrangements may change when the person with dementia is no longer able to live alone. Language impairments combine with cognitive decline to make communication more difficult. More importantly, the increase in behavioral issues associated with moderate dementia exacerbates caregiver burden at this stage. Clyburn et al. (2000) reported that the higher the number of problem behaviors, the more likely the family caregiver is to become depressed, and that these behaviors are a more reliable predictor of caregiver burden than either cognitive or functional impairment. As the person with dementia progresses to the severe stage, caregiving becomes an around-the-clock responsibility. Although caregiving does change in the event of institutionalization, families frequently continue to provide care and support and report the same or increased levels of stress and depression (Schulz et al., 2004).

The consequences of caregiving can continue even after death of the individual with dementia. Berg-Weger, Rauch, Rubio, and Tebb (2003) reported that former family caregivers continued to experience stress and depression at levels comparable to current caregivers and at much higher levels than those associated with noncaregivers. There are also data to suggest the opposite; bereaved families often report lower levels of depression compared with active caregivers and caregivers who have placed a family member in a nursing home (Schulz et al., 2001, 2003). Clearly, caregiving is a demanding role that requires the understanding and support of family, friends, and professionals. Table 3.2 provides an overview of caregiving demands and caregiver needs at each stage of the disease process.

The framework developed by Aneshensel, Pearlin, Mullan, Zarit, and Whitlatch (1995) provides one way to understand family caregiving. They described family caregiving as a career that changes with the trajectory of the disease, from diagnosis, to in-home assistance, to nursing home placement, and finally to death. These phases resemble those of a professional career in that they have patterns of predictability and shared experiences with other caregivers.

Like the progression of dementia, entry into the family caregiver role is often gradual, insidious, and unplanned. Aneshensel et al. (1995) described caregiving role enactment as occurring in three stages, each with its own characteristics. Preparation for and acquisition of the role of caregiver is the first stage and often happens so subtly that the family member may not realize that he or she has become a caregiver until he or she is fully enmeshed in the role. During this stage, the caregiver witnesses the decline of a loved one while performing work that is largely invisible to society, as well as socially isolating. Throughout the second phase of role enactment, the family member continues to provide substantial care to the person with dementia to meet caregiving tasks and responsibilities. The third stage of the caregiving career, role disengagement, typically occurs after the death of the individual with dementia, although it may occur earlier for some caregivers if other family members assume caregiving responsibilities. For many caregivers, this is a time of grief, relief, and social readjustment as they reenter the workforce, deal with health changes resulting from caregiving demands, and reenter society after a period of relative isolation.

Context of the Disease Process

Occupational therapists understand and value the importance of context in occupational functioning. Nowhere is this perspective and skill more critical than in work with individuals with dementia and family caregivers. The ESP process is explicit in recognition that service delivery is embedded within multiple contexts, including the cultural environment of the family and the physical and social environment of the home and community. Many factors influence the performance of individuals with dementia (Woods, 2001); the same is true for the performance of families. These factors, which form part of the context of the disease process, include neuropathology, social environment, the individual's personality and life experiences, physical health, medication regimen, and medication side effects. We argue that, with the exception of neuropathology, these factors are equally influential in the performance of family caregivers and the quality of the caregiver–care recipient dyad.

Edwards and Baum (1996) observed that neuropsychological tests do not correlate neatly with functional performance and that people with dementia may be more or less functional than would be expected given their cognitive stage or disease state. In a small study with 60 Black clients who lived alone in an urban environment, they found that those individuals whose routines before the onset of dementia were more simplified and rote seemed to be able to continue to function at a higher level than those with lives less characterized by routine. Additionally, support systems were able to provide adequate assistance to enable individuals to remain in their own homes longer than would be expected based on cognitive status test scores. This study suggests the importance of evaluating the context in which the functional performance of individuals with dementia occurs, including the cultural, social, and physical environments of daily living and the capacity, values, and beliefs of the family system.

Managing Dementia Across the Disease Trajectory

Bullock and Hammond (2003) identified three key areas of intervention to enable effective management of dementia and maximize quality of life: (1) the treatment of coexisting medical conditions, (2) the management of problematic behaviors, and (3) the provision of meaningful activities. Although the role of the occupational therapist may be minimal in the treatment of coexisting conditions, he or she may serve the individual with dementia and the family caregiver by suggesting that additional medical services may be necessary and providing information to help the family seek those services. The occupational therapist plays a greater role in the second area by helping the caregiver identify triggers for disruptive behaviors and exploring environmental strategies for their management. Likewise, the occupational therapist offers important expertise in the third area regarding the simplification and downgrading of meaningful activities to engage participation of the person with dementia for as long as possible.

Bullock and Hammond (2003) identified three key areas in which intervention for effective management of dementia can have an impact on quality of life: the treatment of coexisting medical conditions, the management of problematic behaviors, and the delivery of meaningful activities. Additionally, the NIA (2003a) identified treatment and caregiving as one of the priorities for federally supported AD research. Although the role of the occupational therapist may be minimal in the treatment of coexisting conditions, he or she may serve as a resource to the individual with dementia or the family caregiver, or both, in suggesting that additional medical services may be necessary and the family should seek those services. However, the occupational therapist has a greater role in assisting the caregiver in identifying triggers for disruptive behaviors and exploring environmental strategies for their management. Occupational therapists offer expertise in the simplification and downgrading of meaningful activities to engage participation of the person with dementia as long as possible. Occupational therapy can also provide caregivers with training and education to better meet the evolving demands of caregiving, from the need to provide supervision, verbal cueing, and visual cues to the delivery of a range of physical assistance from minimal to total care.

The role of caregiving is not static. Instead, it is a role that evolves over time, an ever-dynamic process, as dementia robs the affected individual of cognitive functioning and the ability to perform ADL. Occupational therapists have a role in assisting caregivers to anticipate and plan for future caregiving demands.

CONCLUSION

Dementia is a growing concern that will continue to have a substantial impact on the lives of increasing numbers of older adults and family members. Although researchers have made important progress in determining the neuropathology associated with the dementias and in developing treatments to slow the rate of progression of some forms of dementia, there currently are no effective treatments to reverse the disease process. Family caregivers assume responsibility for most of the daily care involved and are susceptible to many negative consequences of this role.

This chapter provided a basic understanding of the etiology of the disease, treatments of choice, and the impact of the disease on families. When working with families, it is important to be familiar with current scientific understanding and to be comfortable with explaining the disease process, because many families lack access to basic information and are uninformed. Providing education about the disease, its stages, and its treatment approaches is an important component of any intervention with families and is the basis from which all other strategies of ESP proceed.

Additionally, occupational therapists have valuable expertise in understanding the relationship between the context and occupational performance at each stage of the disease process. Families are routinely informed about what their loved ones cannot do, but they may not fully comprehend their preserved capabilities. Thus, the occupational therapist has a critical role in helping families attain the right balance of support and autonomy.

REFERENCES

Alzheimer's Association. (2003). *Stages of Alzheimer's disease.* Retrieved February 2, 2004, from http://www.alz.org/AboutAD/Stages.htm

Alzheimer's Disease Education and Referral Center. (2004a). *Donepezil may have short-term benefit for mild cognitive impairment: More analysis needed to assess clinical implications of new data.* Retrieved August 16, 2004, from http://www.alzheimers.org/nianews/nianews68.html

Alzheimer's Disease Education and Referral Center. (2004b). *Studies suggest people with early AD can still learn.* Retrieved August 16, 2004, from http://www.alzheimers.org/nianews/nianews67.html

American Psychiatric Association. (2000). *Diagnostic and statistical manual of mental disorders* (4th ed.). Washington, DC: Author.

Aneshensel, C. S., Pearlin, L. I., Mullan, J. T., Zarit, S. H., & Whitlatch, C. J. (1995). *Profiles in caregiving: The unexpected career.* New York: Academic Press.

Berg-Weger, M., Rauch, S. M., Rubio, D. M., & Tebb, S. S. (2003). Assessing the health of adult daughter former caregivers for elders with Alzheimer's disease. *American Journal of Alzheimer's Disease and Other Dementias, 18,* 231–239.

Bullock, R., & Hammond, G. (2003). Realistic expectations: The management of severe Alzheimer disease [Electronic version]. *Alzheimer Disease & Associated Disorders 17*(Suppl. 3), 80–85.

Clyburn, L. D., Stones, M. J., Hadjistavropoulus, T., & Tuokko, H. (2000). Predicting caregiver burden and depression in Alzheimer's disease. *Journal of Gerontology: Social Sciences, 55B,* S2–S13.

DeKosky, S. (2003). Early intervention is key to successful management of Alzheimer disease [electronic version]. *Alzheimer Disease & Associated Disorders, 17*(Suppl. 4), 99–104.

Doody, R. S., Stevens, J. C., Beck, C., Dubinsky, R. M., Kaye, J. A., Gwyther, L., et al. (2001). Practice parameter: Management of dementia (an evidence-based review) [Electronic version]. *American Academy of Neurology, 56,* 1154–1166.

Edwards, D. F., & Baum, C. M. (1996). Functional performance of inner city African-American older persons with dementia. *Topics in Geriatric Rehabilitation, 12,* 17–27.

Edwards, D. F., Deuel, R. K., Baum, C. M., & Morris, J. C. (1991). A quantitative analysis of apraxia in senile dementia of the Alzheimer type: Stage-related differences in prevalence and type. *Dementia, 2,* 142–149.

Ernst, E. (2002). The risk–benefit profile of commonly used herbal therapies: Gingko, St. John's Wort, ginseng, echinacea, saw palmetto, and kava. *Annals of Internal Medicine, 136,* 42–53.

Family Caregiver Alliance. (2001). *Fact sheet: Selected caregiver statistics.* Retrieved July 1, 2004, from http://www.caregiver.org/caregiver/jsp/content_node.jsp?nodeid=439

FDA approves memantine (Namenda) for Alzheimer's disease. (2003). Retrieved February 2, 2004, from http://www.fda.gov/bbs/topics/NEWS/2003/NEW00961.html

Fleming, K. D., Adams, A. C., & Petersen, R. C. (1995). Dementia: Diagnosis and evaluation. *Mayo Clinic Proceedings, 70,* 1093–1107.

Griffith, H. R., Belue, K., Sicola, A., Krzywanski, S., Zamrini, E., & Harrell, L., et al. (2003). Impaired financial abilities in mild cognitive impairment: A direct assessment approach. *Neurology, 60,* 449–457.

Hake, A. M. (2002). The treatment of Alzheimer's disease: The approaches from a clinical specialist in the trenches. *Seminars in Neurology, 22,* 71–74.

Haley, W. E., Wadley, V. G., West, C. A. C., & Vetzel, L. L. (1994). How caregiving stressors change with severity of dementia. *Seminars in Speech and Language, 15,* 195–205.

Hebert, L. E., Wilson, R. S., Gilley, D. W., Beckett, L. A., Scherr, P. A., Bennett, D. A. et al. (2000). Decline of language among women and men with Alzheimer's Disease. *Journal of Gerontology: Psychological Sciences, 55B,* P354–P360.

Herbert, L. E., Scherr, P. A., Bienias, J. L., Bennett, D. A., & Evans, D. A. (2003). Alzheimer disease in the U.S. population. *Archives of Neurology, 60,* 1119–1122.

Holtzer, R., Tang, M. X., Devanand, D. P., Albert, S. M., Wegesin, D. J., Marder, K., et al. (2003). Psychopathological features in Alzheimer's disease: Course and relationship with cognitive status. *Journal of the American Geriatrics Society, 51,* 953–960.

Knopman, D. S., Boeve, B. F., & Petersen, R. C. (2003). Essentials of the proper diagnoses of mild cognitive impairment, dementia, and major subtypes of dementia. *Mayo Clinic Proceedings, 78,* 1290–1308.

Loewenstein, D. A., Acevedo, A., Czaja, S. J., & Duara, R. (2004). Cognitive rehabilitation of mildly impaired Alzheimer disease patients on cholinesterase inhibitors. *American Journal of Geriatric Psychiatry, 12,* 395–402.

Lustig, C., & Buckner, R. L. (2004). Preserved neural correlates of priming in old age and dementia. *Neuron, 42,* 865–875.

Lyketsos, C., Lopez, O., Jones, B., Fitzpatrick, A., Breitner, J., & DeKosky, S. (2002). Prevalence of neuropsychiatric symptoms in dementia and mild cognitive impairment: Results from the Cardiovascular Health Study. *Journal of the American Medical Association, 288,* 1475–1483.

Martin, C. O. (2001). Neurology: Dementia. In M. A. Graber & M. L. Lanternier (Eds.), *University of Iowa family practice handbook* (4th ed., chap. 9). Retrieved June 24, 2004, from http://www.vh.org/adult/provider/family_medicine/FPHandbook/Chapter09/02-9.html

McKeith, I. G., Galasko, D., Kosaka, K., Perry, E. K., Dickson, D. W., Hansen, L. A., et al. (1996). Consensus guidelines for the clinical and pathologic diagnosis of dementia with Lewy bodies (DLB): Report of the consortium on DLB international workshop. *Neurology, 47,* 1113–1124.

Merriam-Webster Online. (2004). *Dementia.* Retrieved July 8, 2004, from http://www.m-w.com

National Institute of Neurological Disorders and Stroke. (2004). *The dementias: Hope through research.* Retrieved June 24, 2004, from http://www.ninds.nih.gov/health_and_medical/pubs/dementias.htm

National Institute on Aging. (2003a). *2001–2002 Alzheimer's disease progress report* (NIH Publication No. 03-5333). Silver Spring, MD: Author.

National Institute on Aging. (2003b). *Alzheimer's disease: Unraveling the mystery* (NIH Publication No. 02-3782). Silver Spring, MD: Author.

National Institute on Aging (2004). *2003 Progress report on Alzheimer's disease* (NIH Publication No. 04-5570). Silver Spring, MD: Author.

Neumann, P. J., Araki, S. S., Arcelus, A., Longo, A., Papadopoulos, G., Kosik, K. S., et al. (2001). Measuring Alzheimer's disease progression with transition probabilities: Estimates from CERAD. *Neurology, 57,* 957–964.

Petersen, R. C. (2000). Aging, mild cognitive impairment, and Alzheimer's disease. *Neurologic Clinics, 18,* 789–805.

Prigerson, H. G. (2003). Costs to society of family care giving for patients with end-stage Alzheimer's disease [Electronic version]. *New England Journal of Medicine, 349,* 1891–1892.

Reisberg, B. (1984). Stages of cognitive decline. *American Journal of Nursing, 84,* 225–228.

Reisberg, B., Ferris, S. H., DeLeon, M. J., & Crook, T. (1982). The global deterioration scale for assessment of primary degenerative dementia. *American Journal of Psychiatry, 139,* 1136–1139.

Rymer, S., Salloway, S., Norton, L., Malloy, P., Correia, S., & Monast, D. (2002). Impaired awareness, behavior disturbance, and caregiver burden in Alzheimer disease [Electronic version]. *Alzheimer Disease and Associated Disorders, 16,* 248–253.

Sadik, K., & Wilcock, G. (2003). The increasing burden of Alzheimer disease [Electronic version]. *Alzheimer Disease & Associated Disorders, 17*(Suppl. 3), 75–79.

Santillan, C. E., Fritsch, T., & Geldmacher, D. S. (2003). Development of a scale to predict decline in patients with mild Alzheimer's disease. *Journal of the American Geriatrics Society, 51,* 91–95.

Schneck, M. K., Reisberg, B., & Ferris, S. H. (1982). An overview of current concepts of Alzheimer's disease. *American Journal of Psychiatry, 139,* 165–173.

Schulz, R., Beach, S. R., Lind, B., Martire, L. M., Zdaniuk, B., Hirsch, C., et al. (2001). Involvement in caregiving and adjustment to death of a spouse: Findings from the Caregiver Health Effects Study [Electronic version]. *Journal of the American Medical Association, 285,* 3123–3129.

Schulz, R., Belle, S. H., Czaja, S. J., McGinnis, K. A., Stevens, A., & Zhang, S. (2004). Long-term care placement of dementia patients and caregiver health and well-being [Electronic version]. *Journal of the American Medical Association, 292,* 961–967.

Schulz, R., Mendelsohn, A. B., Haley, W. E., Mahoney, D., Allen, R. S., Zhang, S., et al. (2003). End-of-life care and the effects of bereavement on family caregivers of persons with dementia [Electronic version]. *New England Journal of Medicine, 349,* 1936–1942.

Souder, E., Chastain, J. R., & Williams, R. D. (2002). Dementia in the new millennium. *Medsurg Nursing, 11,* 61–69.

Tariot, P. N., & Federoff, H. J. (2003). Current treatment for Alzheimer disease and future prospects [Electronic version]. *Alzheimer Disease & Associated Disorders, 17*(Suppl. 4), 105–113.

Vogel, A., Stokholm, J., Gade, A., Andersen, B. B., Hejl, A. M., & Waldemar, G. (2004). Awareness of deficits in mild cognitive impairment and Alzheimer's disease: Do MCI patients have impaired insight? [Electronic version]. *Dementia and Geriatric Cognitive Disorders, 17*, 181–187.

Wolfson, C., Wolfson, D. B., Asgharian, M., M'Lan, C. E., Ostbye, T., Rockwood, K., et al. (2001). A reevaluation of the duration of survival after the onset of dementia [Electronic version]. *New England Journal of Medicine, 344*, 1111–1116.

Wong, A. C., Smith, M., & Boon, H. S. (1998). Herbal remedies in psychiatric practice. *Archives of General Psychiatry, 55*, 1033–1044.

Woods, R. T. (2001). Discovering the person with Alzheimer's disease: Cognitive, emotional and behavioural aspects. *Aging and Mental Health, 5*(Suppl. 1), 7–16.

Zubenko, G. S., Zubenko, W. N., McPherson, S., Spoor, E., Marin, D. B., Farlow, M. R., et al. (2003). A collaborative study of the emergence and clinical features of the major depressive syndrome of Alzheimer's disease [Electronic version]. *American Journal of Psychiatry, 160*, 857–866.

Caregiving as a Cultural Activity

Mary A. Corcoran, PhD, OTR/L, FAOTA
Tracey Vause Earland, MS, OTR/L
Rosalyn S. Lipsitt, MHL, OTR/L
Susan Toth-Cohen, PhD, OTR/L

It's not the men's job. The men's job was to go out and work in the old days. So when they become caregivers, they really don't know why or what to do. They give up. They would have to. They haven't had the experience.

—Caregiving Styles Study (Corcoran) NIA R29-AG13019 10002#2:1005–1014

Caregiving is very important to me. It is very absorbing now. It's something I do with my heart for my husband as well as with my two hands.

—Caregiving Styles Study (Corcoran) NIA R29-AG13019 10013#2:497–451

I think as far as skills are concerned, [the occupational therapist] needs to have effective communication skills and have a cultural sensitivity when entering this role, respecting the [families'] values and understanding where they're coming from. I think that's critical. More so than knowing all the intervention strategies that you have to know.

—Toth-Cohen, #2 Text Unit 110, *Dissertation Abstracts*, 61(1-A), July 2000

When one enters the home of a new client with dementia, it is immediately apparent that the referral information—such as stage of disease and client's age and gender—is inadequate for understanding the occupational performance issues present in the home. For all occupational therapy clients, but especially for those with cognitive problems and the family members providing ongoing care, the context of the home environment is a critical component of the occupational therapy process. As stated in the *Occupational Therapy Practice Framework*, "context is an overarching, underlying, embedded influence on the process of service delivery" (American Occupational Therapy Association [AOTA], 2002, p. 614). Thus, the context, as it affects and is affected by the family and client, is an essential aspect of the goals and outcomes of occupational therapy, in general, as well as of the Home Environmental Skill-Building Program (ESP), especially because intervention with families and people with dementia occurs in the home.

Context can be conceptualized as both external factors, such as the physical surroundings in the home, and internal attributes, such as personal and spiritual contexts (AOTA, 2002). In ESP, both the internal and external attributes of the environment (or context) are part of and contribute to the intervention process. Specifically, in ESP the occupational therapist teaches the caregiver to identify and modify physical and social attributes of the environment and activity demands to promote the functioning of the person with dementia and ease the family member's burden of care. Additionally, the cultural context, which includes the caregiver and family's internalized values and beliefs, contributes significantly to ESP by guiding the occupational therapy process.

In ESP, the occupational therapist uses knowledge of the ways in which family members define their roles as caregivers and of the ways in which caregiving is enacted in the home to communicate effectively with the family, make culturally appropriate and relevant recommendations for adaptations to the home, and teach specific communication and task simplification skills so that strategies fit the values and lifestyle of the family. Understanding the culture of the home—in other words, the underlying rules, values, and beliefs that guide caregivers' thoughts and actions—is fundamental to the success of the intervention and to improving quality of life for both caregiver and care recipient.

The purpose of this chapter is to examine in detail the notion of culture, the cultural influences on caregiving, and implications for assessment and intervention. We begin by discussing an approach to understanding culture and the fundamental perspectives on which ESP is based—the view of caregiving as a cultural activity and caregivers as "lay practitioners" (Hasselkus, 1988). We next examine the influence of specific cultural dimensions, such as the structural elements of race or ethnicity, gender, and filial affiliations, on the caregiving experience and on decisions about who assumes the caregiver role in a family system and why. Additionally, we examine the cultural dimensions that refer to process elements, or how the caregiver makes care decisions and how he or she carries out care. Because dementia is a progressive disease and as such involves continual changes and transitions with time, we will examine the adjustments families make to emerging and worsening symptoms and changing capacities. Adjustments over time provide a window into the active enactment of culture and reveal how culture emerges to influence care strategies and family relationships. Finally, we focus on the clinical implications of culture for occupational therapists' work with individuals with dementia and their families.

WHAT IS CULTURE?

Culture is a complex phenomenon and is difficult to define. Anthropologists, psychologists, and sociologists have traditionally used a descriptive approach or a rules approach, or both, to elaborate on definitions of culture. According to Bonder, Martin, and Miracle (2004), a descriptive approach is designed to establish a set of observable characteristics of a specific group, while a "rule approach" focuses on the cognitive realities of the group in terms of expectations for shared beliefs and behaviors. These approaches can serve as a starting point from which to recognize differences among groups in a general sense. Culture facts, such as ethnicity or heritage, may give one a basic understanding of behavior patterns and rules for a particular group. However, these approaches fail to recognize the vast individual variations within a particular socially constructed category, such as race or ethnicity, and can create inaccurate generalizations and stereotypes.

Occupational therapists have proposed various definitions of culture, as well. In 1997, Christiansen and Baum (1997) described culture as "the values, beliefs, customs and behaviors that are passed on from one generation to the next" (p. 61). The *Occupational Therapy Practice Framework* further defines culture as "customs, beliefs, activity patterns, behavior standards, and expectations accepted by the society of which the individual is a member" (AOTA, 2002, p. 623). These viewpoints reflect a static model of culture within a particular group; in contrast, ESP conceptualizes culture as a dynamic, evolving concept that is part of the context of daily life.

In ESP, culture is recognized as a dynamic process grounded in the everyday interactions of individuals and enacted and changed by individual actions. Bonder et al. (2004) referred to this view as "culture emergent" and accentuated both group patterns and the individual's unique patterns of behavior, which are based on an array of influences within a given place and time. Individuals have new experiences, new roles, and new information throughout their life spans that shape their unique, individualized culture and affect how group expectations and patterns actually become integrated and played out in daily life. This "culture in action" evolves through time to shape new patterns of behavior.

In the home environment, occupational therapists can observe how individuals' everyday caregiving decisions enact or transform household culture; this is especially true after the caregiver receives new information, education, or skill training. It is important for occupational therapists to recognize that how culture is enacted is highly individualized. It is also important to understand the cultural factors that shape care and, ultimately, the acceptance or rejection by families of occupational therapy intervention.

KEY CULTURAL CONCEPTS IN WORK WITH CAREGIVERS

Caregiving is an activity and a culture in and of itself. Caregiving is enacted within the framework of a household and is shaped by societal institutions. The notion of family caregiving as a cultural activity (Able, 1991) emerged in the late 1980s and early 1990s based on a series of ethnographic studies of caregivers that were designed to provide an understanding of burden and responsibility (Gubrium, 1986, 1991). *Cultural activity* refers to the enactment of a role based on customs, beliefs, standards, and expectations that are generally accepted by the society of which the individual is a member. Caregiving as a cultural activity therefore reflects the social roles, shared history, traditions, customs, rituals, and routines of the family members who are engaged in daily care.

As a cultural activity, caregiving reflects highly particularized actions that are rooted in each family's unique history. Additionally, caregivers as a whole tend to share a common way of talking about their caregiving experiences that suggests that caregivers have a shared culture by virtue of their role (Albert, 1990). Thus, caregiving reflects many layers of culture including the unique and emergent cultural patterns within the household, and larger cultural influences shaped in part by the role itself and by social structural considerations (e.g., availability of health services, organization of service delivery, and access to services). The household, as the life space and microcultural context in which caregiving occurs, provides a recognizable and relevant framework within which caregiving proceeds and occupational therapy using the ESP approach is conducted.

Vital to the perspective of caregiving as a cultural activity is an understanding of the pinnacle role of the primary family caregiver. As the central figure in the household who makes care decisions, shapes daily caregiving routines (e.g., enacts culturally based decisions), and bears responsibility for the health-related quality of life of the person with dementia, the role of the family caregiver is much like that of a health care provider. For this reason Hasselkus (1988), among others, has referred to primary family caregivers as lay practitioners to underscore the fact that most caregivers develop expertise about the care recipient and have first-hand information about the person's past and current occupational profile. In addition, the caregiver intimately understands the physical and social contexts of the home and is aware of the meanings associated with attributes of these contexts. The knowledge of the lay practitioner also includes an ongoing assessment (albeit an informal one) of which strategies work to promote function and to ease care and which do not.

The contextual knowledge and skills of the lay practitioner differ in some ways from the more technical expertise of the occupational therapist. The occupational therapist is trained in the broad scientific basis of occupation, the neuropathology of the disease, and the theoretical implications for assessment and intervention. Those with experience have practical knowledge to share with the caregiver, but no occupational therapist can approach the contextual expertise of the caregiver. Therefore, in ESP the occupational therapist strives to collaborate with the caregiver to blend cultural or contextual knowledge with technical knowledge. As will be discussed in Chapter 6, this collaboration is a powerful partnership that promotes the caregiver's role as a lay practitioner. However, such a partnership depends on the degree to which the occupational therapist understands the cultural influences on caregiving in the home; these influences may include ethnic, gender, and filial differences in how the caregivers define and enact caregiving.

Although ESP is focused on the micro level of culture (i.e., as it exists within individual households) and the view of the caregiver as a lay practitioner, it is useful now to turn to a discussion of macro-level cultural concepts as a way of understanding further the practices of the lay provider. Research has shown that social structural factors at the macrocultural level, including ethnic, gender, and filial categories, influence who provides care and how care is enacted, thus exerting important influences at the micro level of the individual household (Haley et al., 2004).

Cultural Influences of Ethnicity on Caregiving

Who becomes the primary caregiver in a family tends to vary across ethnic groups. For example, White families typically turn to, in descending order of preference, a spouse, daughter, daughter-in-law, son, and other relatives or friends (Litwak, Jessop, & Moulton, 1994; Walker, 1992). The preference order followed by other ethnic and cultural groups is different; in Korean families, the eldest son and his wife are typically the primary caregivers, and in Black families the primary caregiver may be more than one person who may or may not be kin (Gallagher-Thompson et al., 2003; McCann et al., 2000). Moreover, in most ethnic groups, secondary and tertiary caregivers may consist of fictive kin who are informal caregivers but not relatives. In these homes, friends, neighbors, or other individuals who have been associated with the caregiver over many years (such as domestic workers or formal caregivers) may provide care (Tennstedt, McKinlay, & Sullivan, 1989). The caregiver involves fictive kin based on culturally relevant attributes, such as similar care priorities, connections over time, and specialized knowledge consistent with the care needed in the home. Cantor (1991) suggested that the primary caregiver chooses helpers based on a perceived match with his or her preferences and needs and the candidate's willingness to provide the amount and type of care needed.

Nkongho and Archbold (1995) reported that Black caregivers tended to identify three categories of reasons for caregiving: (1) familial (duty to care for one's own, integrity of extended family), (2) relational (reciprocity, affection, respect for elderly people in general), and (3) personal (religious beliefs). The extended family, along with informal support networks, is a key factor in the care provision of Black elderly people (Richardson, 1990). Caregiving is viewed as a customary expectation rather than as a disruption of the life course (Haley, Roth, Coleton, Ford, & West, 1996). According to Richardson (1990), "Black elders are believed to be entitled to reciprocity for the care they have provided their children and grandchildren when they were young and unable to care for themselves" (pp. 39–40), suggesting that reciprocity of shared goods and services is characteristic of Black cultural values.

Caregivers from traditional Asian and Pacific Islander backgrounds tend to place a strong cultural value on harmony and unity of the family. There is a sense of familial obligation toward elderly people and a belief that caregivers within the family unit should provide their care (Braun & Browne, 1998). Asian families traditionally value social interaction, interdependency, hierarchical relationships, and empathy. These strong family values tend to make caregiving a family affair, because family members share the responsibilities (Schulz, 2000). Filial piety is a recognized value among Asian and Pacific Islander families. However, as Asian families acculturate into Western society, they find it increasingly difficult to honor this responsibility in traditional forms, in part because of conflict with Western values of independence and autonomy (Morioka-Douglas & Yeo, 1990).

Aranda and Knight's (1997) research provided a basis from which to understand caregiving among Latino people. As they cautioned, the term *Latino* is problematic, given the vast intragroup differences based on country of origin. Thus, there are more cultural differences than similarities among populations whose families originated in Mexico, Puerto Rico, Cuba, and Central and South America. Nevertheless, these groups face similar challenges in that they typically care for family members who are at higher risk of poor health and functional problems and who may have pre-existing co-morbid problems. Within the Latino community, Aranda and Knight found the biggest differences in caregiving perceptions and responses in Mexican Americans and Cuban Americans, possibly as a result of contextual variables such as immigration status, educational background, and current socioeconomic status.

Strong family ties are the foundation for caregiving of Latino elderly people in the United States. *Familismo,* which refers to the primary importance of family over the individual, is instilled early in life and is used as the context within which values such as mutual assistance are taught (Villa, Cuellar, Gamel, & Yeo, 1993). Many Latino caregivers believe in the priority of family relative to the individual. Therefore, children of elderly Latinos may feel a filial obligation to participate in the caregiving role. Additionally, Latinos with strong religious views may view responsibility for the elderly person's care as a spiritual effort and may see caregiving as an opportunity to redeem themselves before God (Gallagher-Thompson et al., 2003). The emphasis on *familismo* may explain in part why Latino caregivers tend to underutilize extended care facilities such as nursing homes, residential care homes, and in-home care compared with other ethnic groups (Villa et al., 1993).

Cultural Influences of Gender on Caregiving

There is now a substantial body of research showing that men and women traditionally experience and enact caregiving in very different ways. In the current cohort of individuals older than age 65, both husbands and wives tend to provide care out of a sense of commitment and reciprocity, but they report key differences in the way they carry out the role of caregiver. Older caregiving husbands spend less time involved in care tasks and arrange for more help than do older caregiving wives, and they focus their efforts on money management and household chores (Corcoran, 1992; Hirsch, 1996; Metropolitan Life Insurance Company [MetLife], 2003; National Alliance for Caregiving & American Association of Retired Persons, 1997). In contrast, older wives spend more time with personal care, tend to engage in multitasking, and choose certain approaches because they are beneficial on several levels (Corcoran, 1992; MetLife, 2003; National Alliance for Caregiving & American Association of Retired Persons, 1997; Rose-Rego, Strauss, & Smyth, 1998). For example, a caregiving wife who sets out her husband's clothing, hands him the items to be donned in a correct sequence, and praises his efforts realizes multiple benefits. Although it would be easier for her simply to dress her husband, she values the opportunity to help him feel productive and appreciated.

There is evidence to suggest that these gender differences in caregiving are changing; recent researchers are reporting fewer gender-related differences than found in studies of the 1980s and early 1990s. Contemporary thinking is that men engage in caregiving as a labor of love and fully commit themselves to the role, performing any care tasks that need to be done (Hirsch & Newman, 1995). The remaining gender differences appear to involve a tendency for men to use a number of strategies that help them avoid feeling trapped by their negative responses to caregiving. For instance, DeVries, Hamilton, Lovett, and Gallagher-Thompson (1997) described men's use of a problem-solving style of coping that helps them approach caregiving as a series of resolvable issues, thereby reducing anxiety. Mac Rae (1998) and Perkinson (1995) described the men in their studies as attentive to their own needs in an effort to avoid role overload.

Gender differences are particularly difficult to identify in subgroups of care-givers, such as working caregivers (Harris, 1998; Thompson, Tudiver, & Manson, 2000). Half of all working caregivers are men (Galinsky, Bond, & Friedman, 1993), and male caregivers are just as likely as their female counterparts to modify their working schedules or take leave to provide caregiving (MetLife, 2003). Working male caregivers also report more instances of needing to forgo work-related trav-el and more conflict overall as they attempt to balance the demands of work and caregiving (Marks, 1998). Men are less likely than women to discuss caregiving with their coworkers or to seek emotional support (Kramer & Thompson, 2002), but with regard to knowledge about available benefits, there seem to be no gen-der differences. In one study of 1,386 employees of three Fortune 500 companies, approximately two-thirds of working caregivers did not know about existing cor-porate elder care benefits (MetLife, 2003). Although this study was limited by a small response rate (5%) and the sample does not represent the workforce in gen-eral, this research found an alarming lack of awareness at a time when elder care benefits may be expanding in response to the needs of aging baby boomers. This picture of subgroup gender differences suggests the need to use screening tools, not assumptions, to identify working caregivers at risk of role conflict.

Cultural Influences of the Filial Role on Caregiving

A sense of filial obligation often shapes the decisions of sons and daughters to assume a caregiving role. This obligation includes a sense of duty to the family and indebtedness for the parent's efforts and sacrifices in the past. In addition, sons and daughters often model their parents' approach to child care and, when applicable, elder care. Gender differences are notable in parent care, with sons tending to support a caregiving sister; to buy help for their impaired parents; or to focus exclusively on instrumental tasks, such as finances, home chores, or gro-cery shopping (MetLife, 2003; Ingersoll-Dayton, Starrels, & Dowler, 1996; Stoller, 1990). Daughters and daughters-in-law provide hands-on assistance with meal preparation, cleaning, and self-care (Coward & Dwyer, 1990).

As with gender differences in general, the differences in the ways that sons and daughters conduct care appear to be shrinking with each generation (Barnett, 1998; Spillman & Pezzin, 2000). The MetLife (2003) study reported that caregiving daughters and sons were similar in terms of being the primary caregiver for a par-ent or parent-in-law, being responsible for a full range of daily help, providing financial support, and experiencing the negative consequences of care. Reflecting the literature on gender differences in general, caregiving sons in the MetLife study were less likely than caregiving daughters to provide personal care.

Beyond Macrocultural Influences

When working with caregivers, regardless of gender or culture, it is important for the occupational therapist to understand the factors that motivate them to take on and continue in the caregiving role. Furthermore, it is critical that the occupational therapist understand how caregivers appraise their roles in order to help them build appropriate skills. Occupational therapists can use strategies (discussed later in this book) to gain such an understanding, including unstructured interviewing and collaborative techniques. It may also be beneficial for the occupational therapist to help the caregiver examine his or her own motivations for caregiving for the purpose of reinforcing or expanding those motivators, a particularly salient activity as the disease progresses and the challenges facing the family change.

CAREGIVING OVER TIME: A DYNAMIC CULTURAL PROCESS AS DEMENTIA PROGRESSES

The influences on the care relationship are complex and dynamic, shaped by the qualities and personalities of those involved, the level of care recipient disability, and the degree of reciprocity (Clipp & George, 1990; Walker, Pratt, & Oppy, 1992). Over time, the progressive nature of dementia introduces many factors, such as emerging disability, that can alter the caregiving relationship. As the individual with dementia experiences a change in capacity, family members must redefine their image of the person and of their relationships with that person. The person with dementia will, with time, require more assistance, give up certain roles within the family, and behave in ways that are contrary to the family's image of that person. How caregivers interpret, adapt to, and respond to such changes over time depends largely on cultural processes.

As the disease progresses, caregivers must constantly redefine the nature and meaning of their relationship with care recipients. Caregivers construct meaning in their relationship by reconciling discrepancies between their images or expectations and new realities, and in so doing they develop one of three types of relationships (Chesla, Martinson, & Muwaswess, 1994):

1. *Continuous relationship:* The caregiver who maintains a continuous relationship with the care recipient interprets certain behaviors as characteristic of the care recipient, even as they recognize the extensive changes in the person. The caregiver typically watches for and is comforted by these familiar behaviors. For example, a wife caring for a husband who was in the terminal stages of dementia watched for familiar facial expressions and interpreted them as affection or understanding.

2. *Continuous but transformed relationship:* With this type of relationship, the caregiver considers the person he or she formerly knew to be dead and expresses

grief at the loss of his or her loved one. However, the caregiver continues to notice and comment on ambiguous or brief signs of the care recipient's former personality. These fleeting glimpses of the loved one's former self help the caregiver remain strongly committed to the care recipient, who has become, in essence, a stranger.

3. *Discontinuous relationship:* In a discontinuous relationship, the care recipient is unrecognizable as his or her former self and may possibly even be an affront to the caregiver's memories of the care recipient before memory problems developed. For example, a wife described her husband as being very proper, diplomatic, and sensitive to the feelings of others before the onset of dementia. In the middle stages of the disease, he began to tell immature jokes in public that were often sexist or racist. The wife knew that her husband would be horrified at his own behavior if the disease had not diminished his judgment. In these relationships, caregivers may claim to no longer know the care recipient because of the personality changes associated with the progression of the disease. They may describe feeling that the former person is gone, and they may have a more detached relationship with the care recipient.

Consistent with the idea of an evolving role, several authors have explored caregiving as a career (Pearlin & Aneshensel, 1994; Seltzer & Li, 1996). This concept is consistent with Hasselkuss's (1988) idea of caregivers as lay practitioners. Transition points in the caregiving career are (1) entry into the role, (2) exit from caregiving, and (3) postcaregiving. Perhaps more importantly, the caregiving career literature examines the changes in social involvement, family support, and psychological well-being brought on by transitions, especially for wives. For example, the initial introduction to caregiving disrupts social involvement because the wife's primary social and marital partner is cognitively impaired. These transitions are often very salient to caregivers and have been referred to as turning points in their career course (Corcoran, 2003).

Complementary to the notion of caregiving as a career is the conceptualization of caregiving in terms of a trajectory of care. The transitions in a trajectory may be related to the level of disability in the care recipient (Clipp & George, 1990). As time advances and circumstances change, a trajectory model suggests that the caregiver adjusts his or her focus of caregiving in predicable ways. For example, early caregiving is characterized by the need to find information and resources that will help minimize the effects of the disease. In later stages, however, the focus of care may shift to end-of-life issues and validation. Similarly, Wuest, Ericson, and Stern (1994) examined the changing levels of intimacy in family relationships involving dementia and identified three transitional phases: (1) dawning, (2) holding on, and (3) letting go. Finally, Farran, Miller, Kaufman, and Davis (1997) developed a "finding meaning" trajectory whereby the caregiver moves over time from struggling to facing reality and then to finding meaning in the caregiving role. Wuest et al. (1994) and Farran, Collins, and Isobe (1997) proposed that caregivers do not necessarily complete all phases of the trajectory and that progress may halt at any point. However, it is crucial that occupational therapists consider caregivers' current needs and priorities as occupying one point on a care trajectory.

CLINICAL IMPLICATIONS OF A CULTURE-EMERGENT PERSPECTIVE

For occupational therapists to work effectively with caregivers, they must understand caregivers' subjective appraisal of the caregiving role and incorporate this knowledge into skills training programs. In this book, we provide information to help occupational therapists identify caregivers' perspectives and make critical adjustments to the methods and goals of intervention.

The perspective we adopt here—that caregiving is a cultural activity—requires that the occupational therapist work to support the caregiver in the role as it is defined in that particular household. To uncover the cultural underpinnings of how the caregiver provides care, the occupational therapist must regard the caregiver as a lay practitioner whose contextual-based knowledge and daily expertise are vital to the success of the intervention. The premise of ESP is that knowledge of the culture emergent is critical to the success of the program. That is, the occupational therapist designs the intervention to provide a caregiver with skills that empower him or her to enact the role more effectively and easily in ways that are compatible with the culture of the home (Gitlin, 2003).

UNDERSTANDING THE CULTURE OF THE HOME

To understand the culture of the home, the occupational therapist must observe the physical, task, and social dimensions of the home environmental context through direct observation of object placement and task performance and through interviews with the caregiver and other family members to obtain information about their personal and spiritual inner lives. Table 4.1 summarizes strategies for obtaining information about the home environmental context.

It is also important for the occupational therapist to listen carefully to how the caregiver refers to his or her relationship with the family member since the onset of dementia. Caregivers often provide numerous indicators of the status of their relationship as (a) continuous, (b) continuous but transformed, or (c) discontinuous. In a continuous relationship, the caregiver is likely to support a number of strong preferences that the care recipient formerly demonstrated. For example, a woman may dress her spouse in the type of clothing he traditionally wore, even if those clothes making dressing him difficult. Other indicators of a continuous relationship include frequent demonstrations of affection; a tendency to make conversation with the person who has dementia (even if the conversations are one sided); and obvious attempts to make sense out of movements, sounds, or

TABLE 4.1. Strategies for Obtaining Information About the Context of the Home

Strategy	Context	Information Obtained
Interview primary caregiver	Personal	Level of education Age and place of birth Occupational status Socioeconomic status
	Social	Values and beliefs: Definition of dementia, attitudes toward caregiving Important family traditions Personal and symbolic meaning of objects and spaces Social resources (e.g., other caregivers, adult day care) Club and organization involvement Relationships with others and emotional support
	Temporal	Length of time caregiving Stage of life (e.g., approaching retirement)
	Spiritual	Religious or spiritual beliefs and practices Sources of inspiration and motivation
Observe interactions among caregiver, care recipient, and other family members	Social	Patterns of caregiving Styles of interaction Approaches to coping and caring
Observe features of the physical environment	Physical	Object placement Safety hazards (e.g., lighting) Adaptations Level of orientation Comfort (e.g., presence of meaningful items, privacy, noise level)

gazes. For example, one man stated that he could tell when his wife wanted to be turned because she "coughed" at him. Another woman dressed her husband in a tie and dress shirt daily and claimed that he communicated with his eyes (e.g., that he was anxious when looking around the room but content when looking at her).

Clinical implications for a continuous relationship focus on helping the caregiver avoid exhausting himself or herself trying to maintain the former routines and habits of the care recipient. The occupational therapist must help such caregivers maintain the identity of the care recipient while reducing the burden of care by simplifying the care tasks. For example, the woman who dressed her husband in a tie and dress shirt may be willing to use more casual attire (something her husband may have worn on weekends), forgo the tie altogether, or use a clip-on tie. We recommend that the occupational therapist *not* try to convince the caregiver that the care recipient is unable to communicate; such perceived communication is an important part of the caregiver's effort to maintain his or her loved one's identity.

In a continuous but transformed relationship, the caregiver may refer to the care recipient as a baby or a shell. The caregiver may claim that there has been a personality change and that his or her loved one is gone. Displays of affection and conversations may also characterize the continuous but transformed relationship, but these are less frequent, and the caregiver may use them to produce a different outcome. For instance, affection in a continuous relationship may be a display of love and tenderness, but affection in a continuous but transformed relationship is more likely to be for the purpose of keeping the care recipient calm and focused on the caregiver. Clinical implications for a continuous but transformed relationship involve providing some activities that reestablish a relationship. For example, activities that sharpen the memories of the caregiver about the person with AD, such as creating a photo album together, may help add continuity to the relationship. Another approach is to suggest activities to create a brand-new relationship between the caregiver and care recipient; choices are numerous and should include anything the dyad can do to work together and have fun.

Finally, in a discontinuous relationship, the caregiver talks about the family member as if he or she were a stranger or mentions how horrified the care recipient would be if he or she were aware of his or her behavior. In this type of relationship, the caregiver may accuse the care recipient of engaging in malicious behavior that is purposely intended to annoy. A discontinuous relationship can compromise the quality of care if the caregiver has little motivation or sense of commitment to an individual who is so different from how he or she once was. Clinical implications for a discontinuous relationship may include the need for more respite for the caregiver and for strategies to avoid confrontation and annoyances. The caregiver may also benefit from reminders not to take the care recipient's behavior personally. The occupational therapist may also suggest bonding activities to help the caregiver establish a new relationship with the care recipient.

CASE ILLUSTRATIONS

The following two case illustrations demonstrate how the culture-emergent process works. In both of these illustrations, observing the context of the home, and especially its individualized culture, allowed the occupational therapist to tailor the intervention to the caregiver's needs. Cultural exploration led to openness, collaboration, rapport, and trust between occupational therapist and caregiver, ensuring acceptance of needed environmental interventions.

Mr. C

Mr. C is a 67-year-old Black Philadelphian who took early retirement 3 years ago to care for his wife, who is now 70 years old. Mrs. C is in the moderate to severe stage of Alzheimer's disease (AD) and exhibits balance and mobility decline, poor visual skills, and difficulties with communication and self-care. Mr. C owns his modest row house in Philadelphia; his socioeconomic status is lower working class. Mr. C has a high school education, worked in factories most of his career, and has been married for more than 40 years (there are no children).

The occupational therapist obtained an understanding of the cultural values and beliefs of this family by listening to Mr. C's experiences (narrative history), asking probing questions (e.g., What is important to you regarding Mrs. C's care?), observing caregiver and care recipient interactions, and observing the physical environment of the home. Mr. C demonstrated that the relationship was continuous in the way he spoke to and about his wife. Mr. C understood the importance of maintaining a clutter-free, safe environment. He valued the importance of self-educating and learning as much as he could about AD. Mr. C, through his questioning and curiosity, demonstrated that he was open to hearing new ideas and adaptations.

Nursing home placement was not an option for this caregiver. Mr. C did not view caregiving as a disruption of his life; he said on one occasion, "She would do the same for me if it was the other way around." Mr. C dutifully coordinated nursing aide care, medical appointments, and visitation of friends and family. He maintained a relationship with his church family and believed that his faith in God and the support he received from his church family were important to his inspiration and motivation for caregiving.

Mr. C spoke gently and quietly to his wife, giving simple, one- or two-step instructions and patiently waiting for a response. He provided a light physical touch to direct her. He consistently encouraged her to do as much as she could independently. For instance, self-feeding was a priority to Mr. C. He intervened only when necessary, preferring that she perform the task independently. Based on the contextual factors of the household, the occupational therapist, in collaboration with the caregiver, identified acceptable strategies to address the problem of self-feeding. To help Mr. C with cleanup issues, the occupational therapist provided a color-contrast Dycem Pad (Dycem Limited, 83 Gilbane Street, Warwick Central Industrial Park, Warwick, RI 02886) to prevent sliding, soft vinyl bibs, and a divider dish to reduce spilling. During mealtimes, Mrs. C would become distracted by twirling her hair. The occupational therapist suggested donning a scarf during mealtime. The caregiver instantly remarked, "She has a drawer full of colorful scarves upstairs—she always wore scarves!" The use of a colorful turban preserved Mrs. C's self-image, was culturally appropriate, and reduced distraction during mealtime.

Mrs. Z

Mrs. Z was providing care for her father in a three-bedroom suburban apartment, where she lived with her toddler son and husband. Mrs. Z's father had recently moved in with her after his wife died and their home was sold. Although her father appeared to be in the mild stages of AD, Mrs. Z was overwhelmed with caring for him. During the first two sessions, she spent much time crying and complaining about how her father was trying to "work her to death."

Mrs. Z's father was independent in all self-care but could not perform any IADL. Furthermore, Mrs. Z did not trust her father's judgment when he was home alone. On one occasion he barricaded himself in the apartment and went to bed, and the family had had to summon the fire department to enter the apartment. On another occasion, Mrs. Z's father turned the thermostat up to 90 degrees during the night, causing her son to become dangerously overheated. Mrs. Z complained that her father made a mess in the bathroom, would not retrieve anything for himself, and expected her to wait on him "hand and foot." He was not the helpful, calm, happy man she remembered, and their relationship appeared to be discontinuous.

After working with the occupational therapist, Mrs. Z decided that she wanted some daily time away from her father, that she did not want to supervise him closely when he was home, and that she wanted him to create less of a mess. The first strategy was to get Mrs. Z's father into a day program; the proceeds from the sale of Mr. Z's home facilitated this step. Next, the occupational therapist helped Mrs. Z get materials to educate her about AD and the nature of her father's disruptive behaviors. These materials provided the basis for a strategy that involved environmental modifications to the home.

Mrs. Z caught on very quickly, because she was in the process of baby proofing the apartment, so items such as a thermostat cover and cabinet locks were very acceptable. In fact, Mrs. Z was such a quick learner that, on her own, she decided to paint the door to her father's bathroom a bright color and to place his picture on the door. She installed a mechanism to automatically shut the doors to both the bathroom and his bedroom, allowing her to avoid dealing with the messes her father made until she was ready. To prepare for the possibility that her father would barricade himself in the apartment, Mrs. Z asked her husband to install a keyed window lock on one window. Mr. and Mrs. Z kept the key to the lock on their key ring and could always get in, even if the door was blocked. The last strategy was to use supervised child care activities, especially play time, to establish a relationship between Mrs. Z and her father.

In the case of Mrs. Z, the therapist's observations of the caregiver's expectations about belief and behavior (rules approach) suggested that Mrs. Z was already "baby-proofing" her home and so may therefore be willing to apply the same approach to her father's behavior (relying on physical adaptations to mitigate or eliminate problems).

CONCLUSION

This chapter examined the role of culture in caregiving at home for people with dementia. We adopt the term *culture emergent* to reflect the often ambiguous, shifting, and implicit roles, values, beliefs, and decisions that guide dementia caregiving in the home. A family's cultural profile is composed of a unique constellation of gender roles and ethnic background; the beliefs, values, roles, and expectations of the societal group; and family members' history, routines, patterns, education, and knowledge. People are not just passive products of such structural elements as ethnicity and educational background but rather are active interpreters and transmitters of culture through day-to-day caregiving and decision making.

Caregiving actions and decisions reflect the culture of the household, as well as the attributes of the setting in which care is provided, the characteristics of the person for whom care is provided, and the skills and capacities of the caregiver. Caregivers may take on this difficult and complex role based on attitudes of reciprocity and commitment and on expectations that stem from cultural norms. In turn, caregivers shape and enact the requirements of the role based on how they define caregiving, disease, health, and other concepts; again, the occupational therapist draws from a cultural foundation to do so. Thus, although caregivers have a shared culture as a consequence of the commonalities of the experience itself, each household also presents as a unique cultural entity.

REFERENCES

Able, E. (1991). *Who cares for the elderly? Public policy and the experiences of adult daughters.* Philadelphia: Temple University Press.

Albert, S. (1990). Caregiving as a cultural system: Conceptions of filial obligation and parental dependency in urban America. *American Anthropologist, 92,* 319–331.

American Occupational Therapy Association. (2002). Occupational therapy practice framework: Domain and process. *American Journal of Occupational Therapy, 56,* 609–639.

Aranda, M. P., & Knight, B. G. (1997). The influence of ethnicity and culture on the caregiver stress and coping process: A sociocultural review and analysis. *Gerontologist, 37,* 342–354.

Barnett, R. C. (1998). Toward a review and reconceptualization of the work/family literature. *Genetic, Social, and General Psychology Monographs, 124,* 125–183.

Bonder, B. R., Martin, L., & Miracle, A. W. (2004). Culture emergent in occupation. *American Journal of Occupational Therapy, 58,* 159–168.

Braun, K. L., & Browne, C. V. (1998). Perceptions of dementia, caregiving, and help seeking among Asian and Pacific Islander Americans. *Health and Social Work, 23,* 262–274.

Cantor, M. H. (1991). Family and community: Changing roles in an aging society. *Gerontologist, 31,* 337–346.

Chesla, C., Martinson, I., & Muwaswess, M. (1994). Caregiving: Continuities and discontinuities in family members' relationships with Alzheimer's patients. *Family Relations, 43,* 3–10.

Christiansen C., & Baum C. (1997). *Occupational therapy: Overcoming human performance deficits* (2nd ed.). Thorofare, NJ: Slack.

Clipp, E. C., & George, L. K. (1990). Caregiver needs and patterns of social support. *Journal of Gerontology, 45*(3), S102–111.

Corcoran, M.A. (1992). Gender differences in dementia management plans of spousal caregivers: Implications for occupational therapy. *American Journal of Occupational Therapy, 46*, 1006–1012.

Corcoran, M. A. (2003). Strategies and styles of caregiving spouses. In K. Doka (Ed.), *Living with grief: Alzheimer's disease* (pp. 167–181). Washington, DC: Hospice Foundation of America.

Coward, R. T, & Dwyer, J. W. (1990). The association of gender, sibling network composition, and patterns of parent care by adult children. *Research on Aging, 12*, 158–181.

DeVries, H. M., Hamilton, D. W., Lovett, S., & Gallagher-Thompson, D. (1997). Patterns of coping preferences for male and female caregivers of frail older adults. *Psychology and Aging, 12*, 263–267.

Farran, C. A., Collins, R. P., & Isobe, T. L. (1997). Theoretical perspectives concerning positive aspects of caring for elderly persons with dementia: Stress/adaptation and existentialism. *Gerontologist, 37*, 250–256.

Farran, C. J., Miller, B. H., Kaufman, J. E., & Davis, L. (1997). Race, finding meaning, and caregiver distress. *Journal of Aging & Health, 9*, 316–333.

Galinsky, E., Bond, J., & Friedman, D. (1993). *The changing workforce: Highlights of a national study.* New York: Families and Work Institute.

Gallagher-Thompson, D. E., Haley, W., Guy, D., Rupert, M., Arguelles, T., Zeiss, L. M, et al. (2003). Tailoring psychological interventions for ethnically diverse dementia caregivers. *Clinical Psychology: Science and Practice, 10*, 423–438.

Gitlin, L. N. (2003). Conducting research on home environments: Lessons learned and new directions. *Gerontologist, 43*, 628–637.

Gubrium, J. (1986). *Oldtimers and Alzheimer's: The descriptive organization of senility.* Greenwich, CT: JAI Press.

Gubrium, J. (1991). *Mosaic of care: Frail elderly and their families in the real world.* New York: Springer.

Haley, W. E., Gitlin, L. N., Wiszniewski, S., Mahoney, D. R., Coon, D. W., Winger, L., et al. (2004). Well-being, appraisal, and coping in African-American and Caucasian dementia caregivers: The REACH study. *Aging and Mental Health, 84*, 316–329.

Haley, W. E., Roth, D. L., Coleton, M. I., Ford, G. R., & West, T. L. (1996). Appraisal, coping, and social support as mediators of well-being in black and white family caregivers of patients with Alzheimer's disease. *Journal of Consulting & Clinical Psychology, 64*, 121–129.

Harris, P. B. (1998). Listening to caregiving sons: Misunderstood realities. *Gerontologist, 38*, 342–352.

Hasselkus, B. R. (1988). Meaning in family caregiving: Perspectives on caregiver/professional relationships. *Gerontologist, 28*, 686–691.

Hirsch, C. (1996). Understanding the influence of gender role identity on the assumptions of family caregiving roles by men. *International Journal of Aging and Human Development, 42*, 103–121.

Hirsch, C., & Newman, J. L. (1995). Microstructural and gender role influences on male caregivers. *Journal of Men's Studies, 3*, 309–333.

Ingersoll-Dayton, B., Starrels, M. E., & Dowler, D. (1996). Caregiving for parents and par-
    ents-in-law: Is gender important? *Gerontologist, 36*, 483–491.
Kramer, B. J., & Thompson, E. H. (2002). *Men as caregivers: Theory, research, and service
    implications* (Springer Series: Focus on Men). New York: Springer.
Litwak, E., Jessop, D. J., & Moulton, H. J. (1994). Optimal use of formal and informal sys-
    tems over the life course. In E. Kahana, D. E. Biegel, & M. L. Wykle (Eds.), *Family
    caregiving across the lifespan: Vol. 4. Family caregiver applications series* (pp. 96–130).
    Newbury Park, CA: Sage.
Mac Rae, H. (1998). Managing feelings: Caregiving as emotion work. *Research on Aging,
    20*, 137–160.
Marks, N. F. (1998). Does it hurt to care? Caregiving, work-family conflict, and midlife
    well-being. *Journal of Marriage and the Family, 60*, 951–966.
McCann, J. J., Herbert, L. E, Beckett, L. A., Morris, M. C., Scherr, P. A., & Evans, D. A.
    (2000). Comparison of informal caregiving by black and white older adults in a com-
    munity population. *Journal of the American Geriatrics Society, 48*, 1612–1617.
Metropolitan Life Insurance Company Mature Market Institute. (2003). *The MetLife study
    of sons at work: Balancing employment and eldercare.* Westport, CT: Author.
Morioka-Douglas, N., & Yeo, G. (1990). *Aging and health: Asian/Pacific Island American
    elders.* Stanford, CA: Stanford Geriatric Education Center.
National Alliance for Caregiving, & American Association of Retired Persons. (1997,
    June). *Family caregiving in the U.S.: Findings from a national study.* Washington, DC:
    Authors.
Nkongho, N. O., & Archbold, P. G. (1995). Reasons for caregiving in African American
    families. *Journal of Cultural Diversity, 2*(4), 116–123.
Pearlin, L. I., & Aneshensel, C. S. (1994). Caregiving: The unexpected career. *Social Justice
    Research, 7*, 373–390.
Perkinson, M. A. (1995). Socialization to the family caregiving role within a continuing
    care retirement community. *Medical Anthropology, 16*, 249–267.
Richardson, J. (1990). *Aging and perceived rewards of health: Black American elders.* Stanford,
    CA: Stanford Geriatric Education Center.
Rose-Rego, S., Strauss, M. E., & Smyth, K. A. (1998). Differences in the perceived well-
    being of wives and husbands caring for persons with Alzheimer's disease.
    Gerontologist, 38, 224–230.
Schulz, R. (2000). *Handbook on dementia caregiving: Evidence-based intervention for family care-
    givers.* New York: Springer.
Seltzer, M. M., & Li, L. W. (1996). The transitions of caregiving: Subjective and objective
    definitions. *Gerontologist, 36*, 614–626.
Spillman B. C., & Pezzin L. E. (2000). Potential and active family caregivers: Changing net-
    works and the sandwich generation. *Milbank Quarterly, 78*, 347–374.
Stoller, E. P. (1990). Males as helpers: The role of sons, relatives, and friends. *Gerontologist,
    30*, 228–235.
Tennstedt, S., McKinlay, J., & Sullivan, L. (1989). Informal care for frail older persons: The
    role of secondary caregivers. *Gerontologist, 29*, 677–683.
Thompson, B., Tudiver, F., & Manson, J. (2000). Sons as sole caregivers for their elderly
    parents. *Canadian Family Physician, 46*, 360–365.
Villa, M. L., Cuellar, J., Gamel, N., & Yeo, G. (1993). *Aging and health: Hispanic American
    elders.* Stanford, CA: Stanford Geriatric Education Center.

Walker, A. J. (1992). Conceptual perspectives on gender and family caregiving. In J. W. Dwyer & R. T. Coward (Eds.), *Gender, families, and elder care* (pp. 34–46). Newbury Park, CA: Sage.

Walker, A. J., Pratt, C. C., & Oppy, N. C. (1992). Perceived reciprocity in family caregiving. *Family Relations: Journal of Applied Family and Child Studies, 41*(1), 82–85.

Wuest, J., Ericson P. K., Stern, P. N. (1994). Becoming strangers: The changing family caregiving relationship in Alzheimer's disease. *Journal of Advanced Nursing, 20,* 437–443.

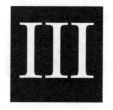

Fundamentals of
the Intervention

5

Conceptual Foundations of the Home Environmental Skill-Building Program

Laura N. Gitlin, PhD
Mary A. Corcoran, PhD, OTR/L, FAOTA

My daughter sent me to a wonderful dentist, her dentist. He was really neat. And I'm not crazy about dentists or dentistry, but he was an awfully nice man. One day I was driving along, and I said, "Oh, I have to go to Dr. M this afternoon." And when I went in, I said, "You know, I was looking forward all day to coming up here," and I said—all of a sudden I said to myself, "B, you're in a bad way when the biggest joy in your day is looking forward to sitting in the chair and letting Dr. M drill your teeth." But I said, "You're so nice, and you're taking care of me, and that's what I need."

—Corcoran, Styles Study # NIA R29-AG13019 10061#1:1044–1057

The Home Environmental Skill-Building Program (ESP) is based on several important theoretical frameworks and principles. These conceptual underpinnings provide the rationale for the structure and processes of the intervention and the specific strategies that occupational therapists implement. Additionally, these frameworks provide the basis for an understanding of why the ESP is beneficial and for whom. Given the dual focus of ESP—quality of life and occupational performance in both the caregiver and care recipient—the occupational therapist draws on different but complementary theories to support or frame each aspect of the intervention. This chapter describes the basic theoretical tenets that frame ESP and explains the underlying mechanisms by which it succeeds.

STRESS–HEALTH PROCESS MODEL

We begin by placing ESP within traditional or mainstream theoretical assumptions that have guided caregiver intervention studies as a way to identify the unique contribution of occupational therapy to dementia care. Thus, we start with a discussion of the broad stress process model commonly used to describe the stressful impact of dementia on families and how and why interventions may be beneficial (Ballard, Lowery, Powell, O'Brien, & James, 2000). Although numerous stress models exist, we use the stress–health process model that was adapted by the National Institutes of Health multisite initiative called REACH (Resources for Enhancing Alzheimer's Caregiver Health; Schulz, Gallagher-Thompson, Haley, & Czaja, 2000). The REACH investigators adapted the basic stress process model by extending it to include environmental stressors and their impact on caregiver health.

According to the REACH stress–health process model, the primary stressors in caregiving are external to the caregiver. Primary stressors in dementia caregiving include events and conditions within the home, the functional capacity and behaviors of the person with dementia, social environmental considerations (e.g., the presence and roles of other family members and formal providers, multiple role demands on the caregiver), and physical environmental features (e.g., level of stimulation, hazards, accessibility). Caregivers evaluate the extent to which these events or conditions place demands that pose a potential threat to their own well-being and that of their family members and whether they have sufficient coping capabilities to manage those threats. Thus, when an event occurs—for example, the care recipient is agitated in the morning and resists being bathed and groomed—the caregiver appraises this external stressor in two ways. First, he or she makes attributions related to the meaning of the event (e.g., my husband must shower every day; this is what he has always done throughout his life). Second, he or she makes personal evaluations of his or her ability to manage the situation (e.g., I can't keep struggling with my husband to get him into the shower, my back hurts too much, and I don't know what to do).

As shown in Figure 5.1, if caregivers perceive external demands as threatening and their coping resources as inadequate, they may experience significant upset or burden. In turn, the appraisal of stress may contribute to negative behavioral responses or ineffectual coping strategies (e.g., excessive eating, smoking, drinking, yelling, experiencing increased anxiety) that place the caregiver at increased risk for psychiatric conditions (e.g., clinical depression), physical conditions, and possibly mortality (Schulz & Beach, 1999).

The REACH expansion of the basic stress process model to include the physical and social environment highlights the importance of factors external to the caregiver that may serve as a source of stress. These external factors are of utmost importance in ESP, in that they are modifiable. Thus, the model underscores factors that the occupational therapist can manipulate or modify to minimize negative caregiver outcomes. The model also provides a basis for understanding the mechanism by which an intervention involving environmental redesign can positively disrupt the stress process cycle.

As shown in Figure 5.1, ESP targets three points along this stress–health process model. The primary target of the intervention is the external demands placed

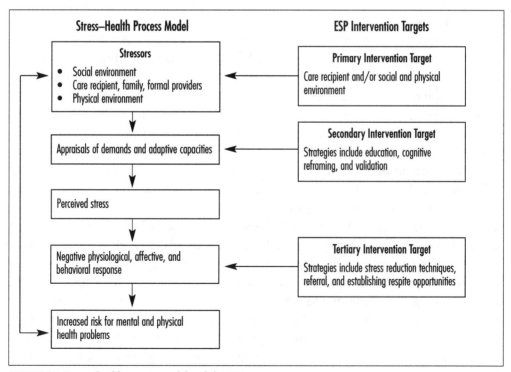

FIGURE 5.1. Stress–health process model and the ESP.

Note. From *Handbook on Dementia Caregiving: Evidence-Based Interventions for Family Caregivers* (p. 56), by R. Schulz and M. Ory, 2000, New York: Springer. Copyright © 2000 by Springer Publishing Company, Inc., New York, NY 10012. Adapted by permission.

on caregivers by the social environment (e.g., a caregiver's management and communication style, presence of disruptive behaviors) and by the physical environment (e.g., clutter, accessibility problems). Consequently, a primary goal of ESP is to provide caregivers with specific skills (e.g., communication techniques, environmental adaptations) to minimize or control external stressors.

The secondary target of ESP is the caregiver's appraisals of his or her situation, including cultural and knowledge-based attributions of the disease process and of his or her role as a caregiver (e.g., cultural explanations of the disease; cultural expectations as to who becomes primary caregiver). The occupational therapist can help the family to understand the disease process (e.g., observed behaviors are due to the disease and are not purposeful or conscious efforts to be stubborn, resistant, or negative) and to reframe the family's situation effectively. Targeting these appraisals enhances the family's coping resources by altering expectations (e.g., the disease is not going to go away) and allowing consideration of changes in caregiving (e.g., it may not be possible or necessary to bathe a care recipient daily). If occupational therapists can teach caregivers specific skills (problem-solving, communication, task simplification, and hands-on techniques) to effectively manage behaviors and other external events, they will experience less upset, have greater self-confidence in their own ability to manage complex care issues and, as a consequence, experience fewer burdens.

The third component of the stress–health process model that is targeted by ESP is the caregiver's perceived stress. In ESP, occupational therapists provide caregivers with basic stress reduction strategies (e.g., deep breathing, counting to 10 slowly forward or backward) to break the cycle of chronic muscle tension and stress. Helping caregivers reduce their own stress levels may also contribute to establishing a calming environment that can help reduce care recipients' disruptive behaviors.

Most previously tested caregiver intervention programs haven been psychoeducational; they primarily address caregiver appraisals (e.g., by helping families cognitively reframe situations) or caregiver-perceived stress (e.g., through counseling, stress reduction; Kennet, Burgio, & Schulz, 2000). Only a few studies have tested an intervention that provides caregivers with specific problem-solving skills to manage or reduce external stressors (e.g., Burgio, Stevens, Guy, Roth, & Haley, 2003), an approach now widely recognized as an important component of programs designed to help families provide quality care at home. Thus, ESP adds an important dimension to caregiver intervention research and interventions in the stress–health process spiral. It targets three critical points along this model with the expressed goal of helping both caregiver and care recipient. Consequently, ESP provides a basis for testing whether an intervention approach that targets factors external to the caregiver makes a measurable difference in quality of life in comparison to an emotion- or cognitive-oriented approach.

TRIADIC MODEL

To better illustrate how the external stressors on caregiving, the status of the person with dementia, and approaches to managing care influence the behavioral manifestations of dementia, we draw on a simple three-pronged model. The model, shown in Figure 5.2, suggests that care recipient behaviors secondary to dementia, such as resistance to care, wandering, and repetitive questioning, may represent excess disability or disablement over and above the underlying pathology or level of cognitive impairment. The prevailing thinking is that dementia-related behaviors are a product of a three-way interaction among risk factors that are modifiable associated with the care recipient, the caregiver, and their physical and social environment (Cohen-Mansfield, 2001; Colenda, 1995; Reisberg et al., 1987). Modifiable factors related to the care recipient may include medical status (e.g., the presence of an underlying infection); polypharmacy; pain; discomfort; fatigue; or other internal states such as anxiety, sadness, or confusion. Modifiable factors related to the caregiver include knowledge about and understanding of the disease, communication patterns, and his or her approach to providing care. Environmental factors may include the level of clutter (physical and auditory), barriers to navigation in or access to rooms, and the impact of the presence of others.

This model suggests that care recipient behaviors are triggered by one or more of these factors and that an approach to managing behaviors must be multicomponent, addressing each potential trigger. Occupational therapists implementing the ESP treatment process focus on each of the three domains by

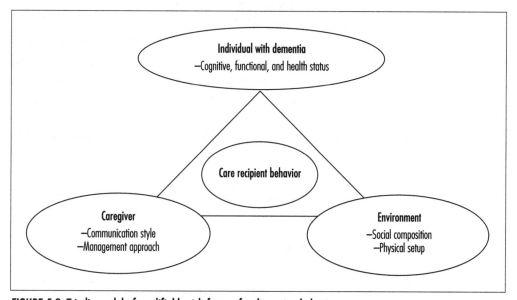

FIGURE 5.2. Triadic model of modifiable risk factors for disruptive behaviors.

1. Providing caregivers with knowledge about medical conditions that may exacerbate dementia-related behaviors and teaching effective communication skills to caregivers,
2. Referring care recipients with exacerbated behaviors to their physicians for medical follow-up, and
3. Implementing environmental modifications.

Additionally, when appropriate, this tripartite model can be introduced to caregivers as a heuristic instructional tool to help them problem solve regarding the particular triggers of the presenting targeted behavior.

ENVIRONMENTAL MODELS

ESP attempts to enhance the coping repertoire and resources of caregivers by introducing a range of strategies that modify the physical and social environment. To understand and frame the specific environmental strategies that occupational therapists introduce as part of ESP, we draw on several environmental frameworks.

Competence–Environmental Press Framework

First, we begin with a basic understanding of the relationship of people to their living environment by drawing on the work of Lawton and Nahemow (1973) and their competence–environmental press framework. This conceptual framework highlights the powerful influence of the environment in promoting positive behaviors or contributing to negative outcomes, particularly for individuals with reduced competencies. According to this framework, the interaction of an individual's competence (e.g., biology, function, cognition, time use, and social behavior) with the "press" (environmental supports and restrictions) of his or her living environment shapes behavior, as depicted in Model 5.1 (Lawton, 1982). A match or fit between individual capabilities and environmental demands supports adaptive behavior, whereas a poor fit may result in maladaptive behaviors. Applied to the context of dementia care in the home, this framework suggests that as cognitive competencies decline, the individual with dementia may have increasing difficulty deciphering environmental cues. The

MODEL 5.1. The interaction of an individual's competence with the press of the environment shapes behavior.

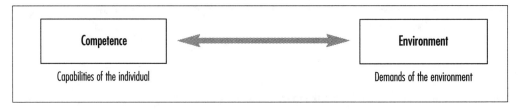

care recipient may ignore, misinterpret, or confuse the meaning of common household objects, contributing to his or her disorientation and agitation (Borell, Ronnberg, & Sandman, 1995).

Thus, adjusting the press of the environment by, for example, labeling objects or posting pictures depicting how they are used may help a person with reduced cognitive competencies to successfully navigate the environment. Studies conducted in institutional settings suggest that environmental adaptations might benefit people with dementia in multiple ways. For example, environmental strategies have been shown to control such behaviors as wandering, agitation, and restlessness (see Gitlin, Liebman, & Winter, 2003, for a review of this research).

The competence–environmental press framework drives ESP and is the basis for examining and explaining the complex interactions between the capabilities of an individual with dementia and the external environmental demands for performance. However, we must draw on other models to help conceptualize the particularities of the home environment and its relation to dementia behaviors and to derive specific environmental strategies to support the efforts of caregivers in the home.

Progressively Lowered Threshold

Hall and Buckwalter (1987), working within an environment–behavior tradition, suggested that people with dementia experience a progressively lowered stress threshold because of their declining abilities to cope. Thus, people with dementia experience their environments with increasing anxiety, one consequence of which is inappropriate behaviors. Therefore, minimizing the demands or press of the environment and preventing the buildup of negative effects from a demanding environment may effectively prevent, reduce, or minimize disruptive behaviors.

Environmental Hierarchy

To describe the home environment, we adopt a model developed in occupational therapy (Barris, Kielhofner, Levine, & Neville, 1985) that conceptualizes the environment as consisting of four hierarchically arranged and interacting layers (see Model 5.2):
1. Objects (tools or items in the home),
2. Tasks that compose daily life routines (e.g., dressing, bathing, and toileting),
3. Social groups and their organization (household composition and other social resources), and
4. Culture (values and beliefs that shape the provision of care in the home).
Based on this model and an understanding of dementia, we have derived 12 environmental principles, listed in Table 5.1, that guide the development of specific

MODEL 5.2. Model in which the environment consists of four hierarchically arranged and interacting layers.

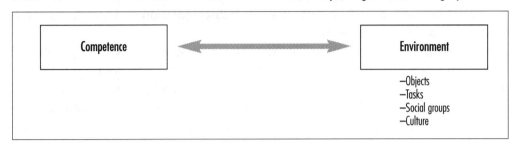

environmental strategies in ESP (Corcoran & Gitlin, 1991). As shown, there are four principles that guide the development of specific strategies at the object layer, four principles at the task layer, three principles at the social layer, and one principle at the cultural layer. The strategies derived from each principle involve low-cost manipulations of the arousal (degree of stimulation) and press (demands for performance) that result from the objects, tasks, social interactions, and cultural aspects of the environment.

Strategies at the object layer involve manipulating existing objects—for example, disabling appliances to increase safety; removing clutter to increase way finding; removing unnecessary objects to decrease confusion and agitation; and installing assistive devices such as grab bars, safety locks, commodes, tub benches, stair glides, or monitoring systems to increase safety, mobility, and self-care performance. Other object layer modifications involve alterations to the

TABLE 5.1. Basic Environmental Principles Guiding Dementia Management Strategies in the ESP

Layer	Principle
Objects	1. Make needed items available. 2. Simplify surroundings. 3. Clarify expectations about use of objects. 4. Use age- and gender-appropriate objects.
Tasks	1. Reduce complexity of tasks. 2. Follow a predictable routine, with rests. 3. Clarify criteria for task performance. 4. Eliminate negative consequences.
Social groups	1. Help family members meet their own needs. 2. Collaborate with caregivers. 3. Empower caregivers.
Culture	1. Incorporate family norms

structure of the home such as widening doors, reconstructing rooms, or installing ramps or stair rails to improve safety, facilitate mobility, and provide comfortable areas in a residence. The principle of object availability refers to the need for objects to be present and accessible at the time they are required in order for a person with dementia to be able to perform a task. Based on this principle, occupational therapists can instruct caregivers in a number of strategies, such as placing all grooming aids that are necessary for a given grooming task in a marked container.

Strategies at the task layer represent no-cost solutions that minimize the complexity of an environment and its demands by modifying the ways in which the caregiver and care recipient perform daily routines. Task layer strategies include instructing caregivers in the use of verbal coaching and written and tactile cueing to downgrade the complexity of a task by prompting the initiation and sequencing skills that are required in performance. For example, by placing a short list of instructions in the bathroom (e.g., 1. ᴿ   , 2. Wash face, 3. Shave), the caregiver may provide the necessa   t the person with dementia needs to initiate, organize, and sequ   rooming tasks.

Strategies at the social layer of the envirc   the occupational therapist helping caregivers develop con   een home and adult day care, involve others in daily care ro   utines to conserve their own energy. The purpose of any o   environmental strategies in each layer is to enable caregive   tch between the care recipient's level of competence and th   n his or her behavior.

Collaborative Framework and the Environment

Although ESP does not directly manipulate or   r of the environment for change, this layer informs the co   n. The cultural l   beliefs and   ay that caregiver   , and solicit   in the care of an individu   rategies that c   nge the other environmental layers m   rm to the cultural elements or value context in which a   Understanding of and sensitivity to the values and nee   w they are expressed within the care environment is a   e intervention for caregivers that involves environment   4 and 7).

ESI   cultural layer of the environment through the process   pters 6 and 7), as depicted in Model 5.3. In a collaborati   ip, the occupational therapist views the caregiver as a la   a partnership in which both share their perspectives on   d the influence of the environment (Hasselkus,

MODEL 5.3. A collaborative therapeutic relationship.

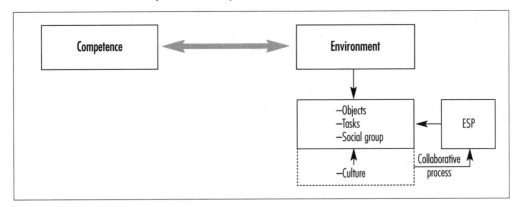

1988). In ESP, the occupational therapist's challenge is to develop environmental strategies that are relevant to the particular concerns of a caregiver and that are consistent with the caregiver's personal values and beliefs. In this way, an environmental strategy that may require personal change or alterations to a valued object or preferred way of performing a task can be made more appropriate and useful. A collaborative approach to building skills in environmental change is particularly effective in working with caregivers who, through daily experiences, have preferred approaches to providing care and hold values and beliefs that differ from those of formal providers.

PERSONAL CONTROL THEORY

Unlike other environmental interventions, ESP was designed to address issues that add to caregiver burden, such as fatigue, frustration, and lack of information. Recent advances in personal control theory provide a foundation for understanding the role and value of behavioral actions and cognitive motivational framework that support the use of strategies such as environmental manipulations to mitigate the negative effects of caregiving. Maintaining personal control is an inherent drive that involves two classes of mechanisms: primary mechanisms that refer to active, behavioral attempts to control one's life space or environment and secondary mechanisms that refer to cognitive orientation and appraisal of one's situation in support of activation (Schulz & Heckhausen, 1999). ESP cognitively orients caregivers to gain control over troublesome aspects of caregiving through use of primary mechanisms of control (e.g., modifying the environment to make caregiving easier, learning about resources, and learning how to effectively communicate with formal providers). The effective use of what is referred to as engagement control primary strategies has been associated with improved self-efficacy and reduced upset, particularly in female caregivers (Gitlin, Corcoran, Winter, Boyce, & Hauck, 2001).

DISABLEMENT MODEL OF DEMENTIA-RELATED BEHAVIORS

To better understand dementia-related behaviors in relationship to the disease process and the home environment, we adopt a basic disablement model initially proposed by Nagi (1965) in sociology, Katz (1983) in medicine, and subsequently reformulated by others (Verbrugge & Jette, 1994). Despite variations, the disablement model essentially proposes a pathway or trajectory from pathology (a disease state) to distinct but related and measurable consequences. This model is a useful conceptual scheme for understanding the manifestation of dementia-related behaviors and different assessment and treatment approaches involving environmental strategies. Although the disablement model has been subsequently expanded by the World Health Organization (WHO) to include a health model (as opposed to an impairment and disability model), titled the *International Classification of Functioning, Disability, and Health* (ICF), for our purposes, we use a disablement perspective to examine the complexities of a neurologically based disorder that has progressive behavioral manifestations for the individual and profound implications for his or her immediate social system. Both the American Occupational Therapy Association and the American Occupational Therapy Foundation have embraced the ICF as an important way of conceptualizing the health-related benefits of occupation and occupational therapy.

For our immediate purposes here, the focus of the NCMRR model on impairment and disability provides a mechanism for understanding the full range of effects related to a disease process. This model is especially useful for helping occupational therapists understand the role of ESP within a rehabilitative framework and the complexities of a neurologically based disorder that has progressive behavioral manifestations in the individual which also has profound implications for his or her immediate social system.

A wide range of functional, cognitive, and psychiatric behavioral problems have been documented as an integral part of the progressive deterioration associated with dementia (Cohen-Mansfield & Billig, 1986). The disablement model differentiates impairment, functional limitations, disability, and social limitations as four distinct but related consequences of an underlying disease process or pathological condition, as shown in Model 5.4. Although the model portrays the impact of pathology such as dementia in a linear fashion, each level may have multiple consequences for any or all of the other levels.

The disablement model defines *pathology* as an interruption of or interference in normal physiological and developmental processes resulting in neurological or physiological deficits. In an individual with dementia, the pathological or structural changes of the brain result in neuronal loss and amyloid plaques. The primary consequence of pathology or a disease process is *impairment,* defined as an abnormality at the organ level that affects a cognitive process, motor perception,

MODEL 5.4. Disablement model.

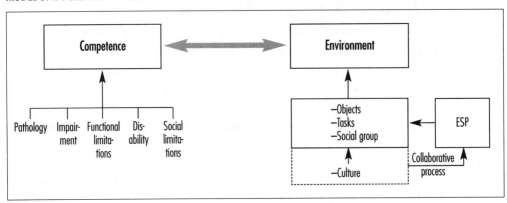

sensory process, or psychological function. The pathology of dementia results in a range of impairments in cognitive performance, such as memory loss and disorientation; in psychosocial performance, such as defective self-regulation, aggression, and affective lability; and in motor performance, such as loss of fine motor control. The pathology also has functional consequences, such as the inability to make judgments or to initiate, attend to, or participate in a sequenced task.

As the disease progresses, impairment and functional limitations increase and affect the individual's ability to perform self-care and instrumental tasks. At this disability level, individuals with dementia become confused by the meaning and purpose of everyday objects and tasks, and thus become resistive, uncooperative, or extremely agitated as the caregiver attempts to implement care routines. Other behaviors symptomatic of dementia, such as wandering, catastrophic reactions, or incontinence, may also reflect the model level of disability. Finally, pathology results in deficits at the social level when individuals with dementia have difficulties enacting prescribed social roles (e.g., family member, spouse, employee). An inability to continue involvement in work and leisure activities may also result in the individual experiencing excessive boredom and disengagement, further contributing to disability-level behaviors such as restlessness, excessive agitation, and wandering.

This approach to grouping and assessing behaviors with regard to levels of disablement can guide the selection of a treatment or a combination of treatment approaches. For example, mood swings, physical outbursts, and memory loss, which are behaviors at the impairment level, may be amenable to treatment with pharmacological agents. Resistance to self-care and wandering, which are behaviors at the disability level and thus may not be amenable to pharmacological solutions, may more effectively be addressed with an environmental strategy. An individual who manifests excessive agitation would perhaps respond to a combination of treatments, such as a pharmacological approach concurrent with the removal of clutter from the home environment.

Excess Disability and Behavioral Disturbances

Within the model of disablement, disability and social limitations are the central components that represent the confluence or interaction of the environment with pathology and impairment. That is, this model suggests that disability—that is, the inability to perform activities of daily living (ADL)—may be a consequence of the interplay among internal factors (e.g., loss or abnormality of mental, emotional, or physiological structures and functions) and extrinsic factors (e.g., physical and social environments). In individuals with dementia, loss of ADL function and excessive maladaptive behaviors may thus be the outcome of both the cognitive impairment that underlies dementia and components of the environment that impose too much demand or complexity for the individual. Likewise, loss of social role performance may be a consequence of both the underlying impairment and factors in the environment that act as barriers to engagement in meaningful leisure or work activities.

The concept of excess disability is particularly important at this level of the disablement model. *Excess disability* refers to dysfunction that is disproportional to the degree of cognitive impairment (Mace, 1990; Reifler & Larson, 1989). Excess disability implies that factors other than the pathology, such as comorbid illness or environmental features, may exacerbate the effects of cognitive impairment. These factors represent treatable or manageable components of the disease process, and their addition to the ESP model is depicted in Model 5.5.

An environmental intervention directly targets the disability and social levels that are affected by the disease process. The primary purpose of an environmental strategy is to remove or minimize barriers that create excess disability or

MODEL 5.5. Factors other than pathology may exacerbate the effects of cognitive impairment but are treatable or manageable components of the disease process.

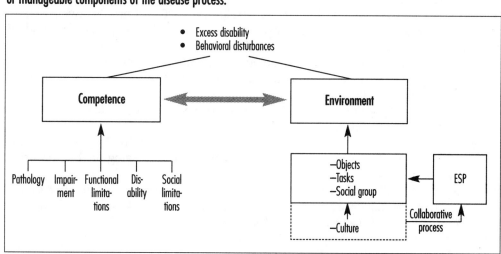

hinder task performance and social role enactment. Environmental strategies may also have an indirect impact on impairment and functional limitations in that such strategies may reduce the risk of fall-related morbidity, prevent the worsening of psychopathological conditions, and support the level of function that still exists.

CONCLUSION

Theories and frameworks are basic tools that guide treatment and enable an understanding of why a particular intervention strategy may or may not be effective. We have presented here various related theories and conceptual frameworks to provide the foundation for understanding the therapeutic benefits of ESP. Each framework offers a slightly different lens through which to examine the home care situation, the role of the family caregiver, the caregiver's motivation to adopt new strategies and seek potential benefits, the impact of environmental features, and potential triggers of behaviors and excess disability in people with dementia. The environmental models that support the role of ESP in providing a functional maintenance program for people with dementia heighten this program's potential to be a reimbursable service under current Medicare Part B guidelines (see Chapter 12).

REFERENCES

Ballard, C., Lowery, K., Powell, I., O'Brien, J., & James, I. (2000). Impact of behavioral and psychological symptoms of dementia on caregivers. *International Psychogeriatrics, 12*(1), 93–105.

Barris, R., Kielhofner, G., Levine, R. E., & Neville, A. (1985). Occupation as interaction with the environment. In G. Kielhofner (Ed.), *A model for human occupation* (pp. 42–62). Baltimore: Williams & Wilkins.

Borell, L., Ronnberg, L., & Sandman, P. O. (1995). The ability to use familiar objects among patients with Alzheimer's disease. *Occupational Therapy Journal of Research, 15,* 111–121.

Burgio, L., Stevens, A., Guy, D., Roth, D. L., & Haley, W. E. (2003). Impact of two psychosocial interventions on White and African American family caregivers of individuals with dementia. *The Gerontologist, 43,* 568–579.

Cohen-Mansfield, J. (2001). Nonpharmacologic interventions for inappropriate behaviors in dementia: A review, summary, and critique. *American Journal of Geriatric Psychiatry, 9,* 361–381.

Cohen-Mansfield, J., & Billig, N. (1986). Agitated behaviors in the elderly. *Journal of the American Geriatric Society, 34,* 711–721.

Colenda, C. C., III. (1995). Agitation: A conceptual overview. In B. A. Lawlor (Ed.), *Behavioral complications in Alzheimer's disease* (pp. 3–17). Washington, DC: American Psychiatric Press.

Corcoran, M. A., & Gitlin, L. N. (1991). Environmental influences on behavior of the elderly with dementia: Principles for intervention in the home. *Occupational Therapy and Physical Therapy in Geriatric Care, 9*(3 & 4), 5–21.

Gitlin, L. N., Corcoran, M. A., Winter, L., Boyce, A., & Hauck, W. W. (2001). A randomized, controlled trial of a home environmental intervention: Effect on efficacy and upset in caregivers and on daily function of persons with dementia. *Gerontologist, 41,* 15–30.

Gitlin, L. N., Liebman, J., & Winter, L. (2003). Are environmental interventions effective in the management of Alzheimer's disease and related disorders? A synthesis of the evidence. *Alzheimer Care Quarterly, 4,* 85–107.

Hall, G. R., & Buckwalter, K. C. (1987). Progressively lowered stress threshold: A conceptual model for care of adults with Alzheimer's disease. *Archives of Psychiatry Nursing, 1,* 399–406.

Hasselkus, B. R. (1988). Meaning in family caregiving: Perspectives on caregiver/professional relationships. *Gerontologist, 28,* 686–691.

Kennet, J., Burgio, L., & Schulz, R. (2000). Interventions for in-home caregivers: A review of research 1990 to present. In R. Schulz (Ed.), *Handbook on dementia caregiving: Evidence-based interventions for family caregivers* (pp. 61–125). New York: Springer.

Lawton, M. P. (1982). Competence, environmental press, and the adaptation of older people. In M. P. Lawton, P. G. Windley, & T. O. Byerts (Eds.), *Aging and the environment: Theoretical approaches* (pp. 33–59). New York: Springer.

Lawton, M. P., & Nahemow, L. E. (1973). Ecology and the aging process. In C. Eisdorfer & M. P. Lawton (Eds.), *The psychology of adult development and aging* (pp. 619–674). Washington, DC: American Psychological Association.

Mace, N. L. (1990). The management of problem behaviors. In N. L. Mace (Ed.), *Dementia care: Patient, family, & community* (pp. 74–112). Baltimore: Johns Hopkins University Press.

Nagi, S. (1965). Some conceptual issues in disability and rehabilitation. In M. B. Sussman (Ed.), *Sociology and Rehabilitation* (pp. 100–113). Washington, DC: American Sociological Association.

Reifler, B. V., & Larson, E. (1989). Excess disability in dementia of the Alzheimer's type. In E. Light & B. D. Lebowitz (Eds.), *Alzheimer's disease treatment and family stress: Directions for research* (pp. 340–362). Rockville, MD: U.S. Department of Health and Human Services.

Reisberg, B., Borenstein, J., Salob, S. P., Ferris, S. H., Franssen, E., & Georgotas, A. (1987). Behavioral symptoms in Alzheimer's disease: Phenomenology and treatment. *Journal of Clinical Psychiatry, 48,* 9–15.

Schulz, R., & Beach, S. (1999). Caregiving as a risk factor for mortality: The caregiver health effects study. *Journal of the American Medical Association, 282,* 2215–2219.

Schulz, R., Gallagher-Thompson, D., Haley, W. E., & Czaja, S. (2000). Understanding the intervention process: A theoretical/conceptual framework for intervention approaches to caregivers. In R. Schulz (Ed.), *Handbook on dementia caregiving: Evidence-based interventions for family caregivers* (pp. 33–60). New York: Springer.

Schulz, R., & Heckhausen, J. (1999). Aging, culture and control: Setting a new research agenda. *Journal of Gerontology: Psychological Sciences, 54B,* P139–P145.

Verbrugge, L. M., & Jette, A. M. (1994). The disablement process. *Social Science & Medicine, 38,* 1–14.

World Health Organization. (2001). *International classification of functioning, disability, and health (ICF).* Geneva, Switzerland: Author.

6

Collaboration as a Core Principle and Method for Working With Families in the Home

Susan Toth-Cohen, PhD, OTR/L
Rosalyn S. Lipsitt, MHL, OTR/L
Tracey Vause Earland, MS, OTR/L
Laura N. Gitlin, PhD

Collaboration doesn't really come naturally to everybody. I [used to] think as a traditional occupational therapist, where I did more of the directive kind of prescriptive treatment once upon a time. I really have to stop and close my mouth, listen to their ideas, and it's a give-and-take. So I think even in the style of communicating, having a collaborative model really changes my style of communicating with that caregiver. I will ask key questions or probing questions and pose something: "What do you think?"

—From Toth-Cohen, Text Unit 7, Interview 2, Participant 3

And this dealing with the whole social psychological caregiver thing, you know, the doctor gives you the diagnosis and just says yeah, you better take care of yourself too, and I'm like, yeah, and that means what? I mean, what am I? There's nothing coming from the doctors, and we have good doctors.

—Caregiving Styles Study (Corcoran) NIA R29-A613019 10411#1:437–440

Collaboration is a core principle of occupational therapy that is central to professional practice and that involves working effectively with individuals to help them regain the ability to engage in meaningful occupations (American Occupational Therapy Association [AOTA], 2002; Peloquin, 1990, 1993, 1995). Collaboration is also at the center of the therapeutic process of the Home Environmental Skill-Building Program (ESP), as shown in Figure 6.1. The ESP approach requires occupational therapists to base their interventions on the caregiver's priorities. It is through a collaborative process that the caregiver–occupational therapist team identifies specific problem areas and develops and customizes strategies. This approach to working with people is critical to the skill-building goals of ESP (Corcoran & Gitlin, 2001).

Thus, collaboration is the basis from which occupational therapists work with caregivers of people with dementia in their homes, and it serves as the primary method of delivering ESP intervention. This chapter closely examines the

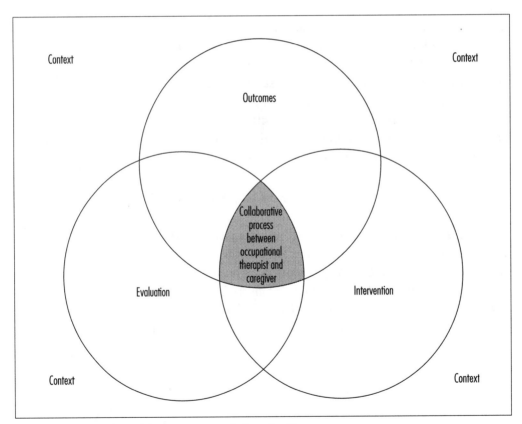

FIGURE 6.1. The occupational therapy process as the basis for ESP.

Note: From "Occupational Therapy Practice Framework: Domain and Process," by the American Occupational Therapy Association, 2002, *American Journal of Occupational Therapy, 56,* p. 614. Copyright © 2002 by the American Occupational Therapy Association. Adapted with permission.

concept of collaboration and describes five key components of this process that are essential in the delivery of ESP.

COLLABORATION AS A TOOL

Collaboration refers to occupational therapists and clients working jointly to identify problem areas and a treatment plan (AOTA, 1995). This approach requires occupational therapists to adopt a particular stance toward a client—in ESP, the family caregiver. This stance includes the following components:

- Collaboration requires the occupational therapist to view the caregiver as a "lay practitioner" (Hasselkus, 1988; see Chapter 4) who has important and valuable knowledge about the care situation that informs the therapeutic process.
- Occupational therapists must value the caregiver's perspective and elicit his or her input and participation in all phases of treatment (assessment, problem solving, implementation, and evaluation of strategies).
- Occupational therapists must demonstrate respect for a caregiver's values and belief structure regarding care provision and must evaluate how these shape a family's readiness to participate in the treatment process and to accept strategies requiring behavioral change (Gitlin, Corcoran, & Leinmiller-Eckhardt, 1995).
- Occupational therapists can use active listening as an effective tool the occupational therapist can use to demonstrate respect, gain important information, and promote collaboration is active listening. This tool enables the occupational therapist to elicit key information about the caregiving experience from which to proceed therapeutically.

In a collaborative relationship, the occupational therapist regards the caregiver as an equal partner in the therapeutic process. Collaboration is characterized by a mutual give-and-take between occupational therapist and family member as they engage in positive negotiations about problem areas to target, treatment goals to achieve, and strategies to implement. Nevertheless, although it is a mutual process and a shared relationship, the occupational therapist shapes the therapeutic process, and there may be wide variation in the extent to which caregivers participate as partners in the process. Of utmost importance is the occupational therapist's commitment to "doing with" rather than "doing for" or "doing to" (Mosey, 1981). Given that there is no "magic bullet" or one care solution that will solve a caregiver's daily challenges, the involvement of caregivers in the process of identifying approaches to care is critical.

The concept of collaboration sounds simple and appears on the surface to be a natural part of any therapeutic relationship. This is not the case, however. A collaborative approach represents a form of treatment that is very different from traditional practice with adults. Traditional practice (excluding the family-centered care approach typical of pediatrics) usually focuses on the patient as the primary recipient of services, and within that framework occupational therapists may offer education and therapeutic information prescriptively to families. That is, in traditional practice, the occupational therapist adopts the role of expert whose job it is to instruct patient and family about what they should do to address specific problems. This process often occurs with little input from either patient or family.

In contrast, collaboration is based on an approach in which the caregiver's perspective is considered equal to that of the occupational therapist and helps to direct the treatment process (Law, 1998). Additionally, the occupational therapist perceives collaboration as different from traditional practice, because he or she must work hard to ensure that the caregiver's perspective is adequately represented in the intervention process and that the occupational therapist's values and beliefs about what is appropriate care do not overshadow those of the caregiver. Collaboration can be particularly challenging when occupational therapist and caregiver disagree over particular treatment goals—for example, the occupational therapist may see safety as the main concern, whereas the caregiver might prefer to direct more effort to preserving the family member's sense of personhood and dignity. Table 6.1 contrasts elements of the collaborative and traditional approaches in work with adults.

An occupational therapist's ability to collaborate depends in part on his or her ability to communicate effectively and to engage in a reflective clinical reasoning process. The occupational therapist must continually elicit feedback and input from the caregiver and must also process the information received.

TABLE 6.1. Comparison of the Collaborative and Traditional Approaches

Collaborative Approach	Traditional Approach
Rapport and empathy:	Directive:
Demonstrates interest and concern for the caregiver and care receiver	Focuses narrowly on limited aspects of care (e.g., medical issues) or focuses only on the needs of the care recipient
Listens when caregiver speaks	Discourages caregiver communication that is not directly related to the occupational therapist's goals
Promotes the caregiver's comfort	
Indicates that he or she has been thinking about the caregiver's problems	Does not pay adequate attention to easing the burden of care
Uses communication strategies	Makes communication errors
Elicits the caregiver's perspective	Misses opportunities to elicit caregiver perspective
	Talks too much
Uses lay terms	Communicates using technical language or other language that is difficult for the caregiver to understand
Uses affirming body language—for example, maintains eye contact, leans forward, and nods head periodically	Uses body language that conveys lack of interest or support

Reflection is critical in occupational therapy practice: The therapist must view his or her own professional and personal values and concerns in relationship to those expressed by the caregiver and be on guard against imposing his or her own personal, medical, or professional preference.

In work with families in their homes, collaboration is a highly desirable and advantageous approach for several reasons (Toth-Cohen, 2000). First, treatment occurs in the home or living space of the family. The occupational therapist enters the world of the family member, rather than the reverse, which typically occurs in a medical or clinical setting. Second, families are typically long-term caregivers, having been involved in the care of their loved one for many months or years. They have everyday knowledge of the family's needs and preferences and the best care approaches (Gitlin & Gwyther, 2002) and thus are lay practitioners with expertise in providing care to their family member. During the collaborative process, the occupational therapist elicits the important knowledge families have about the care situation and combines this knowledge with his or her own expertise to develop strategies that fit the particular context and that hence are potentially more effective.

A further advantage of collaboration is that, because it is the family caregiver who implements the therapeutic strategies in his or her own home, independent of the occupational therapist, the caregiver's buy-in and input are essential to ensure appropriate follow-through and treatment effectiveness. Finally, caregivers must manage day-to-day care on their own following intervention, making adjustments as the disease progresses. Thus, it is important for occupational therapists to provide caregivers with the skills they will need to handle future care challenges.

In a collaborative approach, the power driving the direction and focus of the intervention does not reside with the health professional. Rather, the collaborative approach supports the caregiver as pivotal in the treatment process and as a valued decision maker. This empowerment can be a powerful therapeutic tool that supports the caregiver in his or her capacity as care provider.

FIVE ELEMENTS OF COLLABORATION

How do occupational therapists build and sustain collaborative relationships with family caregivers? There are five elements in enhancing the ability of caregiver and occupational therapist to collaborate successfully. As summarized in Table 6.2, these elements include building rapport (e.g., listening to the caregiver's story), identifying the caregiver's priorities (e.g., asking directly what the caregiver is having difficulty with), finding the "way in" (e.g., a strategy for immediate use by the caregiver), developing and targeting strategies to the caregiving situation, and facilitating the caregiver's active problem-solving abilities (Toth-Cohen, 2000).

TABLE 6.2. Elements of Effective Collaboration With Caregivers

Elements	Behaviors
Building rapport	Communicate empathy Use the caregiver's language Validate the caregiver's strategies
Identifying the caregiver's priorities	Use active listening strategies Probe for the caregiver's concerns Use a semistructured interview Be aware of the caregiver's difficulties in identifying his or her own priorities
Finding the way in	Identify a concrete strategy based on the caregiver's priority that can be used immediately
Developing and targeting strategies to the caregiving situation	Suggest ways for the caregiver to expand on existing strategies Be aware of the caregiver's values and beliefs that influence acceptance of strategies
Facilitating the caregiver's active problem-solving abilities	Target approach to the caregiver's level of skill and knowledge in caregiving Prompt the caregiver rather than providing answers right away Ask questions to elicit the caregiver's thoughts about why a particular task or management area is difficult Share stories of successful strategies used by other caregivers

Building Rapport

As in other areas of practice, developing rapport is essential in work with care-givers in their homes. The rapport-building process begins at the first contact with the caregiver and continues throughout intervention. The initial focus of rapport building is to communicate empathy and find ways to connect with the caregiver in a way that facilitates the gathering of information on important care-giver priorities and provides an effective basis for developing the caregiver's knowledge and skills. Specific techniques for building rapport include using the caregiver's language and finding common ground with the caregiver. For example, if the caregiver refers to the hired companion as "the sitter" and to resistive behavior as "the mood," it is important for the occupational therapist to use these terms as well.

Validation is another important strategy for building trust and rapport. Validation involves supporting the caregiver's actions and decisions when appropriate and praising his or her efforts. Caregivers rarely receive feedback about the difficult job they do and often are unable to evaluate whether their approaches are effective or beneficial. The use of validation serves to reinforce the caregiver as a skilled person who is in charge.

For example, Mrs. H cared for her 78-year-old brother-in-law in a three-story home. When she first consulted with the occupational therapist, Mrs. H appeared apologetic when describing how she locked doors throughout the house to prevent her brother-in-law from wandering into off-limit areas. The occupational therapist reassured Mrs. H that this technique was valuable in keeping her brother-in-law safe, as well as in helping to maintain her peace of mind. This purposeful validation by the occupational therapist helped to make Mrs. H feel comfortable, empowered her, reaffirmed her expertise as a caregiver, and extended her understanding of why her approach was effective.

Listening is another important aspect of rapport building. The occupational therapist should listen carefully as caregivers tell their stories. The therapist must be fully present and totally focused on what the caregiver says the problems are and what the caregiver believes is important. The occupational therapist needs to display an attitude of empathy in understanding the caregiver's world and to try to enter into the experience of the caregiver; this has been referred to as an *action of empathy* (Peloquin, 1995). On one hand, the occupational therapist aligns his or her feelings and beliefs with those of the caregiver to enhance their connection. On the other hand, the occupational therapist is able to step back from the connection to see the big picture, allowing him or her to prioritize while simultaneously collaborating on care management solutions (Peloquin, 1995).

Identifying the Caregiver's Priorities

Two important approaches to identifying the most important issues for caregivers are to ask open-ended or probing questions and to administer a semistructured clinical interview (Gitlin & Corcoran, 1997). Using various probes to facilitate dialogue allows the caregiver to expand on his or her thoughts and serves as a springboard for discussion of key priorities, as well as further establishing rapport and trust between the caregiver and the occupational therapist. The following are examples of open-ended probes to explore priorities and problem areas:

- "Tell me how you manage a typical day."
- "Tell me more about _____."
- "What are your feelings about the future?"
- "What most worries or concerns you?"
- "How do you feel about doing _____?"
- "How is it now vs. before _____?"
- "Could you tell me more about that?"
- "How has doing _____ changed anything?"

In addition to open-ended probing questions, use of the Caregiver Assessment of Management Problems, a tool developed by ESP investigators, can help elicit caregiver perspectives and structure the clinician's dialogue. This assessment elicits caregivers' appraisals of the difficulty of specific management areas and is discussed further in Chapter 8.

Many occupational therapists may need to make some effort to resist responding to identified problems by immediately proposing a solution. Caregivers frequently need time to express themselves. Therefore, the occupational therapist needs to refrain from impulsively responding and offering quick advice or solving the problem or dilemma immediately without giving the caregiver sufficient time to reflect. In clarifying priorities, the occupational therapist should engage in active listening using restatement, reflection, and clarification techniques as needed (Davis, 1998). Statements such as "It sounds like you are disappointed and apprehensive about your future" indicate to the caregiver that the occupational therapist is hearing the underlying emotion and not just the words.

Active listening is designed to help the caregiver know that the occupational therapist hears what he or she is saying. It is not intended to solve the problem or dilemma being described; rather, it involves offering feedback to confirm what the caregiver is expressing. Therapist responses used in active listening include the following:

- "It sounds as though that really upset you."
- "So you're saying that when _____ happens, you get so frustrated you could just scream."
- "I bet that makes you mad!"
- "It's just not fair that _____."
- "You must feel exhausted at the end of the day."

It is also helpful for the occupational therapist to validate what the caregiver has expressed. For example, in response to a caregiver statement, the occupational therapist could say, "Yes, it would be important to learn how best to deal with what's happening. Let's talk about some of these challenges and see which ones we should address first. That way I'll understand what is happening, and together we can solve the things that are a priority for you."

Finding the Way In

One of the most challenging aspects of working with family caregivers has been called "finding a way in," also referred to by ESP occupational therapists as a "hook," "connection," or "foot in the door." The way in may be found through recommending a simple environmental strategy that provides a concrete and simple way for caregivers either to enhance their ability to manage caregiving demands or to adopt a different mindset that enables them to deal with a caregiving problem more effectively (Toth-Cohen, 2000). For example, a catalog of adapted equipment served as a catalyst for a caregiver who was initially reluctant to become involved in the intervention. The occupational therapist described this process as follows:

> He hadn't really tried the strategies. It was very difficult for him to focus. I struggled with, "How can I get that hook? What can I get his interest in that is not so much demand on his energy level, on his mind—that will work?" That's when I pulled out the catalog. I felt like at that moment he was able to focus on something. It was really weird because . . . he was in a real complaint mode at that point in time and did not know how [the intervention] was going to help him at all. And that just kind of re-directed him. I don't know what made me do that. But I said [to myself], "Well, let me get something like a catalog that's concrete that we can begin to look at." And from there we began to identify some things, and they were successful items, and it worked. (Toth-Cohen, 2000, p. 57)

Ways in are not limited to physical devices; they can also be conceptual tools that guide the caregiver to view current circumstances in new ways or to reframe the situation (Schon, 1987). For example, one 80-year-old caregiver had great difficulty being assertive with his wife, who was in the beginning stages of Alzheimer's disease. He disliked having to tell her what to do, but this became increasingly necessary because she refused to take important medicines and to perform other tasks that affected the family's well-being. The hook for this caregiver, which the occupational therapist and the caregiver's daughter devised together, was to think about caregiving as a job. The caregiver's daughter expressed this strategy to her father as follows:

> It's your job, and you are allowed to tell somebody what to do when it's your job. Sometimes you have to do things that aren't pleasant. But keep doing it, and it gets easier. (Toth-Cohen, 2000, p. 57)

This strategy was successful because it provided a link between the caregiver's previous role as worker, with which he could identify, and his current role as caregiver.

Developing and Targeting Strategies to the Caregiving Situation

Developing an effective strategy is a multistep process. One approach that an occupational therapist can try is to initially identify a strategy that a caregiver is already using effectively and then help the caregiver understand why it works. The following communication between an occupational therapist and a caregiver illustrates this strategy:

> *Occupational therapist:* I see that laying out your Mom's clothes for her really helps. That's great. Why do you think it has worked so well?
> *Caregiver:* I could see how confused she would get looking into her closet, knowing that she had to get dressed but being unable to pick things out.

Sometimes she would just walk away and not get dressed at all. I realized that there were too many things to look at, and it was too hard to make a decision, so I decided to choose for her. Seeing her clothes on the bed with nothing else on it made the task of dressing more doable for her.

The interventionist next focused on the caregiver's concern about her mother's difficulty with brushing her teeth. When the occupational therapist asked the daughter how she could use her dressing strategy with toothbrushing, the daughter was able to transfer her strategy for dressing; she decided to declutter the bathroom vanity, lay out the toothbrush and toothpaste, and then verbally cue her mother, as she did with dressing.

As with identification of priorities, strategy development and refinement are not always clear-cut. Working with caregivers to develop and refine strategies to fit within the family's culture, beliefs, perspectives, and lifestyle is often challenging. For example, one caregiver made it clear to the occupational therapist that the intervention process and any strategy that was introduced could not refer in his wife's presence to the fact that she had dementia. The occupational therapist agreed not to mention dementia or to discuss his wife's deficits when she was present. Complying with this preference was difficult, because the caregiver's wife was present at most intervention visits. The occupational therapist circumvented this constraint by writing down strategies for the caregiver and giving copies of the strategies to his daughter. The therapist also made suggestions for communication strategies by framing them as techniques that were "good for all couples," regardless of health status; the therapist suggested to the caregiver techniques for assisting his wife with word finding and ways to respond when she became verbally abusive.

Facilitating the Caregiver's Active Problem-Solving Abilities

Because caregivers, as lay practitioners, are experts about their family members' likes, dislikes, and care needs, it is critical for occupational therapists to help them develop their problem-solving skills in order to enhance their ability to provide continued and effective care. Problem-solving skills offer caregivers an enduring technique for managing newly emerging problems after a formal intervention is completed.

As may be expected, caregivers begin intervention with varying levels of problem-solving ability. A caregiver's health, emotional response to caregiving, and expertise in the caregiving role influence his or her problem-solving abilities. For this reason, approaches to help caregivers develop or refine their problem-solving abilities must be very flexible. One strategy is to prompt caregivers to explore potential solutions by giving them ideas instead of by providing answers. Additionally, it is helpful for the occupational therapist to ask questions that elicit the caregiver's thoughts about why a particular task or management area is difficult. Discussing their own experience helps caregivers identify specific ways to address the problem. One occupational therapist explained the effectiveness of this technique:

> It happened through a lot of prompting. Holding back from giving answers. I did a lot of "What do you think about this? Would you think about trying something else?" and giving her ideas but not telling her to do things.
>
> I think I do that with everybody. I try not to tell them what they should do, because I don't know what's going to be best for them. I try to give them ideas to think about. [For example,] we were talking and problem solving about clothing for [the person with AD] to wear because of the whole toileting issue. I asked [the caregiver] questions like, "How is this going to make it better?" or "What is it about this situation as it is now that makes it difficult?" Getting her to identify those things. Then . . . you could almost see [the caregiver] start to think, "This is what makes it difficult. So, if I change to using a hospital gown, that eliminates that problem."

In problem solving, occupational therapists may encounter some caregivers who are skeptical about the potential effectiveness of a strategy. In these situations, sharing stories about strategies that worked for other caregivers may prove beneficial. A concrete example of how a particular strategy worked to address a similar problem for another caregiver often reinforces and validates the approach that the occupational therapist is offering. For example, one caregiver desperately needed respite breaks for a few hours per week but did not have support systems available to care for her husband. Asking family members or neighbors was out of the question, because she couldn't "burden them with such a request." The occupational therapist shared the way other caregivers used a university-based program that offered low-cost respite and home support services for caregiving families. She noted that the program allowed these other caregivers to go to the beauty shop, attend a religious study group, or just window shop. Providing an actual example opened the caregiver's eyes to other possibilities and facilitated brainstorming as to the possible strategies that would work for her. Thus, the technique of using a concrete example contributed to problem solving for this caregiver about approaches to obtaining respite.

Another strategy that may be useful is to help the caregiver solve the problem of why a particular challenging behavior occurs. For example, a caregiver indicated that she was upset by her husband's constant questioning and following her around the house, which prevented her from having time for herself. The occupational therapist discussed potential underlying causes or triggers for the shadowing and repetitive questioning behaviors and helped the caregiver identify her husband's sense of loss of control, generalized anxiety that she would leave him alone, and possible boredom. Based on an assessment of these potential triggers, the occupational therapist offered several solutions, including meaningful activities to engage her husband and techniques to reassure him and address his underlying anxiety.

In introducing the use of meaningful activity, the occupational therapist most likely will need to show caregivers how to engage care recipients in an effective way. Most caregivers know what their family member cannot do, but they may not be fully aware of his or her preserved capabilities. For example, caregivers may not fully understand that their loved one can participate in an activity such as preparing a light meal if the caregiver initiates the task and provides some level of cueing to help with sequencing the components of the activity. It is often difficult for caregivers to recognize that their family member is unable to initiate an activity but can still be engaged in a meaningful task with appropriate cueing. In addition, caregivers may impose unrealistic requirements for activity performance or have difficulty relaxing the rules, and they may need help to understand that it is the process of participating in an activity that is important, and not the end product.

Along with presenting strategies and ideas, it is important that the occupational therapist work actively to help caregivers continue to identify priorities and develop or refine their problem-solving skills. This approach is important because the ultimate aim of the process is to enhance caregivers' quality of life and empower them in their caregiving roles. Facilitating caregivers' problem

TABLE 6.3. Caregiver Behaviors as Markers of Positive Engagement

Behaviors Indicating Positive Engagement	Behaviors Indicating Lack of Positive Engagement
Conveys the impression that occupational therapist is welcome to contact them and return to the home Invites the occupational therapist to share in a meal or other family activity	Appears bored or disinterested during session
Engages in the therapeutic process Actively discusses care issues with the therapist Shares his or her own knowledge with the occupational therapist Offers feedback when occupational therapist makes a suggestion Asks questions, demonstrates curiosity, and expresses need for more information	Resists attempts to develop a therapeutic relationship Appears reluctant or unwilling to reveal information Appears unwilling to explore intervention options Focuses on problems rather than solutions Rejects suggestions
Appears to be using the environmental strategies	Does not follow through on strategies agreed upon during previous visit
Expresses feelings of mastery or self-efficacy in handling daily problems	Expresses feelings that nothing can help them or the situation

solving, instead of just providing solutions, enables caregivers to continue their efforts after the intervention has ended.

JUDGING SUCCESS IN COLLABORATION

Occupational therapists working with family caregivers may benefit from a systematic approach to evaluating the extent to which they have formed a positive relationship built on collaborative principles. Table 6.3 provides examples of key behaviors of caregivers that serve as markers that reflect the quality of the therapeutic relationship.

Behavioral markers of caregiver engagement in a positive therapeutic relationship include the overall attitude conveyed toward the occupational therapist and the intervention, the level of engagement in the therapeutic process, the degree to which there is follow-through with intervention strategies discussed and agreed on, and changes in the caregiver's perceived mastery or self-efficacy regarding specific aspects of the caregiving role.

Occupational therapist–based behavioral markers can be categorized according to three interrelated aspects: rapport and empathy, communication strategies, and use of a caregiver-as-expert approach. The occupational therapist may use these markers to guide a self-assessment of his or her skills in creating a collaborative relationship. For difficult or more challenging cases, occupational therapists may find it helpful to audiotape a treatment contact (with the caregiver's permission). Reviewing the recording later provides a means for self-reflection, enabling the occupational therapist to analyze and improve on his or her communication patterns.

FREQUENTLY ASKED QUESTIONS ABOUT COLLABORATION

As we have noted, collaboration is challenging; it involves obtaining the right balance between shaping and directing the intervention and enabling meaningful participation by the caregiver. There are numerous issues in finding this balance, and the following questions and answers address a few of these:

1. *What should the occupational therapist do if he or she observes unsafe conditions that the caregiver does not want to work on?*

   This is a common dilemma and reflects a potential conflict between a lay and professional perspective. Although it is important for the occupational therapist to help caregivers understand why a particular situation may be unsafe, it is equally important for the occupational therapist to explore and reflect further as to why the caregiver does not perceive the situation in the same way. It may be because the caregiver lacks an understanding of the disease process, or is more concerned with upholding normalcy in the household, or is working from a way of looking at the caregiving situation that is not congruent with that of the caregiver.

2. *What should the occupational therapist do if the caregiver identifies a problem that is misleading or that is not the "real" problem?*

   Sometimes a caregiver identifies a problem that is not the true problem, at least as the occupational therapist sees it. As in every case, occupational therapists must listen carefully to understand how caregivers frame problems and why they identify certain areas as problematic.

   For example, Mrs. T wanted an ESP interventionist to help her set up a technology system in the home to monitor her husband, who had moderate dementia, while she was at work all day. She wanted her husband to call her every 2 to 3 hours to check in with her. Although he had been capable of using the telephone in the early stages of the disease process, he was not able to remember to contact her, and he got confused about how to use the phone even with instant dialing. More importantly, he was home all day alone and unable to safely prepare meals or snacks. Thus, the occupational therapist believed that the "real" problem was not that Mr. T did not check in with his wife during the workday, but that Mrs. T believed that he was capable of doing this.

   To work on this problem, the occupational therapist began by educating Mrs. T about the disease process and about Mr. T's current capabilities. In response, Mrs. T revealed that she was having great difficulty adjusting to his decline and was fearful that she could no longer continue to work outside the home, which was critical to their financial stability. Following this revelation, the occupational therapist began to discuss care options such as adult day care and other arrangements that Mrs. T could make to keep Mr. T safe at home, as well as ways to prepare adequately for further declines.

3. *What if the caregiver does not like to talk or cannot identify a problem area?*

   Collaboration is based on mutual give-and-take and on the caregiver's active participation in the assessment, treatment, and implementation process. However, some caregivers are so overburdened that they perceive ESP as too much effort—they just want someone to tell them what to do to make life better. With such caregivers, it is important for the occupational therapist to recognize and appreciate the stress of caregiving and to refrain from imposing any additional burden. It is helpful for the occupational therapist to explain that, although there is no magic bullet or one single way in which a particular care problem can be solved, there are techniques that the occupational therapist can teach the caregiver to help resolve some of the pressing issues he or she confronts. For the overwhelmed caregiver, it is important to start and move slowly and to begin by introducing an easy-to-use strategy (e.g., deep breathing to reduce caregiver stress) that provides an immediate reward.

CONCLUSION

A collaborative approach is essential to the occupational therapist's conduct of the ESP intervention with family caregivers of people with dementia. The emphasis in ESP goes beyond the level of collaboration typically found in traditional practice. In ESP, occupational therapists must view the caregiver as a lay practitioner, elicit the caregiver's input and participation in all phases of treatment, and demonstrate respect for the caregiver's values and belief structure and the ways in which these shape intervention.

In ESP, the essential elements of collaboration are establishing rapport, identifying the caregiver's priorities, finding the way in, and targeting strategies that fit the family's unique situation; the final stage of collaboration involves preparing the caregiver to problem solve independently, without further reliance on the occupational therapist's guidance. Thus, the ultimate goal of the collaboration process is to facilitate caregivers' active problem solving and to provide a basis for continued strategy development and use after intervention has ended. Behavioral markers indicating caregiver engagement in a positive collaboration enable occupational therapists to assess the strength of the collaborative relationship. Occupational therapists also must reflect on their own behaviors to determine ways in which they may be helping or hindering collaboration.

REFERENCES

American Occupational Therapy Association. (1995). Concept paper: Service delivery in occupational therapy. *American Journal of Occupational Therapy, 49,* 1029–1031.

American Occupational Therapy Association. (2002). Occupational therapy practice framework: Domain and process. *American Journal of Occupational Therapy, 56,* 609–639.

Corcoran, M., & Gitlin, L. N. (2001). Family caregiver acceptance and use of environmental strategies in occupational therapy intervention. *Physical & Occupational Therapy in Geriatrics, 19,* 1–20.

Davis, C. M. (1998). *Patient practitioner interaction.* Thorofare, NJ: Slack.

Gitlin, L. N., & Corcoran, M. C. (1997). *Intervention documentation: Home Environmental Skill-Building Program* (Manual for Philadelphia REACH, a project funded by the National Institutes on Aging Grant IR01-AG133265-01A1). Philadelphia: Thomas Jefferson University, College of Health Professions.

Gitlin, L. N., Corcoran, M. C., & Leinmiller-Eckhardt, S. (1995). Understanding the family perspective: An ethnographic framework for providing occupational therapy in the home. *American Journal of Occupational Therapy, 49,* 802–809.

Gitlin, L. N. & Gwyther, L. P. (2002). In-home interventions: Helping caregivers where they live. In D. Coon, D. Gallagher-Thompson, & L. Thompson (Eds.), *Innovative interventions to reduce caregiver distress: A clinical guide* (pp. 139–160). New York: Springer.

Hasselkus, B. R. (1988). Meaning in family caregiving: Perspectives on caregiver/professional relationships. *Gerontologist, 28,* 686–691.

Law, M. (1998). *Client-centered occupational therapy.* Thorofare, NJ: Slack.

Mosey, A. (1981). *Occupational therapy: Configuration of a profession.* New York: Raven Press.

Peloquin, S. (1990). The patient–therapist relationship in occupational therapy: Understanding visions and images. *American Journal of Occupational Therapy, 44,* 13–22.

Peloquin, S. (1993). The patient–therapist relationship: Beliefs that shape care. *American Journal of Occupational Therapy, 47,* 935–942.

Peloquin, S. (1995). Fullness of empathy: Reflections and illustrations. *American Journal of Occupational Therapy, 49,* 24–31.

Schon, D. A. (1987). *Educating the reflective practitioner.* San Francisco: Jossey-Bass.

Toth-Cohen, S. (2000a). The influence of context on clinical reasoning of occupational therapists providing intervention for caregivers of persons with dementia (Doctoral dissertation, Temple University, 2000). *Dissertation Abstracts International Section A: Humanities & Social Sciences, 61(1-A),* 100.

Toth-Cohen, S. (2000b). Role perceptions of occupational therapists providing education and support for caregivers of persons with dementia. *American Journal of Occupational Therapy, 54,* 509–515.

7

Assessing the Collaborative Process

The Therapeutic Engagement Index

Yeon Kyung Chee, PhD
Laura N. Gitlin, PhD

I said, "What do you think about, instead of getting a whole new recliner, putting a firm cushion in the recliner?" She said, "Oh, I never thought about that." I said, "Well, would you be willing to try it out?" [She said,] "Yeah, I'll give it a try." And it's this give and take. And the follow-up of that is just that: follow-up of how did it work. And . . . I must also be willing to say, "If she doesn't like it, we'll move on to something else, or we'll look at another option." So that's where collaboration is very much a skill and an art, and it needs to be developed. And you have to be patient with it. And you have to set your—your, uh, bossiness aside, or your authoritativeness aside, to make it work.

—Toth-Cohen NIA Grant #K07 AG00998, Text Unit 9, Interview 2, Participant 3

A collaborative approach to working with family caregivers is caregiver centered—that is, the caregiver's values, preferences, and target goals are central
to the health care decision-making and treatment processes (Holman & Lorig,
2000; Stewart, 2001; Von Korff, Gruman, Schaefer, Curry, & Wagner, 1997). As
described in Chapter 6, the ability to develop a positive relationship and to
engage the caregiver fully in the treatment process is essential to implementing
the Home Environmental Skill-Building Program (ESP) and obtaining desired
intervention outcomes.

The importance of using a collaborative approach in ESP is supported by
previous research in health care showing collaboration to be effective in achieving positive health outcomes, including increased adherence to treatment,
improvement in health status and role performance, and satisfaction with medical care (DiMatteo, 1994; Greenfeld, Kaplan, & Ware, 1985; Stewart, 2001). Within
the primary care setting, for example, research on physician–patient communication patterns (e.g., active listening) has consistently shown that health care
providers who successfully involve patients in the treatment process obtain better health outcomes (Roter, 2000). In a similar way, research studies on the psy-
chotherapeutic relationships highlight the critical role of building a therapeutic
alliance with clients, suggesting that it is the relationship, and not necessarily the
content of, a particular intervention that has the beneficial effect on various psychological and behavioral problems (Frieswyk et al., 1986; Horvath, Gaston, &
Luborsky, 1993). Finally, based on such evidence, a report from the Institute of
Medicine (2001) strongly advocated for health professionals to use a patient-
centered approach and collaborative strategies, declaring this approach central to
the delivery of effective health services.

Despite increased recognition of the importance of evaluating caregiver–
therapist interactions, the quality of the engagement process among service
providers and family caregivers has not been systematically evaluated. This gap
in the research is due in large part to the lack of an adequate assessment tool to
help occupational therapists examine this process, particularly as it pertains to
family caregivers.

This chapter describes a measure—the Therapeutic Engagement Index
(TEI)—specifically developed for ESP. The purpose of this scale is to provide
occupational therapists with a concise and easy-to-use approach to gauging the
progress of family caregivers' therapeutic engagement as it unfolds in home
intervention visits.

ASSESSMENT OF THE THERAPEUTIC PROCESS

It is important for several reasons to understand and evaluate the extent to which
families are engaged in ESP. First, as has been discussed in previous chapters, the
vast majority of individuals with dementia are cared for by families at home who

typically provide daily, hands-on assistance, particularly in the middle stage of the disease process (Haley & Bailey, 1999). Thus, families are inextricably involved in managing the disease and are vital to helping occupational therapists to understand the most effective strategies that can be implemented to manage difficult or challenging behaviors. The effectiveness of ESP is based on a partnership between the therapist and the family caregiver that involves active engagement of the caregiver in the assessment–treatment process. Caregivers must feel comfortable enough to reveal information that is sometimes intimate, and their knowledge of the care situation from which occupational therapists can then develop customized strategies. Evaluation of the extent to which a caregiver is engaged in the therapeutic process can help the occupational therapist determine whether the caregiver feels comfortable enough to reveal the information and knowledge necessary for developing appropriate strategies.

Because of wide variations in the progression of the disease and resulting impairment, and thus the challenges that families face, customization is a crucial feature of services for caregivers of people with dementia. This is an important point that is supported by research showing that an intervention approach that actively engages caregivers in the process (e.g., hands-on-training vs. didactic or written materials) and that tailors strategies to their specific needs is very effective at reducing caregiver burden and at preventing premature nursing home placement (Mittelman, Roth, Coon, & Haley, 2004; Pusey & Richard, 2001). The occupational therapist's ability to customize a strategy is enhanced by a relationship with the caregiver that is built on trust and mutual respect and the full engagement of the caregiver in the therapeutic process.

Another reason to systematically evaluate the extent to which caregivers are engaged in ESP is to ensure that families are able to disclose the personal and intimate details of daily life that serve as a major source of stress and that may be appropriate to address in the intervention. For instance, some caregivers may initially be embarrassed or reluctant to reveal details related to the toileting issues or sexually inappropriate behaviors of their family members. Thus, a collaborative process based on trust and empathy, as discussed in Chapter 6, is crucial to the occupational therapy process in general and to helping caregivers deal with the sensitive issues of caring for a person with dementia (Peloquin, 1998). The TEI is a brief measure that helps therapists systematically evaluate the collaborative process.

Assessing the extent to which the caregiver is engaged in the therapeutic process is particularly critical when providing intervention in the home setting. The home, as the life space of individuals, differs significantly from traditional medical settings in which health providers deliver services. In the home, the occupational therapist is an invited guest, so to speak, and so must be guided by the family's cultural norms and personal preferences (e.g., best time to meet, presence of others; Gitlin & Gwyther, 2003). Systematically evaluating the strength of a caregiver's involvement in the collaborative process enables occupational therapists to reflect on their success or lack thereof in effectively assisting a family caregiver (Peloquin, 1998).

THERAPEUTIC ENGAGEMENT INDEX

Development

The TEI, composed of 14 items, was initially developed with 10 occupational therapists and 99 caregivers who participated in ESP (Gitlin, Corcoran, Winter, Boyce, & Hauck, 2001). The tool was then modified by the research team, and the modified version was subsequently evaluated with an additional 6 occupational therapists who worked with 118 caregivers participating in the ESP study (Gitlin et al., 2003). The occupational therapists who helped test the TEI were registered and licensed and had a minimum of 3 years' postgraduate clinical training and home care experience. Also, the occupational therapists were familiar with dementia care and had used a collaborative therapeutic framework in other treatment settings.

The items developed for the TEI were designed to measure provider perceptions of the nature of engagement with family caregivers, which can inform providers about the extent to which a collaborative therapeutic relationship with family caregivers has been established. An initial pool of items was developed to represent both verbal and nonverbal caregiver behaviors that might suggest the development of positive therapeutic engagement. These items were generated in three ways: (1) through a systematic review of existing research and clinical publications on therapeutic alliance, management of dementia, and home care; (2) in focused meetings with the 10 occupational therapists involved in home care; and (3) through consultation with key researchers in occupational therapy and informal caregiving. Occupational therapists and researchers with expertise in this area then reviewed each item.

Table 7.1 presents the final set of 14 items that compose the TEI. The items reflect concepts of patient-centered care, caregiving for people with dementia, and ethical considerations in caregiving, and they are behavioral markers or indicators of positive therapeutic engagement. For each item, occupational therapists rate their appraisal of the caregiver's participatory behavior on a 5-point scale (0 = *not at all* to 4 = *extremely*, with negative items reverse coded). A total TEI score is derived by summing the score for each of the 14 items. A higher score indicates greater caregiver engagement in the treatment process.

Domains

Chee, Dennis, and Gitlin (in press) evaluated the psychometric properties of the TEI in detail and showed that the TEI is a valid and internally consistent tool

TABLE 7.1. Domains, Items, and Score Ranges of the Therapeutic Engagement Index

Domain	Item	Score Range
	During today's contact, to what extent did this caregiver:	
Openness	1. Resist the therapeutic relationship?	0–20
	2. Reject suggestions?	
	3. Appear bored?	
	4. Seem reluctant to reveal information?	
	5. Indicate that future contacts are canceled?	
Connectedness	6. Make the interventionist feel welcomed?	0–20
	7. Involve the interventionist in family activity?	
	8. Do most of the talking?	
	9. Disclose relevant information?	
	10. Share knowledge with the interventionist?	
Involvement	11. Ask questions?	0–16
	12. Offer feedback?	
	13. Express the need for more information?	
	14. Indicate that contact was useful?	
	Total score range	0–56

Note. Response scores: 0 = *not at all*, 1 = *a little*, 2 = *moderately*, 3 = *very much*, 4 = *extremely*.

consisting of three distinct but related domains: (1) therapist appraisal of the caregiver's receptiveness to suggestions and willingness to share information, referred to as *openness*; (2) therapist appraisal of the caregiver's ability to connect with the occupational therapist on a personal basis, referred to as *connectedness*; and (3) therapist appraisal of the caregiver's willingness to seek help from others, referred to as *involvement*.

Of clinical interest is the way in which each domain is associated with different characteristics of caregivers and care recipients. Openness was associated with the occupational therapist's evaluation of the caregiver's level of readiness to make changes in caregiving routines and style of care (see Tool A-5 in Appendix A), suggesting that caregivers who do not appear ready to change their behaviors (e.g., who are not willing to change the way they communicate to the care recipient) or to adapt new methods of caregiving may not be receptive to the intervention and specific strategy recommendations made by the occupational therapist. Thus, low readiness to change, at least as perceived by the occupational therapist, may mean that these caregivers are at risk of not fully engaging in ESP, which is a behaviorally demanding intervention. Connectedness is related to the occurrence of troublesome behaviors in the dementia patient. That is, caregivers who manage challenging behaviors appear to be able to connect to the therapeutic process better than those who are not managing such behaviors. Finally, Involvement, Domain 3, is related to caregivers who are ready to change, who report anxiety and having to manage problem behaviors. Additionally, we found that caregivers who exhibited readiness to change and anxiety related to problem behaviors scored high in the Involvement domain, suggesting that these caregivers may be motivated to seek help (e.g., by asking questions or offering feedback on suggestions) as a way to manage or cope.

Interestingly, caregiver depressive symptoms were related to higher scores in the Involvement domain but not necessarily in the Connectedness domain. Emotionally distressed caregivers were able to express their needs for more information and provided input into the intervention, but there was no association between depressive symptoms and ability to bond with interventionists or openness to the treatment process in ESP. It is unclear why caregivers with depressive symptoms were willing to seek information without necessarily seeking personal connectedness with interventionists. It may be that caregivers with depression perceived establishing a personal relationship with the occupational therapist as requiring greater levels of personal energy than eliciting desired information.

None of the three domains was associated with level of care recipient physical and cognitive impairments. The various patterns of associations between the three domains of TEI and caregiver affect and care recipient problem behaviors suggest that the development of therapeutic engagement and the factors that influence it are complex and nuanced.

PROGRESS OF THERAPEUTIC ENGAGEMENT

The active phase of ESP (as described in detail in Chapters 8 and 9) consists of five home visits and a telephone contact. Thus, it is important to know how many contacts are necessary for caregivers to become actively engaged in the therapeutic process. We found the TEI to be sensitive in that it differentiated between caregivers who completed all intervention contacts and those who did not. Figure 7.1 shows the average TEI scores obtained from each home visit for both completers and noncompleters of the ESP active phase, including the score from the final (fifth) visit for caregivers who completed the intervention. As shown for completers, the most significant increase in the level of therapeutic engagement occurred from the initial visit to the second visit, with only small, nonsignificant increases occurring at each following visit. This is very important because it shows that, within two visits, the occupational therapists were able to effectively engage caregivers in the therapeutic process.

In contrast, occupational therapists reported lower levels of engaging behaviors for caregivers who eventually dropped out of the intervention. Moreover, ratings of engagement with noncompleters exhibited a dramatic drop over the course of the intervention. As shown, scores for noncompleters significantly

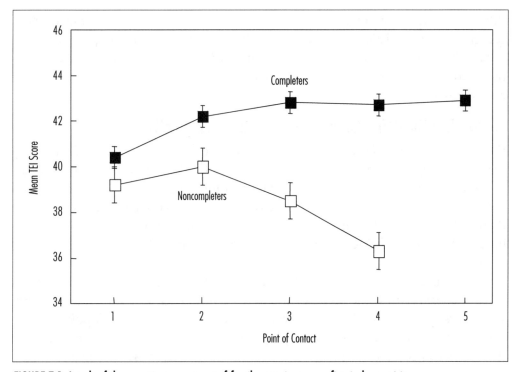

FIGURE 7.1. Levels of therapeutic engagement of family caregivers over five in-home visits.

Note. Completers were those who completed the five visits of the ESP; noncompleters completed fewer than five visits. TEI = Therapeutic Engagement Index.

From "Provider Assessment of Interactions With Dementia Caregivers: Evaluation and Application of the Therapeutic Engagement Index," by Y. K. Chee, M. P. Dennis, and L. N. Gitlin, in press, *Clinical Gerontologist, 28.* Copyright © 2005 by The Haworth Press, Inc. Adapted with permission. Article copies available from The Haworth Document Delivery Service: 1-800-HAWORTH, docdelivery@haworthpress.com.

decreased by the third visit and continued to fall for those who received subsequent visits. Thus, a critical turning point appears to occur by the second visit; there was a sharp decline in noncompleters after two visits compared with completers, who maintained the strong engagement that had been developed by the second visit.

CAREGIVER CHARACTERISTICS AND IMPACT ON ENGAGEMENT

ESP required therapists to consider caregiver characteristics and cultural values and beliefs such that positive engagement should be achievable regardless of caregiver background in terms of age, gender, race, income, education, length of caregiving, and relationship to the care recipient (i.e., spouse vs. nonspouse). That is, if the occupational therapists use collaborative techniques successfully, the characteristics of a caregiver should not influence the level of engagement that can be achieved. We tested this assumption and found that TEI scores did not differ by basic caregiver characteristics for any of the treatment contacts; thus, caregiver characteristics were not associated with therapeutic engagement. The occupational therapists who conducted the ESP intervention were able to develop positive collaborative relationships with caregivers from diverse backgrounds and to engage them successfully in the process.

USE IN THE HOME ENVIRONMENTAL SKILL-BUILDING PROGRAM

We recommend that occupational therapists score and complete the TEI immediately following the conclusion of each home visit. When completing the TEI, the occupational therapist should not refer to the ratings of prior contacts and should rate each item based on the experience of that specific contact. The occupational therapists found it difficult to use the TEI following telephone contacts, perhaps because they were unable to gather via telephone sufficient information about the caregivers' behaviors to assign a score.

The TEI can provide four scores: a total score (the sum of all item scores) and three subscale scores (the sums of the items within each domain; Table 7.1 provides possible ranges). Although at present we cannot offer a cutoff point to indicate if a caregiver is at risk of dropping out from the intervention, occupational therapists can compare a caregiver's overall score with those of completers and noncompleters of the ESP study intervention, shown in Figure 7.1. Furthermore, a drop in scores from Session 1 to Sessions 2 or 3 signals that the caregiver may be at risk of not remaining in treatment.

A caregiver's TEI score can be used as a tool to assist in the clinical reasoning process. If a caregiver is not actively involved in the treatment process, as reflected in a score below about 38, the occupational therapist may need to consider the possible factors that may be contributing to the lack of engagement and may need to change the course of the intervention, try a different approach, or introduce a different set of strategies to match the caregiver's psychological stance (Toth-Cohen, 2000). For instance, clients tend not to inquire about the treatment until a positive climate has been created and they feel encouraged to interact with the occupational therapist (Beisecker & Beisecker, 1990). The occupational therapist may wish to discuss with caregivers how they view the treatment contacts and whether they perceive that the contacts are helpful or are addressing their particular concerns. Asking the caregiver directly which approach he or she might prefer (e.g., supplementary education materials or more opportunities for practicing one strategy) may help facilitate therapeutic engagement.

Additionally, it is important for the occupational therapist to evaluate the degree to which each of the three components of therapeutic engagement—openness to suggestions and sharing, connectedness with the therapist, and involvement with others—develops during the intervention process and contributes to obtaining optimal health outcomes. Although we recommend use of the entire

TEI score, it may also be helpful to examine subscale scores to identify the particular domains or aspects of engagement that are or are not developing positively. Particularly with caregivers who prefer to remain passive throughout the intervention program, the occupational therapist may focus specifically on improving one or two domains of engagement that are the most salient in achieving collaborative treatment.

CONCLUSION

This chapter presents an innovative, brief 14-item scale developed for use by providers in assessing the extent to which caregivers are engaged in ESP. The TEI has been tested using two different caregiver intervention trials, each of which involved multiple in-home visits. To date, we cannot provide a particular cutoff point on the TEI that reflects whether a relationship is failing. Nevertheless, the scale can help guide the occupational therapist in the self-reflective process as to the progress of the intervention and determine whether adjustments in therapeutic style are necessary to achieve desired treatment outcomes.

It is important to note that there are three components to this scale—openness to suggestions and sharing, connectedness with the therapist, and involvement in obtaining information—each of which is associated with a different set of caregiver characteristics. It is also important to note that the extent to which caregivers were engaged in the process was not associated with specific characteristics of the patient with dementia, namely the level of cognitive impairment and functional dependence. The TEI can be a useful tool, especially in an intensive and long-term home intervention, to aid the occupational therapist in evaluating the caregiver's level of engagement and to guide whether adjustments need to be made to ensure treatment adherence.

REFERENCES

Beisecker, A. E., & Beisecker, T. D. (1990). Patient information-seeking behaviors when communicating with doctors. *Medical Care, 28,* 19–28.

Chee, Y. K., Dennis, M. P., & Gitlin, L. N. (in press). Provider assessment of interactions with dementia caregivers: Evaluation and application of the Therapeutic Engagement Index. *Clinical Gerontologist, 28.*

DiMatteo, M. R. (1994). The physician–patient relationship: Effects on the quality of health care. *Clinical Obstetrics and Gynecology, 37,* 149–160.

Frieswyk, S. H., Allen, J. G., Colson, D. B., Coyne, L., Gabbard, G. O., Horwitz, L., et al. (1986). Therapeutic alliance: Its place as a process and outcome variable in dynamic psychotherapy research. *Journal of Consulting and Clinical Psychology, 54,* 32–38.

Gitlin, L. N., Corcoran, M., Winter, L., Boyce, A., & Hauck, W. W. (2001). A randomized, controlled trial of a home environmental intervention: Effect on self-efficacy and upset in caregivers and on daily function of persons with dementia. *The Gerontologist, 41,* 4–14.

Gitlin, L. N., & Gwyther, L. P. (2003). In-home interventions: Helping caregivers where they live. In D. W. Coon, D. Gallagher-Thompson, & L. W. Thompson (Eds.), *Innovative interventions to reduce dementia caregiver distress: A clinical guide* (pp. 139–160). New York: Springer.

Gitlin, L. N., Winter, L., Corcoran, M., Dennis, M. P., Schinfeld, S., & Hauck, W. W. (2003). Effects of the Home Environmental Skill-Building Program on the caregiver–care recipient dyad: Six-month outcomes from the Philadelphia REACH Initiative. *The Gerontologist, 43,* 532–547.

Greenfeld, S., Kaplan, S., & Ware, J. E. (1985). Expanding patient involvement in care: Effects on patient outcomes. *Annals of Internal Medicine, 102,* 520–528.

Haley, W. E., & Bailey, S. (1999). Research on family caregiving in Alzheimer's disease: Implications for practice and policy. In B. Vellas & J. L. Fitten (Eds.), *Research and practice in Alzheimer's disease* (Vol. 2, pp. 321–332). New York: Springer.

Holman, H., & Lorig, K. (2000). Patients as partners in managing chronic disease. *British Medical Journal, 320,* 526–527.

Horvath, A., Gaston, L., & Luborsky, L. (1993). The therapeutic alliance and its measures. In N. E. Miller & L. Lester (Eds.), *Psychodynamic treatment approach: A handbook for clinical practice* (pp. 247–273). New York: Basic Books.

Institute of Medicine. (2001). *Crossing the quality chasm: A new health system for the 21st century.* Washington DC: National Academy Press.

Mittelman, M. S., Roth, D. L., Coon, D. W., & Haley, W. E. (2004). Sustained benefit of supportive intervention for depressive symptoms in caregivers of patients with Alzheimer's disease. *American Journal of Psychiatry, 161,* 850–856.

Peloquin, S. M. (1998). The therapeutic relationship. In E. Crepeau & M. Neistadt (Eds.), *Willard and Spackman's occupational therapy* (9th ed., pp. 105–119). Philadelphia: Lippincott Williams & Wilkins.

Pusey, H., & Richard, D. (2001). A systemic review of the effectiveness of psychosocial interventions for carers of people with dementia. *Aging and Mental Health, 5,* 107–119.

Roter, D. (2000). The enduring and evolving nature of the patient–physician relationship. *Patient Education and Counseling, 39,* 5–15.

Stewart, M. (2001). Towards a global definition of patient centered care. *British Medical Journal, 322,* 444–445.

Toth-Cohen, S. (2000). Role perception of occupational therapists providing support and education for caregivers of persons with dementia. *American Journal of Occupational Therapy, 54,* 509–515.

Von Korff, M., Gruman, J., Schaefer, J., Curry, S., & Wagner, E. H. (1997). Collaborative management of chronic illness. *Annals of Internal Medicine, 127,* 1097–1102.

8

Implementation of the Home Environmental Skill-Building Program

Mary A. Corcoran, PhD, OTR/L, FAOTA
Laura N. Gitlin, PhD

I: Have you puzzled that through and thought about what you might do, or is that something yet to be addressed, as to how to help him know where he is?

S: No. I've just been kind of going along with it, because, as I say—but his name is on his bedroom door. I put that on when we came here, because I knew when we arrived that he would be confused, even though he wasn't as confused in those days. But, you know.

I: So, that says [CR's first name]?

S: [CR's full name]. It's this very official looking thing that was on his desk, in his office. And I had—when we got rid of the office furniture, I had, you know, taken along, kept it. And so, as soon as we assigned the rooms, I stuck this right up on the door just, you know, without even thinking ahead about it. I didn't plan that way. I just said, oh, this is a good place for this. And I don't know if he even notices that anymore, but it probably helps him, because he does read, and he's still very verbal.

I: So, you put that up as a decoration, not as a way to help him find his room?

S: Both. Because—okay, here, this is your room. But he—I don't know, because I put up signs for quite a while about directions.

I: Such as?

S: Such as, I want him to stay out of my bedroom, unless I invite him in, because I often have an ongoing job. I mean, I have my checkbook, I have—I'm sorting, filing, business papers, and don't get it finished, and its spread out on my bed. I don't want him in there; because he has a tendency to think everything is his business, especially if it's on paper.

—Caregiving Styles Study (Corcoran) NIA R29-AG13019 10016#3:200–251

We have arrived at the heart of the matter: This chapter provides a detailed description of the essential elements of the Home Environmental Skill-Building Program (ESP) and its implementation. Previous chapters provided an understanding of the foundation of ESP, but here the focus is on the specifics of implementation: the approach to evaluation, the areas of concern to target, the number of contacts and content of each, the development and implementation of customized strategies, and the evaluation of intervention progress. We begin with a quick overview of the delivery characteristics of ESP and then examine the content of each contact in detail. Brief case examples illustrate the use of selected intervention techniques.

OVERVIEW OF ESP IMPLEMENTATION

The process of educating, building skills, and implementing strategies—the essence of ESP—occurs in two successive phases, active and maintenance, over a 12-month period. The active phase involves six contacts and is the most critical; it occurs over 6 months, although the occupational therapist can implement it in less time depending on caregiver schedule and abilities and reimbursement or service requirements. The goal of the active phase is to build caregiver skill in the use of an environmental approach to resolving management issues in dementia care. In the active phase, the occupational therapist uses standardized assessments and specific approaches to identify, analyze, and resolve caregiving issues that are of concern to family members. These specific concerns are identified through a collaborative process involving negotiation between the occupational therapist and the caregiver.

Table 8.1 lists 13 management areas that can be targeted for intervention and provides examples of specific caregiver issues within each area. The table also reports the percentages of study caregivers who reported difficulty with the management area and who addressed the area in the intervention. Although each household has a unique set of concerns, the pattern of responses shown in Table 8.1 provides an indication of what occupational therapists can expect when implementing ESP. For example, the vast majority of caregivers reported caregiver-centered concerns as one of the most difficult areas to manage; that concern became the focus of intervention for 69% of the caregivers. Safety and mobility were two other areas of concern that caregivers targeted; these concerns were addressed in nearly half of the households.

The occupational therapist and caregiver select approximately three concerns to address in the intervention, although the number of problem areas may vary. For each identified area, the occupational therapist follows a protocol that includes
1. Educating the caregiver about the impact of the environment,
2. Building caregiver skill in manipulating the environment, and
3. Implementing specific environmental strategies.

TABLE 8.1. Targeted Management Areas in ESP and Study Caregivers Who Experienced Difficulty With and Addressed the Area in Intervention

Targeted Area	Examples of Specific Problems	% Caregivers With Moderate to Extreme Difficulty Managing Area	% Caregivers Who Addressed Area in Intervention
Bathing and grooming	CR is resistant to bathing and assistance. CG is unable to physically assist or transfer CR. CG and CR feel unsafe. CG wants CR to bathe more frequently.	43	33
Dressing	CR wears inappropriate clothing. CR is increasingly dependent. CR believes clothing not his or hers or has been stolen. CR disrobes inappropriately.	25	15
Eating	CR becomes distracted and stops eating. CR leaves table or becomes agitated.	21	19
Toileting and incontinence	CR has bowel or bladder accidents. CR wakes at night needing to toilet. CG is unable to physically assist CR. CR cannot reach bathroom in time and is incontinent.	39	32
Leisure	CR does not do anything. CR appears bored or unhappy.	44	48
IADL	CR is unable to prepare simple meals. CG is unable to keep up with housework. CG is unable to leave home for food shopping. CG is unable to transfer CR in and out of car and on and off bed and toilet.	44	48
Safety	CG is unable to leave CR alone. CG is concerned about fire safety and CR access to dangerous objects or substances. CR is still driving.	34	49
Mobility	CR has difficulty ambulating in house. CG is concerned about falling or CR falling. CG is unable to assist in ambulation or transferring.	31	49
Wandering	CG is concerned about elopement (wandering away from the home). CR experiences sundowning (increased confusion late in the day). CR paces excessively in the home.	24	31

(continued)

TABLE 8.1. *(continued)*

Targeted Area	Examples of Specific Problems	% Caregivers With Moderate to Extreme Difficulty Managing Area	% Caregivers Who Addressed Area in Intervention
Communication	CG is unable to understand CR. CR is unable to understand CG. CG is unable to effectively communicate with family members or formal providers.	47	44
Troublesome behaviors	CR has catastrophic reactions. CR engages in repetitive questioning. CR engages in hoarding or rummaging. CR is physically aggressive.	35	27
Caregiver-centered concerns	CG feels guilty. CG does not have time for self. CG needs respite. CG is angry with CR or other family members. CG is unable to take care of self. CG is unable to manage and cope with caregiving role.	66	69
Other	Family is ambivalent about care arrangements and whether nursing home care should be sought. CG travels for work and has difficulty making care arrangements.	50	39

Note. CG = caregiver, CR = care recipient. *Sundowning* refers to excessive agitation or wandering by CR that commonly occurs in early evening.

The goal of the second phase of ESP, maintenance, is to refine the skills developed in the active phase and generalize their use to newly emerging issues. In the maintenance phase, the occupational therapist helps the caregiver reflect on, become familiar with, and reinforce the process used in an environmental approach. The maintenance phase consists of three telephone contacts with the caregiver and one final home visit to review the entire intervention process and obtain closure. Although our research shows that caregivers may need a more intense and ongoing relationship with an occupational therapist to sustain skills and intervention benefits, this minimal contact provides a low-cost approach to supporting families (Gitlin, Hauck, Dennis, & Winter, in press). Table 8.2 provides an overview of the suggested spacing of ESP visits and the content of contacts.

TABLE 8.2. Overview of Intervention Schedule and Content

Month	Contact	Type	Content
1	1	Home visit	Evaluation and negotiation: Build rapport. Assess caregiver-identified problems, care practices, and environmental attributes. List and prioritize perceived care needs.
2–4	2–4	Home visits	Skill building: Educate the caregiver. Use environmental problem solving for three targeted management areas. Adaptive equipment and home modifications: Assess need for adaptive equipment and home modifications. Order needed items or work with caregiver approval.
5–6	5–6	Telephone (1) and home visit (1)	Review and refinement of approach: Modify strategies to improve effectiveness. Reflect on problem-solving process. Generalize problem-solving process to other management issues.
7–12	7–9	Telephone (3)	Review and refinement of approach: Refine strategies. Reinforce use of problem-solving process.
12	10	Home visit	Generalization of strategies: Discuss future use of problem-solving process and strategies.

ESP Treatment Process

Consistent with the *Occupational Therapy Practice Framework* (American Occupational Therapy Association, 2002), ESP follows the occupational therapy process of service delivery, including evaluation, intervention, and outcomes. First, we will introduce the assessment tools used in the ESP evaluation process; the intervention and outcome processes are addressed later in the descriptions of each contact.

Assessment Tools Used in ESP

Occupational therapists implementing ESP use a variety of assessment tools, including open-ended questions, semistructured interview formats, and standardized instruments, to assist in gathering information for use in identifying appropriate problem areas and targeting and customizing strategies. Table 8.3 lists the specific domains assessed, the instruments used, and the schedule of administration; all but one of the instruments used in ESP are included in Appendix A.

Revised Memory and Behavior Problems Checklist

The Revised Memory and Behavior Problems Checklist (RMBPC; from Teri et al., 1992) lists 24 behaviors (9 depressive behaviors, 8 disruptive behaviors, and 7 memory-related behaviors) that are common in people with dementia. Occupational therapists ask caregivers the frequency of occurrence of each behavior in the past week and, if the behavior did occur, how upset the caregivers were by it. This scale is easy to use and provides a systematic way of identifying behavioral disturbances, which are the most difficult aspect of the disease to manage. Additionally, this tool provides an immediate understanding of which behaviors the caregiver finds most upsetting. Even when these behaviors occur infrequently, their occurrence can be acutely burdensome and upsetting and may trigger nursing home placement. Thus, addressing behavioral disturbances can have a positive impact on well-being for both caregiver and care recipient.

TABLE 8.3. Assessment Instruments Used in ESP

Domain	Instrument	Timing
Care recipient abilities and performance problems	Revised Memory and Behavior Problems Checklist (RMBPC; Teri et al., 1992) Caregiver Assessment of Management Problems (CAMP 1)	Contact 1–2
Caregiver-identified management issues	Caregiver upset (CAMP and RMBPC) CAMP 1	Contact 1–2
Caregiver routines, strategies, and environmental attributes for negotiated management areas	Caregiver Readiness Task Management Strategy Index (TMSI) Home Environmental Assessment Protocol (HEAP)	Contact 1–2
Strategy acceptance and integration	Strategies List and Integration Status	Ongoing
Reevaluation of caregiver routines and strategies for negotiated management areas	Caregiver upset (CAMP and RMBPC) RMBPC CAMP 2 (TMSI) Caregiver Readiness	Contacts 6 and 10

Note. Except for the RMBPC, all instruments are provided in Appendix A.

Caregiver Assessment of Management Problems

The Caregiver Assessment of Management Problems (CAMP), a two-part investigator-developed tool, is a semistructured interview designed to elicit the caregiver's perspective on the specific management areas that are difficult to manage (see Tools A.1 and A.2). The CAMP lists the 13 management areas that form the focus of ESP to help the occupational therapist gather information about care practices and identify the problems the caregiver wishes to focus on. CAMP 1 is used during the first and subsequent home visits; for each area, the therapist asks the caregiver to rate the level of difficulty the caregiver is having with managing or handling it, how important it is to him or her to learn new strategies, and the caregiver's perception of his or her effectiveness in handling difficulties. This guided discussion assists the caregiver and therapist in focusing on the truly problematic areas from the perspective of the caregiver and helps to prioritize the areas they will address in the intervention and in what order. CAMP 2 is used after the intervention to help the therapist evaluate its effectiveness and determine whether the areas targeted in the intervention have become less problematic for the caregiver.

Task Management Strategy Index

The Task Management Strategy Index (TMSI; Gitlin, Winter et al., 2002) is a 19-item, easy-to-use tool to assess the task simplification strategies (e.g., visual and tactile cueing, simplifying routines, short instructions) that caregivers use to manage physical dependence and problem behaviors (see Tool A.3). The occupational therapist can assess whether the strategies are in use through either direct observation or discussion with the caregiver. Use of this tool can help the therapist validate and build on the strategies currently in use and provide instruction in strategies not being used.

Home Environmental Assessment Protocol

The Home Environmental Assessment Protocol (HEAP; Gitlin, Schinfeld, Winter, Corcoran, & Hauck, 2002) is a systematic observational checklist of potential hazards and adaptations (e.g., devices, visual cues, home modifications) that may be present in a household (see Tool A.4). It is designed for use by the occupational therapist and the caregiver in conducting a walk-through assessment of the key rooms the care recipient uses. Use of the HEAP provides a basis for the therapist to make equipment and modification recommendations and to gather additional insight as to how the caregiver manages the physical environment to address care issues.

Caregiver Readiness

Assessing the caregiver's level of readiness to make changes in the home or in the ways he or she provides care can be key to the effectiveness of ESP. Caregiver readiness is based on the transtheoretical model that views health behavior change as a process involving a series of stages rather than a single event (Prochaska & Velicer, 1997). After concluding the first contact, the occupational therapist rates his or her initial perception of the caregiver's readiness to try different strategies to help make caregiving easier using a 4-point scale (see Tool A.5):

- 1 = *precontemplation*—the caregiver does not intend to change caregiving behaviors (e.g., he or she is hearing but not listening).
- 2 = *contemplation*—the caregiver intends to change caregiving behaviors in the near future (e.g., he or she is trying to understand the diagnosis).
- 3 = *preparation*—the caregiver intends to take action in the immediate future (e.g., he or she is willing to listen).
- 4 = *action or maintenance*—the caregiver has made changes in caregiving behaviors and actively seeks to continue making changes (e.g., he or she is actively participating in the intervention and modifying strategies).

The Caregiver Readiness score helps the occupational therapist gauge how fast to move through the intervention and how best to begin. For example, a caregiver with a score of 1 may benefit more from education and understanding about his or her role as a caregiver, whereas a caregiver with a score of 3 or 4 will be ready to work hard to learn new action-oriented strategies for a variety of identified problem areas.

Strategies List and Integration Status

The Strategies List and Integration Status (Tool A.6), developed specifically for use in ESP, helps the occupational therapist systematically track each strategy and its use by caregivers. The therapist completes this tool after each contact to record the strategies introduced as well as at follow-up to record whether or not each strategy is still in use and the reasons for nonuse, if applicable. The therapist should complete the Strategies List and Integration Status form as soon as possible, either during the contact or immediately thereafter. The therapist can also use this tool for writing progress notes and tracking the use of specific strategies over several cases. This form is for the therapist's records, although he or she may provide the caregiver with a similar list that is kept in a notebook and that can serve as a simple log of the strategies used to address a particular problem area (we refer to this list as the Caregiver Environmental Strategy List).

Treatment Receipt and Enactment

The Treatment Receipt and Enactment form, developed specifically for use in ESP, assists the occupational therapist in reflecting on whether caregivers received (were willing to consider) and enacted (realized benefits from) the strategies (see Tool A.7). ESP requires a reflective clinical reasoning approach in which the therapist actively evaluates the extent to which his or her efforts with the caregiver are effective. Occupational therapists complete the 16 items for each management area that is addressed. This form is used after each home or telephone contact and provides a gauge as to how well the intervention is unfolding.

ACTIVE PHASE: CONTACT BY CONTACT

The active phase of ESP consists of six contacts—five home visits and one telephone call—over 6 months. The occupational therapist spaces the contacts based on the caregiver's availability and readiness to engage in the intervention; hence, it can be condensed to 3 to 4 months if necessary. The average duration of the home visits in the active phase is 90 minutes, and the telephone call typically lasts 20 minutes; however, the time frame may vary: Some caregivers may be unable to tolerate visits longer than 50 minutes and check-in calls of more than 10 minutes.

The goal of the active phase is to build caregiver skill in using an environmental approach to manage dementia-related behaviors and caregiving dilemmas. The approach provides a method for enhancing the caregiver's ability to

- Identify and define troublesome behaviors related to dementia;
- Specify physical and social environmental factors that have an effect on the management of identified behaviors;
- Set behavioral goals for resolving problem behaviors;
- Modify attributes of the physical and social environment of the home to address current management issues; and
- Evaluate the effectiveness and efficiency of strategies.

During the six contacts of the active phase, the occupational therapist initiates and cultivates a collaborative relationship using the techniques outlined in Chapter 5. This collaborative relationship is the basis for deriving and implementing specific environmental strategies.

During Contact 1, the occupational therapist begins with a set of open-ended prompts, such as "Tell me about a typical day" and "What are your main concerns and challenges?" The therapist then moves on to assess problem areas using the CAMP and RMBPC. Based on the management areas the therapist initially identifies, he or she then engages the caregiver in a discussion of specific problematic performance areas, makes observations in the specific rooms where the problems occur using the HEAP, and observes the caregiver interacting with the care recipient guided by the TSMI. The therapist facilitates discussion by reflecting on his or her own professional perceptions of care needs and how they compare to the caregiver's perspective (Gitlin, Corcoran, & Eckhardt, 1995). The therapist then prioritizes problematic performance areas based on identified risks related to safety and physical and emotional strain for both caregiver and care receiver and asks the caregiver for feedback on these perceptions.

After completion of the first contact, the occupational therapist rates the readiness of the caregiver to engage in behavior change. This rating helps the therapist think about how to proceed in the subsequent contacts. For example, if the therapist rates the caregiver as being at Level 2 (contemplation), he or she might emphasize education, whereas another emphasis would be more appropriate for a caregiver at Level 4 (ready to take action). A caregiver who is considered by the occupational therapist to be at a Level 4 readiness may need only a minimal amount of education regarding the environment and can begin to use that information immediately to devise solutions to specific care issues.

During Contact 2, the occupational therapist and caregiver review the problematic management areas generated during the first visit based on the caregiver's responses to the CAMP and on the therapist's observation of the caregiver's approach to management, the home environment, and the abilities of the person with dementia. They then negotiate their priorities and select on average three specific management areas to address. This negotiation occurs through the use of a dialogue the therapist initiates by presenting his or her perspective on the performance areas that are either unsafe or problematic and his or her rationale for a priority order. The therapist then elicits the caregiver's perspectives and priority order. The therapist and caregiver agree on the final list of management areas to address during intervention and their priority order.

During Contacts 3 through 6 of the active phase, the occupational therapist and caregiver work on each of the three negotiated management areas. For each area, the therapist

- Educates the caregiver regarding the interplay among home environment, behaviors of the person with dementia, and functional performance;
- Enhances the caregiver's ability to manipulate the environment;
- Introduces specific low-cost environmental strategies that manipulate the object, task, and social group layers (see Appendix B for an extensive list of possible strategies for each of the 13 management areas);
- Explores the need for specific assistive devices and home alterations; and
- Practices the use of specific strategies with the caregiver.

The occupational therapist uses a range of therapeutic techniques, depending on their cultural appropriateness, such as demonstration, role-play, observation, and tracking the frequency of care recipient behaviors. The therapist can introduce recording techniques (e.g., calendar recording, journaling, behavior logs) when appropriate to help caregivers identify factors in the home environment that influence care recipient behaviors. Recording techniques can help the caregiver develop and practice skills in evaluating and monitoring the environment.

The occupational therapist also provides two special technical supports when necessary: (1) in-home physical therapy education in use of mobility devices, back protection, and transfer techniques as a task modification strategy and (2) social work consultation via telephone for the purpose of providing information regarding the availability of formal supportive services in the area. The therapist introduces these technical supports for specific conditions such as care recipient mobility difficulties, home safety, and caregiver physical strain. Case Example 8.1 provides a brief illustration of the use of technical supports.

If these technical supports are not readily available in the community, the occupational therapist may decide to provide the content of the physical therapy and social work consultation. We have found, however, that part of the value of having other professionals provide this consultation is the opportunity to reinforce the importance of these techniques and to lend greater credibility to the intervention overall. Caregivers often feel reassured knowing that there is a team of professionals at their disposal who are coordinating their care. Likewise, if the therapist is not able to identify a social worker who can provide information about community resources over the telephone, the therapist may need to become familiar with this information in the caregiver's community. The local Area Agency on Aging or Alzheimer's Association chapter typically are staffed by social workers and others who are extremely knowledgeable about local resources. In addition, local Alzheimer's Association chapters often have educational materials and videotapes available for the caregiver to borrow. Appendix C provides a list of national organizations and their contact information as a further resource for obtaining information.

The following sections provide a detailed description of each intervention contact. We also summarize this description in Figure 8.1 in the form of an easy-to-use checklist. This checklist can help occupational therapists remain on target and organized as they proceed through the intervention contacts. We suggest that,

---

CASE EXAMPLE 8.1. Using Technical Supports in Bathing

The caregiver and occupational therapist identify resistance to bathing as the primary target area and determine that the problem involves the care recipient's poor trunk balance, a cluttered environment that provides confusing cues, and caregiver back strain. The occupational therapist educates the caregiver about the importance of simplifying the environment to promote cue finding and actively involves the caregiver in making a plan to simplify or remove objects in the bathroom (object layer modifications), install assistive devices such as grab bars and a raised toilet seat and alter the shower door (object layer modifications), and set up a routine and task sequence for the performance of bathing (task layer modifications)

   The occupational therapist also recommends a physical therapy home visit to introduce special technical support techniques to enhance the care recipient's balance and decrease back strain for the caregiver (task modification). Additionally, the therapist obtains information from the social worker regarding sources of in-home assistance for bathing. The therapist asks the caregiver to record care recipient behaviors during a bathing routine to monitor and determine the effectiveness of each strategy.

FIGURE 8.1. Checklist of essential activities of ESP intervention.

Caregiver's Name:

Care Recipient's Name:

Contact 1

Explain intervention and purpose.	❑
Use open-ended questions to help caregiver understand management areas.	❑
If possible, tour the home with caregiver as basis for understanding problem behaviors and management issues.	❑
Explore caregiver management issues in the home (see Table 8.3 for appropriate assessment instruments).	❑
Use open-ended questions to explore caregiver priorities.	❑
Begin education about dementia and the environment.	❑
If indicated, record environmental strategies on Caregiver Environmental Strategies List and leave with caregiver.	❑
Close by summarizing the major points covered in contact, what caregiver should practice (if applicable), and next steps.	❑

Contact 2

Introduce purpose of contact.	❑
Complete appropriate assessments.	❑
Negotiate to identify and agree on three management areas to focus on in intervention.	❑
Decide with caregiver which management area or areas to address today.	❑
Conduct in-depth examination of management area or areas, including the nature of problems, strategies used, and care recipient responses.	❑
Educate caregiver about problem behaviors and interactions with environment.	❑
Set behavioral goals for environmental approach.	❑
Develop and record an initial problem-solving approach.	❑
Record environmental strategies on Caregiver Environmental Strategy List and leave with caregiver.	❑
Practice selected aspects of the initial approach.	❑
Consider adaptive equipment needs.	❑
Close by summarizing major points covered in contact, what caregiver should practice (if applicable), and next steps.	❑

Contact 3

Introduce purpose of contact.	❑
Review caregiver use of strategies identified in Contact 2.	❑
Reexamine goals and environmental influences.	❑
Refine or modify environmental approach.	❑
Practice selected aspects of refined approach.	❑
Initiate discussion of any negotiated management areas that have not been addressed.	❑
Record environmental strategies on Caregiver Environmental Strategy List and leave with caregiver.	❑

Discuss adaptive equipment needs. Provide caregiver with ordering information. ❏

Screen to determine need for physical therapy services. ❏

Close by summarizing major points covered in contact, what caregiver should practice (if applicable), and next steps. ❏

Contact 4

Introduce purpose of contact. ❏

Review caregiver use of strategies. ❏

Help caregiver as he or she reexamines goals and environmental influences. ❏

Refine or modify environmental approach. ❏

Use statements that shift decision making to caregiver. ❏

Practice selected aspects of environmental approach. ❏

Record environmental strategies on Caregiver Environmental Strategy List. ❏

If available, teach caregiver use of adaptive equipment. ❏

Use caregiver language to provide feedback to caregiver regarding his or her approach. ❏

Close by summarizing major points covered in contact, what caregiver should practice (if applicable), and next steps. ❏

Contact 5

Introduce purpose of contact. ❏

Review caregiver use of environmental strategies. ❏

Help caregiver reexamine goals and environmental influences. ❏

Refine or modify approach. ❏

Ask caregiver to record environmental strategies on Caregiver Environmental Strategy List. ❏

Use statements that shift decision making to caregiver. ❏

Continue to provide feedback to caregiver on his or her approach. ❏

Close by summarizing major points covered in contact, what caregiver should practice (if applicable), and next steps. ❏

Contact 6

Introduce purpose of contact. ❏

Review caregiver use of environmental approach for all negotiated management areas. ❏

Promote caregiver reexamination of goals and strategies. ❏

Practice selected aspects of environmental approach. ❏

If needed, teach caregiver use of adaptive equipment. ❏

Use open-ended questions to help caregiver summarize his or her approach. ❏

Discuss how caregiver may generalize approach to other care issues. ❏

Explain next phase of intervention. ❏

Close by summarizing major points covered in contact, what caregiver should practice (if applicable), and next steps. ❏

(continued)

FIGURE 8.1. *(continued)*

Contact 7

Introduce purpose of contact. ❑

Review caregiver use of environmental approach for all negotiated management areas. ❑

Promote caregiver reexamination of goals and environmental influences. ❑

Assist caregiver in using Environmental Guidelines to further refine approach. ❑

Remind caregiver to record strategies on Caregiver Environmental Strategy List. ❑

Use open-ended questions to discuss how caregiver may generalize approach to other care issues. ❑

Close by summarizing major points covered in contact, what caregiver should practice (if applicable), and next steps. ❑

Contact 8

Introduce purpose of contact. ❑

Review caregiver use of environmental approach for all negotiated management areas. ❑

Promote caregiver reexamination of goals and environmental influences. ❑

Assist caregiver in using Environmental Guidelines to further refine approach. ❑

Remind caregiver to record strategies on Caregiver Environmental Strategy List. ❑

Explore application of environmental approach to newly emerging care issues. ❑

Close by summarizing major points covered in contact, what caregiver should practice (if applicable), and next steps. ❑

Contact 9

Introduce purpose of contact. ❑

Review caregiver use of environmental approach for all negotiated management areas. ❑

Promote caregiver reexamination of goals and environmental influences. ❑

Assist caregiver in using Environmental Guidelines to further refine approach. ❑

Remind caregiver to record strategies on Caregiver Environmental Strategy List. ❑

Practice selected aspects of refined approach. ❑

Discuss ways that caregiver has generalized and refined approach. ❑

Close by summarizing major points covered in contact, what caregiver should practice (if applicable), and next steps ❑

Contact 10

Introduce purpose of contact. ❑

Summarize what you and caregiver have accomplished in past nine contacts. ❑

Summarize and validate caregiver approach. ❑

Discuss potential issues that may arise and application of approach to these issues. ❑

Close by reviewing all that the caregiver and the occupational therapist have accomplished together,
and thank caregiver for participation. ❑

in addition to using the ESP Road Map provided in Appendix D, the therapist refer to the checklist in Figure 8.1 before and during each contact to help remain on target and focused on the recommended implementation steps.

Each contact begins and ends similarly. To begin, the occupational therapist introduces the specific goals of that particular contact, providing the caregiver with a road map of what the caregiver and therapist can expect and what they will probably accomplish. This road map (Appendix D) helps focus the intervention for caregivers and keep them on track. It serves, in and of itself, as an effective therapeutic and organizational tool. Likewise, the therapist concludes each contact by reviewing the key points covered in the contact and what specific strategies the caregiver should practice, including how many times and where and how practice should occur, and sets the date and time for the next contact. The therapist also indicates what he or she learned from the caregiver that day (e.g., new modifications, special considerations when approaching that particular care recipient, new ideas for future contacts) both as a summary and as an effort to reaffirm the caregiver's own know-how.

Contact 1: Home Visit

The objectives of Contact 1 are to
- Begin the process of building a collaborative relationship,
- Identify behaviors and management areas that are problematic to the caregiver,
- Assess competencies of the care recipient that contribute to the problem, and
- Begin to identify the caregiver's care preferences and needs.

The occupational therapist reviews the purpose and nature of the ESP intervention and emphasizes that it is designed to
- Build and maintain the caregiver's environmental problem-solving skills,
- Focus on making caregiving easier and more effective, and
- Facilitate collaboration between the caregiver and occupational therapist to address the issues that the caregiver determines are important.

The occupational therapist begins to build a common language with the caregiver while explaining the intervention. The therapist informs the caregiver that he or she will develop a plan that will include a combination of environmental strategies to address each of the three management areas. The therapist explains that the caregiver will have an opportunity to practice each strategy and that together they will shape the strategies to fit the caregiver's needs and preferences; in addition, they will record the strategies on the Caregiver Environmental Strategy List, which the caregiver keeps.

The occupational therapist then begins the evaluation process by asking the caregiver open-ended questions (e.g., "Tell me about your day." "What is it like now vs. before?" "What are you having the most difficulty with?"). Then, using the CAMP 1 (Tool A.1) and the RMBPC, the therapist asks the caregiver the specific problems he or she encounters in each targeted area, level of difficulty and effectiveness in managing each specific problem, and the importance of learning new strategies to address the problem. Depending on the number and type of problem areas, it may not be possible to complete the evaluation process during this first contact.

The occupational therapist and caregiver analyze each target management area to briefly name and frame the issues. During this analysis, the therapist affirms the caregiver as the expert and uses active listening in a dialogue about what factors support and detract from the caregiver's ability to manage each area. These factors may reflect the caregiver's needs and preferences, the attributes of the environment, or the nature of the care recipient's behaviors and capabilities.

During this conversation and in subsequent discussions, the occupational therapist elicits the caregiver's

- Perspectives on providing care,
- Perceptions of acceptable care recipient behavior,
- Beliefs about what is "good" caregiving, and
- Recollection of how he or she successfully managed former problems.

The occupational therapist keeps ongoing notes about his or her understanding of the caregiver's perceptions about needs and preferences, frequently validating these impressions with the caregiver. The therapist observes the home environment with the caregiver as the basis for educating him or her about the interplay between dementia and the environment, and together they complete the HEAP (Tool A.4). The therapist also completes the TMSI as he or she observes interactions between the caregiver and care recipient (see Tool A.3). If the therapist introduces strategies during this contact, he or she provides the caregiver with a summary description of each strategy and its use on the Caregiver Environmental Strategy List.

Contact 2: Home Visit

The objectives of Contact 2 are to

- Continue the process of building a collaborative relationship,
- Further explain the intervention's approach to environmental problem solving,
- Improve the caregiver's ability to analyze issues within the targeted management areas,
- Design specific environmental strategies to address specific management issues in the home, and
- Negotiate with the caregiver to choose three management areas they will address in the intervention.

During Contact 2, the occupational therapist continues to expand his or her initial understanding of the caregiver's needs and preferences using open-ended and semistructured interviewing techniques (see Chapters 6 and 7). The therapist also updates the Caregiver Environmental Strategy List initiated during Contact

1. The therapist validates his or her impressions with the caregiver and discusses the caregiver's needs and preferences in relation to environmental solutions. The therapist again uses the CAMP to continue to explore management issues.

The occupational therapist uses negotiation to reach an agreement with the caregiver about which management areas they will address in subsequent visits and telephone contacts. Negotiation is an important aspect of the intervention and involves helping the caregiver identify problems that are appropriate, real, and modifiable. Some issues may reflect the caregiver's own desire not to be the primary caregiver (e.g., "I don't want to do this—how can you help me so I can leave him alone all day while I go to work?") or may reflect a certain level of denial (e.g., "She can go to the store herself—she has always done that by herself"). Although the intervention is caregiver centered, the therapist often needs to help the caregiver focus on a modifiable issue and derive realistic treatment goals. The therapist might say, for instance, "Dementia is a progressive disease, and there is no magic bullet, but we can help make everyday caregiving a bit easier and also introduce activities that may bring you and your family member some pleasure." Exhibit 8.1 provides a suggested script for negotiating the identification of problem areas.

The occupational therapist uses information from observation (HEAP and TMSI) and the CAMP to begin educating the caregiver about dementia and its effects, environmental influences on behavior, and the process of environmental problem solving. The therapist and caregiver identify the first management area to work on. Through dialogue and observation, the therapist gathers details about

- The specific nature of the problem,
- How a typical day proceeds ("Tell me about a typical day in which this problem occurs"),
- Current care strategies in place to handle the identified problem ("What do you do when . . ." or "Let me see how you handle this"), and
- Interactions between caregiver and care recipient.

The occupational therapist presents information relevant to the first negotiated management area as a basis for environmental problem solving. For example, if the management area is wandering, the therapist and caregiver problem solve as to the potential triggers or causes of this problem. The therapist and caregiver conduct an in-depth examination of the factors that influence this management area positively and negatively. The therapist helps the caregiver analyze the problem by identifying some of the factors that may promote and discourage the behavior of wandering, including factors that arise from the caregiver (e.g., approach to communication), from the person with dementia (e.g., confusion or disorientation), and from the physical environment (e.g., auditory or physical clutter). The therapist may offer examples from other families he or she has visited as a way to facilitate this discussion.

EXHIBIT 8.1. Suggested Script for Negotiating Problem Areas

Step 1

Occupational therapist's introduction to the topic:

Mr. or Mrs. _____, let's review what we talked about. Here is a list of the areas you have identified as problematic or for which you would like to learn new strategies. Of these, what is the most important problem for you to deal with? What about this area bothers you the most? What do you want to be done differently? [Caregiver selects one area.]

     I'd like to share with you what I think about this management area. I'm thinking about your well-being, your ability to continue giving good care, and the safety of [care recipient's name]. I think this is an important management area because [provide list of reasons why this management area is important]. What do you think about these reasons? How important is this management area, with 1 being the most important and 10 being the least important?

If occupational therapist and caregiver agree on a score:

Good, we both see the importance of this area in the same way. Let's talk about possible ways of managing this now. [Discussion continues with Step 3 below.]

Step 2

If occupational therapist and caregiver do not agree on a score:

I would have scored it differently. I would have given it a [score] because [clarify reasons]. Tell me more about why this management area is a [caregiver's score] for you and your family.

If occupational therapist and caregiver agree after clarification:

OK, we both agree that [name management area] is important to work on, but we gave it different scores of importance. Let's talk about what we would do to deal with this management area if we both decide to work on it.

Step 3

If we decide to work on this management area, here is a written summary of what we could do to make it better. [The occupational therapist reviews a list of strategies (e.g., a written action plan) with the caregiver and clarifies any questions.]

     [When the action plan has been presented and questions answered, the occupational therapist continues with the standardized script:] Does this sound like a reasonable plan that would work for you? Do you want to work on [name management area] during the next few weeks?

Step 4

OK, so we have decided [to or not to] work on [specific management area]. Let's go on to the next management area that you think is important. [Go on to the next management area until three have been discussed.]

Step 5

Mr. or Mrs. _____, we have identified three caregiving management areas to address. They are [name the three identified management areas]. Is this correct? For each management area, I have given you a written summary of the plan to address it. Do the plans sound OK, or do you have any questions about them?

The occupational therapist and caregiver discuss and agree on specific behavioral, functional, cognitive, or affective outcomes—that is, what the caregiver hopes to achieve by implementing a strategy to address the problem behavior. In the case of wandering, one outcome might be to engage the care recipient in a meaningful activity to decrease his or her attempts to leave the home. Other identified outcomes may be caregiver focused, such as getting an opportunity to take a nap each day.

The occupational therapist and caregiver begin to problem solve through dialogue and demonstration. The therapist may ask the caregiver to demonstrate or role-play how he or she might manage a particular problem area, then use demonstration and role-play to introduce specific possible environmental modifications that may influence the balance of positive and negative forces in that particular management area.

The occupational therapist and caregiver evaluate the potential implications and effectiveness of the strategies on the basis of each strategy's fit with the caregiver's identified needs and preferences. The therapist and caregiver decide on the details of the environmental strategy that they will implement to address this management issue, including actions that both the occupational therapist and the caregiver will take. The therapist develops a written list of agreed on strategies for the caregiver to refer to during the interim between visits and records these strategies on the Caregiver Environmental Strategy List.

The occupational therapist and caregiver practice selected modifications within the agreed-on strategy using demonstration, simulation, and role-play. It is important for the therapist to provide the caregiver with ample opportunities to rehearse and practice each strategy within the context in which it is to be used. Thus, it is optimal to practice strategies related to bathing and grooming in the bathroom the care recipient uses. If appropriate, the therapist can incorporate the care recipient into the contact by directly introducing and modeling strategies for the caregiver.

Following Contact 2, the occupational therapist reflects on the contact to refine his or her understanding of the interplay among management issues, environmental factors, and characteristics of the caregiver and care recipient.

Contact 3: Home Visit

The objectives of Contact 3 are to
- Continue the process of building a collaborative relationship,
- Refine the caregiver's approach to issues in the management area discussed during Contact 2,
- Apply the environmental problem-solving process to a second management area, and
- Improve the caregiver's ability to use the environment in the home to address specific management issues.

During Contact 3, the occupational therapist continues to expand his or her initial understanding of the caregiver's needs and preferences using open-ended questions and updates the Caregiver Environmental Strategy List. The occupational therapist validates his or her impressions with the caregiver and discusses the caregiver's needs and preferences in relation to environmental solutions.

The occupational therapist and caregiver begin by discussing what has happened between contacts. The therapist uses probing questions and active listening to elicit details about the specific strategies the caregiver attempted, the caregiver's perceptions of his or her skill level, and the caregiver's perceptions of the effect of his or her actions on the frequency and severity of the targeted problem behavior.

The occupational therapist and caregiver proceed to refine their understanding of environmental influences on the issues that the caregiver has identified as problematic and wishes to modify. The caregiver and therapist focus on what was effective and ineffective about each strategy and how well it addressed the issues within the management area. The therapist facilitates this process by validating each positive and negative factor influencing the management area with the caregiver. The caregiver and therapist discuss the aspects of the strategy that worked well and those aspects that did not.

The occupational therapist encourages the caregiver to label each component of the environmental strategy that worked well, and the therapist takes the lead from the caregiver about what those labels should be. For instance, an environmental strategy developed for dressing may include components such as laying clothing out in sequence and giving short, simple instructions. The caregiver names each strategy, and throughout the remainder of the intervention the therapist uses the words of the caregiver as a basis for building a shared language. Naming the strategies facilitates their use later for worsening or newly emerging problems. The caregiver and therapist review and refine the approach to issues in this management area and amend the original written environmental strategy recorded on the Caregiver Environmental Strategy List.

As the occupational therapist introduces and develops new modifications, he or she practices each one with the caregiver. Methods for practicing modifications include role-play, with the therapist modeling modifications while narrating what is being done and why, and the caregiver practicing modifications while the therapist observes. These approaches provide an opportunity for both the therapist and the caregiver to observe and comment on the other's performance.

The occupational therapist and caregiver discuss the refined environmental strategy and its advantages, disadvantages, and concerns. For example, to solve the management issue of handling a care recipient's inability to choose appropriate articles of clothing and don them in the correct sequence, the therapist and caregiver may practice the modification of providing verbal cues regarding socially appropriate clothing for the events of the day (social and cultural layers).

This modification becomes part of a refined environmental strategy addressing issues in the management area of dressing. Other modifications may include eliminating extraneous articles of clothing from sight (objects layer) and matching the physical assistance provided in dressing with the care recipient's fluctuating needs (task layer).

The occupational therapist and caregiver review the modifications for this strategy and record them on the Caregiver Environmental Strategy List. Together they discuss each strategy in terms of effectiveness and fit with the family routine, conditions in the home, and special circumstances of the caregiver or care recipient.

The occupational therapist helps the caregiver think about how each modification recorded on the Caregiver Environmental Strategy List may have multiple applications. Case Example 8.2 shows how therapists can expand the caregiver's thinking about modifications to strategies through role-play.

Once the caregiver has mastered or feels comfortable with a strategy, the occupational therapist begins to introduce other strategies. Likewise, once the caregiver has achieved a basic level of mastery and some success with managing the first targeted management area, he or she and the therapist can target the second area. The therapist and caregiver discuss how they might apply strategies used for the first area to this second area. For example, the strategy of using simple commands and a reassuring tone for dressing can be transferred to almost any other management area.

In Contact 3 the occupational therapist begins to consider adaptive equipment and structural renovations that may be needed in the home to address the

---

CASE EXAMPLE 8.2. Use of Role-Play to Facilitate Dressing

The caregiver and occupational therapist identify dressing as a key target area. The caregiver indicates that her mother is somewhat independent but shows a lot of confusion and sometimes puts on the wrong clothing or becomes agitated while dressing. The therapist observes that the caregiver's mother is responsive to verbal cueing, leading the occupational therapist to role-play with the caregiver a set of communication strategies to assist in dressing.

First, the occupational therapist plays the part of the caregiver, and the caregiver takes the part of the care recipient. The therapist (playing the caregiver) says, "Mom, put one foot in the pants, then the other. Now pull your pants up. Great job, Mom. Now put on your sweater. You look very pretty. It's time to go downstairs now." The therapist then explains why simple one-step commands and a calm, reassuring tone are effective. Next, they reverse roles, and the therapist plays the care recipient and the caregiver plays herself to practice the communication sequence. After the role-play, the therapist asks the caregiver how she feels, whether the communication approach was difficult, and whether she believes she will be able to use the new approach and eliminate previously used approaches that were negative and ineffective.

targeted management areas. It is important to allow sufficient time both to order and install the equipment and then to train the caregiver in its use. In developing ESP we were able to use grant funds to purchase and install equipment; in real-world home care, it may be difficult to find funding sources for this aspect of the intervention process. For our research, the average cost of equipment was approximately $400 per caregiver, mostly for bathrooms and handrails. Some caregivers are able to finance such equipment on their own, and consultation with a local Area Agency on Aging may help identify other funding sources for this important aspect of the intervention.

Contact 4: Home Visit

The objectives of Contact 4 are to
- Expand and strengthen the collaborative relationship and understanding of the caregiver's needs and preferences,
- Refine the environmental strategies for the two management areas discussed to date,
- Reinforce and support the caregiver's ongoing use of effective environmental modifications, and
- Validate the caregiver's ability to manage problem areas effectively.

Contact 4 is similar to the previous one, with the occupational therapist working to broaden and enhance the caregiver's understanding of the environmental problem-solving approach and the basic principles behind specific strategies. The occupational therapist initiates a dialogue to see what strategies the caregiver is using and whether they need refinement or modification, and together they update the Caregiver Environmental Strategy List. Additionally, the therapist asks the caregiver to demonstrate the use of key strategies and instructs the caregiver in the use of any assistive devices that have been ordered, installed, or delivered. The caregiver records new strategies that emerge on the Caregiver Environmental Strategy List for future reference.

The occupational therapist continually frames the environmental approach to problem solving, naming and explaining the principles behind each strategy that is introduced and successfully used. This process forms the basis for building skills that can be generalized to newly emerging care issues. A new management area may be addressed following the procedures used in previous contacts—that is, the therapist and caregiver problem solve as to the nature, score, and characteristics of the target area and generate, practice, and refine strategies.

Contact 5: Telephone Call

The objectives of Contact 5 are to
- Refine and modify environmental strategies and modifications,
- Reinforce the need for and importance of practicing using the strategies, and
- Refine the caregiver's understanding of why the strategies are effective.

If necessary, this contact can involve a home visit by a physical therapist or education by the occupational therapist that address the following:
- Teaching the caregiver to use back protection techniques that reduce back strain and sprain,
- Teaching and reinforcing ambulation and transfer techniques,
- Establishing a strengthening and endurance-building regimen for either the caregiver or the care recipient, and
- Providing the caregiver or care recipient with a recommendation for a physician referral to other resources (e.g., physical therapist) for services.

If a physical therapist provides this visit in the home, the occupational therapist reinforces the strategies the physical therapist introduced in the subsequent contact.

The occupational therapist initiates discussion as to whether the caregiver still uses the strategies introduced in previous contacts and whether the problem area has been minimized or is being managed effectively. The contact begins with an update by the caregiver on what strategies he or she tried, whether he or she had to modify the strategies, and the outcomes. The caregiver compares these outcomes to his or her original behavioral and treatment goals. The therapist and caregiver continue their discussion about the steps they took to solve problems as the basis for understanding that process and building generalizable skills.

The occupational therapist elicits newly emerging or unresolved problem behaviors and management issues, including positive and negative factors affecting the issues, and discusses how the caregiver might apply previous problem-solving efforts and specific strategies. The therapist and caregiver problem solve to generate new environmental strategies or refine previous ones. The therapist provides feedback to the caregiver regarding each generated strategy, based on predicted effectiveness and fit with caregiver needs and preferences. The therapist guides the caregiver through an assessment of the skills needed to implement the strategy as compared with skills he or she presently possesses, and together they reflect on how the environmental strategy or specific modifications can be changed to emphasize skills he or she already possesses or how he or she can develop needed skills. The occupational therapist suggests methods for building skills by purposely introducing new skills into the daily routine. The therapist and caregiver decide on skill-building methods, and the caregiver writes them down on the Caregiver Environmental Strategy List to prompt implementation in the interim before the next contact. Case Example 8.3 describes how a caregiver worked to build a new skill needed to assist his mother with dressing.

Contact 6: Home Visit

The objectives of Contact 6 are to
- Facilitate caregiver self-reflection regarding his or her dementia management preferences, skills, and needs;

CASE EXAMPLE 8.3. Avoiding Catastrophic Reactions During Everyday Routines

In a telephone session with a son caring for his mother, the occupational therapist initiates a conversation with a review of the strategies that he is using to address catastrophic reactions. Specifically, the caregiver is attempting to help his mother get through the morning routine of dressing without her becoming upset and agitated. The caregiver complains that his mother is not any better able to dress herself than she was before implementing the strategies, and so he believes they are not working.

The occupational therapist reminds the caregiver that his original goal was that his mother would allow him to help her dress without slapping him or refusing his help, and the therapist asks if this is still a reasonable goal or if he would like to modify it. When asked to clarify, the therapist says, "Well, maybe instead of striving for her to just let you dress her without slapping, the goal should actually be related to how much she can dress herself." The caregiver agrees that this is probably a more satisfying outcome for his efforts.

The occupational therapist asks the caregiver to talk through the way he has approached similar problems and reminds him that he was able to use the placement of objects ("putting stuff just so," as he calls this strategy) to help his mother brush her teeth, comb her hair, and wash her face and hands. The caregiver talks about how this strategy might work with dressing and ways he might approach implementing it. The caregiver's concern, however, is that his mother seems to expect problems whenever he tries to dress her and gets upset before anything happens (he says his mother is "loaded for bear" when he enters her room).

The occupational therapist and caregiver figure out that the strategy will work only if he can calm her down first and then keep her calm throughout the dressing task. Getting his mother to calm down is a skill the caregiver recognizes that he needs to develop, so the therapist helps him plan to practice a new calming strategy every day until he has developed this skill and determined which works best with his mother. Suggested calming strategies include using a pleasant but monotone voice, using "soft" eye contact, giving his mother a hug, stopping when his mother gets agitated, and getting his mother to sing a song. The caregiver records on the Caregiver Environmental Strategy List that he is planning to implement one calming strategy every day before using his strategy of "putting stuff just so" for dressing.

- Generalize the caregiver's environmental problem-solving skills to anticipated problem behaviors;
- Enhance the caregiver's ability to evaluate the effectiveness of strategies and modifications and make further modifications as needed;
- Expand the caregiver's environmental problem-solving skills by applying them to a third negotiated management area; and
- Refine methods for developing effective environmental problem-solving skills.

During Contact 6, the occupational therapist continues to expand his or her initial understanding of the caregiver's needs and preferences using principles for interviewing, and the caregiver updates the ongoing list of strategies recorded on the Caregiver Environmental Strategy Form. When possible, the therapist validates his or her impressions with the caregiver and discusses the caregiver's needs and preferences in relation to environmental solutions.

The occupational therapist and caregiver summarize and detail what they addressed and accomplished in previous contacts and the new skills that the caregiver has learned (e.g., "Let's discuss what we have accomplished and some of the new approaches you have learned to manage everyday caregiving"). Next, the therapist explores which environmental strategies are still in place, which may need refinement, and how comfortable the caregiver is with each. The therapist uses active listening and helps the caregiver reflect on why he or she may be uncomfortable and how he or she can improve the strategies' effectiveness. The therapist may offer other information (e.g., readings or other materials) to supplement the caregiver's knowledge.

The occupational therapist and caregiver brainstorm as to future concerns and behaviors that may occur. The therapist reviews potential strategies that may be helpful in the future and principles for modifying the skills and strategies currently in place.

The occupational therapist encourages the caregiver to make independent, informed management decisions to promote the caregiver's skills and sense of efficacy. For instance, the therapist might ask the caregiver, "Does this way of solving the problem feel right? What is good and not so good about it? How have you considered changing it?" Such encouragement will build the caregiver's confidence in analyzing the effectiveness of his or her environmental strategy and making refinements that are personally satisfying.

The occupational therapist continues to engage in role modeling and information dissemination but begins to shift ownership of management decisions to the caregiver. To do so, the occupational therapist may use a probe such as "It looks like [an environmental strategy or modification] is working. What are you thinking about doing next?"

The occupational therapist helps the caregiver use an environmental problem-solving process to analyze and address issues in the third negotiated management area. The therapist reminds the caregiver of the steps he or she took to solve previous management issues and guides the caregiver in applying this process to the third targeted area.

The occupational therapist engages the caregiver in a discussion of the types of care recipient behaviors he or she might anticipate in the future. The therapist helps the caregiver to sketch out an approach to these behaviors by helping the caregiver

- Identify the process he or she uses to solve a management issue,
- Apply the process to anticipated management issues,
- Outline a possible environmental strategy and modifications to resolve issues in this area, and
- Discuss his or her needs and preferences in relation to the proposed environmental strategy.

The occupational therapist explains the next phase of the intervention, the maintenance phase, and reminds the caregiver that the next two contacts will be by telephone. Case Example 8.4 summarizes the active phase of ESP for one caregiver and her mother and the process they used to improve management of the morning routine.

MAINTENANCE PHASE: CONTACT BY CONTACT

The maintenance phase consists of four occupational therapy contacts that occur in Months 7–12 of the intervention. The goal of the maintenance phase is to reinforce the integration of strategies into daily routines, refine the environmental strategies used by the caregiver, and enable the caregiver to generalize these strategies to newly emerging problems. The four contacts consist of three telephone calls and one home visit. In each contact, the occupational therapist

---

CASE EXAMPLE 8.4. Active Phase of ESP

The caregiver is caring for her 75-year-old mother who is in the moderate stage of Alzheimer's disease. The caregiver works full-time and has arranged for her mother to attend adult day care 5 days a week. The care recipient needs verbal cueing and some physical help from the caregiver for her morning care.

The caregiver must get herself and her mother ready to leave on time every morning; she has scheduled paratransit to pick up her mother at a specific time, and only after the pickup can the caregiver leave for work. The time pressures are a critical factor in the stressful events of most mornings. Usually, the caregiver's attempts to hurry her mother and get ready for work result in the care recipient's resistance to dressing and eating breakfast. Many mornings, the situation escalates to the point where the caregiver is frustrated at her mother's behavior and loses her temper. At this point, the care recipient becomes extremely agitated and upset.

The occupational therapist and the caregiver together develop some strategies during Contacts 1 and 2 that include creating a low-stimulus environment (no TV or radio) and maintaining an established routine that includes a predictable sequence of events. With this routine, the caregiver and her mother can coordinate their morning tasks without confusion or last-minute decisions. These strategies also allow the caregiver to build in more time for her mother to perform self-care and eliminate the need to hurry.

Once this basic structure is in place, the occupational therapist and caregiver begin to explore the benefit of other environmental modifications in Contact 3. They examine the physical help the caregiver provides to her mother and decide on the use of visual cues to reduce the amount of help given. For example, by placing her mother's clothes on the bed, the caregiver can leave the room while her mother dresses. In the telephone contact and subsequent home visit (Contacts 4 and 5), the caregiver also begins to explore the way she uses her voice in speaking to her mother. With practice, the caregiver is able to adopt a calmer and more accepting tone, use reassurances, avoid scolding or criticism, and ignore insignificant but annoying mistakes by Contact 6.

This case demonstrates a multilevel environmental approach to resolving issues. It was an important first step to introduce a predictable, relaxed routine that eliminated the need to hurry. Without a calm atmosphere, other strategies would only add to the stress of the morning. Once the routine was established, the caregiver was able to expand it to include other environmental modifications, such as the use of task breakdown and visual cues.

reviews the process for analyzing and resolving problems identified in the active phase of the intervention and helps the caregiver apply this problem-solving approach to anticipated or newly emerging caregiving difficulties.

Contacts 7–9: Telephone Calls

The objectives of Contacts 7, 8, and 9 include
- Refinement of strategies and modifications,
- Expansion of environmental problem-solving skills, and
- Establishment of a continued plan for skill development.

The occupational therapist initiates discussion with the caregiver of the process and outcomes related to his or her environmental problem-solving efforts. The caregiver begins by reporting on modifications made to the environmental strategies, the reasons for the modifications, and the outcomes. The caregiver then compares these outcomes to his or her original behavioral or affective goals.

The occupational therapist elicits the caregiver's analysis of newly emerging or unresolved problem behaviors using the analytic process used previously throughout the active phase of the intervention. The therapist and caregiver problem solve to develop the caregiver's approach to newly emerging or unresolved management issues. The therapist refers the caregiver to materials that may be relevant to new management areas, such as the Examples of Environmental Strategies for Targeted Management Areas (found in Appendix B). As they consider each potential strategy, the therapist provides feedback to the caregiver regarding how well each might support efforts to resolve the newly emerging management issues based on the therapist's assessment of potential effectiveness and fit with caregiver needs and preferences. The therapist uses guided questions and shares perspectives to shape the caregiver's environmental strategies and modifications, and the caregiver records changes on the Caregiver Environmental Strategy Form.

The occupational therapist and caregiver discuss specific modifications the caregiver has made to the environmental strategies and any new skills he or she needs to enact or modify an environmental strategy. As in Contact 5, the caregiver and therapist compare the skills the caregiver needs with the skills he or she presently possesses, and they discuss how the strategy and modifications can be changed to emphasize current skills or how needed skills can be developed. The therapist suggests methods for skill building by purposely introducing new skills into the daily routine.

Contact 10: Home Visit

The objectives of Contact 10 are to
- Refine the caregiver's use of environmental problem-solving skills;
- Monitor the caregiver's self-reflection on his or her understanding of caregiving preferences, skills, and habits;

- Generalize skills to newly emerging management issues; and
- Wrap up and obtain closure.

The occupational therapist and caregiver use the CAMP as the basis for a discussion of the caregiver's perceptions regarding his or her care difficulties and priorities and the effectiveness of the intervention. This review serves as the basis for a systematic review of the treatment contacts, what worked and what did not, the new skills the caregiver has learned, and ways he or she can generalize these skills.

For each negotiated management area targeted in the intervention, the occupational therapist asks the caregiver to demonstrate or describe how he or she manages it currently. An important task of this final visit is to review, validate, refine, and continue to label the environmental problem-solving process that this caregiver has used to approach problem behaviors. The therapist may begin this summing up by saying, "Because this is our last visit, let me make sure I understand what you were telling me about the steps you take to solve problems." The therapist repeats what he or she understands to be the caregiver's problem-solving process, environmental strategies, and modifications to those strategies and asks, "Did I get it right?"

The occupational therapist asks the caregiver to analyze the environmental approach to each negotiated management area. If indicated, the therapist helps the caregiver fine-tune and make final adjustments to particular modifications and the overall environmental approach, recording changes on the Caregiver's Environmental Strategy Form.

The occupational therapist initiates a discussion that involves the application of the problem-solving process to future problems. This discussion includes a dialogue about how confident the caregiver feels in using an environmental approach. If necessary, the therapist helps the caregiver clarify which adjustments in his or her environmental strategy and modifications may be effective for improving confidence.

The occupational therapist and caregiver review strategies developed during the maintenance phase of the intervention, discussing their effectiveness and routine use by the caregiver. The therapist initiates a discussion regarding the skills the caregiver currently believes he or she possesses and the skills he or she still needs. If possible, the caregiver demonstrates use of these skills through demonstration or role-play. The therapist helps the caregiver analyze the effectiveness of methods used to build skills and, when necessary, refines and expands those methods. The therapist actively works toward closure by reaffirming the skills of the caregiver and discussing what the therapist has learned in the partnership.

PUTTING IT ALL TOGETHER: MR. AND MRS. P

Mr. P cares for his wife with dementia. Both are Black, in their late 70s, and in relatively good health. Mr. P had to quit his part-time job when his wife entered the moderate stage of the disease process about 3 years ago. He is the primary care-giver, and their two sons live far away and so are unable to help provide care, although they provide some financial support. Mr. P is a sensitive and attentive caregiver who must provide constant vigilance throughout the day because his wife has become increasingly agitated, attempts to leave the home, and tends to pace restlessly throughout the home. Recently she has had difficulty eating, tend-ing to leave the table during the course of eating her meal. Additionally, she is having increasingly frequent bladder accidents because she is unable to reach the bathroom on the second story of their row home in time. The accidents trigger emotional distress in Mrs. P, and she becomes disoriented and confused.

Contact 1

In the first visit, the occupational therapist reviewed with Mr. P his typical day and then used the RMBC and CAMP to explore specific areas of concern. These assessment tools revealed that Mr. P was most concerned and upset about Mrs. P's lack of eating. He was concerned that she was not obtaining proper nutrition and was unsure how to handle this. A second concern was her bladder accidents, and he also wanted to learn approaches for calming her and lessening her agita-tion. The therapist's initial perception was that Mr. P was at a readiness level of 3—that is, he recognized that his wife had a progressive disease, he had already tried numerous approaches to engage her and had rearranged his home, and he was ready to listen to suggestions and try new ideas. The therapist and Mr. P agreed to focus on Mrs. P's eating first. The therapist asked Mr. P to take note of what occurred when Mrs. P ate, how long she was able to sit before leaving the table, and which foods she tended to prefer.

Contact 2

In Contact 2, the occupational therapist reviewed the purpose of the contact (e.g., to identify the parameters of the eating behavior and problem solve strategies). The therapist guided Mr. P through a series of questions to identify the potential triggers or antecedents of Mrs. P's leaving the kitchen table. The therapist used role-play to enact what occurred (and used the TMSI to note strategies Mr. P used) and observed the eating area (using the HEAP). The therapist noted sever-al issues and brought them to Mr. P's attention.

The first issue was Mr. P's approach to communication with his wife. He was unclear about what he wanted her to do and offered too many eating choic-es. Additionally, a number of items other than her place setting were on the kitchen table, including the newspaper, the morning mail, and a plant. Third, the occupational therapist discovered through observation that Mrs. P was unable to grasp utensils well and appeared confused about when to use a fork, spoon, and knife. The therapist and Mr. P talked about these potential areas for change, and

Mr. P was willing to explore them all. The therapist started with communication and wrote down specific ways of communicating using short one-step commands. Additionally, the therapist instructed Mr. P to provide Mrs. P with one eating choice (e.g., cereal) and to place the spoon in her hand. The therapist wrote down all of these strategies for Mr. P and also recorded them on the Strategies List and Integration Status (Tool A.6). The therapist concluded the contact with an overview of what they accomplished and the specific strategies Mr. P should try and how often. They then scheduled the next contact.

Contact 3

In Contact 3, the occupational therapist began by reviewing with Mr. P how his week had been, whether he had had a chance to practice the strategies, and what outcomes had resulted. Mr. P used all the strategies and indicated that Mrs. P was much less agitated and left the table only once or twice during a meal. However, she was still playing with her hair and was easily distracted. In reviewing each strategy, Mr. P demonstrated mastery over communicating effectively and serving one type of finger or spoon food. In further exploration of the environment, the therapist recommended that Mr. P place a solid-colored placement (red) on the table to contrast with Mrs. P's white dinner plate. Additionally, the therapist recommended that Mr. P place a turban on Mrs. P's head in the morning when she dressed. Mrs. P had used turbans all her life, and this not only gave Mr. and Mrs. P pleasure, but also prevented her from playing with her hair during mealtime and becoming distracted. Mr. P was excited about trying out these strategies.

Contact 4

During Contact 4, Mr. P reported great success with all of the strategies and felt that he now had mealtimes under control. Mr. P and the occupational therapist moved on to address issues related to toileting and activity engagement. Given the responsiveness of Mrs. P to visual cueing (e.g., color placement), the therapist suggested placing a commode on the first floor and highlighting its contours in red masking tape to cue Mrs. P to use it (see Figure 8.2). This eliminated her need to climb a flight of stairs to use the toilet. The therapist discussed with Mr. P the principle of color contrast and how to generalize its use from one problem area

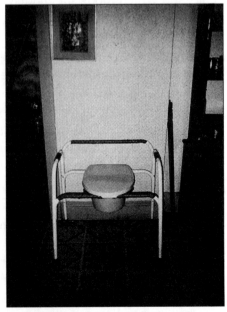

FIGURE 8.2. Use of tape as a visual cue.

to the next. Mr. P in turn came up with the idea of placing a picture of Mrs. P on her bedroom door to cue her that it was her room. The therapist thought this was a great idea and encouraged Mr. P to try it. Additionally, given Mrs. P's responsiveness to wearing the turban, Mr. P and the therapist came up with an activity involving folding colorful materials. Mr. P thought he could take his wife to a store to buy swatches of material, and a bin to keep them in, for her to take out, fold, and put back.

Contact 5

Contact 5 was a telephone call. Mr. P reported that he continued to use all of the strategies and that his idea of the picture on the door had worked well. He had not had time to go to the store with Mrs. P. The therapist problem solved with him about using objects in the household (e.g., towels, clothing, scarves) instead.

Contact 6

In this final contact of the active phase, the occupational therapist guided Mr. P through all of the new skills he had learned (e.g., communication; simplification of tasks; decluttering the environment; setting up the environment; helping Mrs. P initiate and sequence eating, toileting, and participation in activities). They discussed how Mr. P could use these techniques to address problems that might arise in the future.

Contacts 7–10

In the phone calls and final home visit of the maintenance phase, the occupational therapist primarily validated Mr. P's excellent progress and skill development. The therapist also suggested slight modifications or adjustments to the strategies, and they discussed ways to apply them to a new problem: Mrs. P's heightened anxiety when her family came to visit.

CONCLUSION

Although there are multiple steps and processes in both the active and maintenance phases, ESP can be distilled to five core interactive and iterative steps: (1) opening the contact (e.g., building rapport, assessment), (2) negotiating the agenda (e.g., identifying and prioritizing problem areas), (3) exploring cultural dynamics and caregiver readiness, (4) tailoring strategies (e.g., identifying strategies through problem solving and brainstorming and then training in use of acceptable approaches), and (5) closing the contact (e.g., validating caregiver abilities, planning ahead, introducing homework, helping caregiver generalize skills to new areas). These five areas form the ESP Road Map, as graphically portrayed in Appendix D. This ESP Road Map serves as a visual guide of the process and is a quick and easy-to-use reference.

TABLE 8.4. Treatment Implementation Characteristics (N = 116)

Protocol Component	Mean (SD)	Actual Range	Protocol Guidelines
Total number of contacts	5.8 (1.6)	1–10	6
Home visit	4.8 (1.2)	1–7	5
Number of telephone contacts	1.0 (0.9)	0–4	1
Duration of intervention (minutes)	477.2 (145.1)	55–855	480
Home visits			
Total minutes	458.1 (139.8)	55–825	450
Per session minutes	95.8 (18.3)	52.2–151.9	90
Telephone contact			
Total minutes	18.7 (15.8)	0–90	30
Per session minutes	14.9 (14.1)	0–90	30
Number of management areas targeted	4.36 (1.7)	1–12	3–5
Percentage of strategies integrated	54.0 (26.4)	0–100	0–100

Table 8.4 summarizes the data derived from occupational therapist documentation of treatment during the active phase of ESP with 116 caregivers who completed the intervention. The table shows means and ranges for each ESP intervention target, allowing comparison against the protocol guidelines. Although some interventions will inevitably vary from the ESP protocol, the targeted number and duration of contacts are close to the means, indicating that the protocol is achievable in the real world.

REFERENCES

American Occupational Therapy Association. (2002). Occupational therapy practice framework: Domain and process. *American Journal of Occupational Therapy, 56,* 609–639.

Gitlin, L. N., Corcoran, M. A., & Eckhardt, S. (1995). Understanding the family perspective: An ethnographic framework for providing occupational therapy in the home. *American Journal of Occupational Therapy, 49,* 802–809.

Gitlin, L. N., Hauck, W. W., Dennis, M. P., & Winter, L. (in press). Long-term effects of the Home Environmental Skill-Building Program for families caring for persons with Alzheimer's disease and related disorders. *Journal of Gerontology: Medical Sciences.*

Gitlin, L. N., Schinfeld, S., Winter, L., Corcoran, M., & Hauck, W. (2002). Evaluating home environments of persons with dementia: Interrater reliability and validity of the Home Environmental Assessment Protocol (HEAP). *Disability and Rehabilitation, 24,* 59–71.

Gitlin, L. N., Winter, L., Dennis, M., Corcoran, M., Schinfeld, S., & Hauck, W. (2002). Strategies used by families to simplify tasks for individuals with Alzheimer's disease and related disorders: Psychometric analysis of the Task Management Strategy Index (TMSI). *Gerontologist, 42,* 61–69.

Prochaska, J. O., & Velicer, W. F. (1997).The transtheoretical model of health behavior change. *American Journal of Health Promotion, 12,* 38–48.

Teri, L., Truax, P., Logsdon, R., Uomoto, J., Zarit, S., & Vitaliano, P. P. (1992). Assessment of behavioral problems in dementia: The Revised Memory and Behavior Problems Checklist (RMBPC). *Psychology and Aging, 7,* 622–631.

9

Clinical Guidelines for Implementing the Home Environmental Skill-Building Program

Mary A. Corcoran, PhD, OTR/L, FAOTA
Laura N. Gitlin, PhD

The occupational therapist brings out these things, and she showed me some card games, but I don't remember them. It's hard for me.

—Caregiving Styles Study (Corcoran) NIA R29-AG13019 10051#2: 419–421

I started out by thinking activity analysis, [and] the ability to understand things in multiple layers and systems was important. And then I thought, well, it's really the way [occupational therapy] looks at everything. You take a step back and start to do it. Or start to try and figure out, "What am I doing?" You realize you are looking at all these different layers of things. What [ESP] adds to it [is] more than activity analysis; it's this whole view of the person, the environment, the situation, and what's going on . . . it's being open to learning new models and practicing that model within the context of a protocol.

—Toth-Cohen NIA Grant #K07 AG00998, Text Unit 35, Interview 2, Participant 1

The purpose of the Home Environmental Skill-Building Program (ESP) is to enable families to build skills, problem solve independently, use the home environment as an effective management tool, and apply skills to newly emerging and worsening caregiving dilemmas. But how does an occupational therapist manage all of this? Thus far we have addressed the who, what, where, and why of ESP. In this chapter we extend our discussion to *how* to implement this program. We present eight principles that serve as clinical guidelines. These principles enable the occupational therapist to develop strategies that match environmental demands with the capacities of the care recipient and caregiver.

Introducing environmental strategies to families in their homes is a clinical intervention that requires customization and individuation. There is no "magic bullet" or single environmental solution that will work for all families. Families experience caregiving quite differently and have different resources, values, styles of caring, and environmental contexts. Furthermore, the disease process manifests itself in each person in a unique manner. Behavioral manifestations and levels of dependencies differ, even among people at the same stage of the disease process. Thus, tailoring the intervention approach and the types of strategies developed is of utmost importance. For example, a strategy that is effective in one household for wandering behaviors may not work in another with the same concern. Whereas a stop sign placed on the front door may deter elopement for one person with dementia, it may cause confusion and agitation in another. For any problem area, it may be necessary to consider different environmental solutions.

The following principles can help the occupational therapist achieve an effective, tailored approach, one of the tenets of ESP:

1. Observe each room of the home.
2. Evaluate individual capabilities, family concerns, and home environmental features.
3. Involve family members and, if possible, the person with dementia in the evaluation and decision-making processes.
4. Introduce small, incremental changes to the home environment.
5. Use validating statements while re-evaluating with the caregiver what works and doesn't work.
6. Use role-play or demonstration to instruct the caregiver in the use of new strategies.
7. Readjust environmental strategies based on caregiver feedback as to what works best.
8. Provide the family with information about the disease and skills to implement other environmental strategies in the future.

OBSERVATION OF THE HOME ENVIRONMENT

The first principle is to observe each room of the home. In ESP, the home environment is not only the context in which the intervention is delivered but also a primary treatment modality. Thus, an important part of the assessment process is a walk-through assessment of each room the care recipient uses, guided by the Home Environmental Assessment Protocol (HEAP; see Tool A.4 in Appendix A), and dialogue about the types of activities performed in each space. During the home tour, the occupational therapist can solicit the caregiver's assessment of how well each activity (e.g., bathing, meal preparation) is accomplished and whether he or she would like to see change in some aspect of the activity.

For example, in the bathroom the occupational therapist can ask about self-care activities, the care recipient's performance history with these activities, and adaptive equipment in use. As the caregiver discusses routines, the therapist can probe as to whether any aspect of the routines is not satisfying or effective, what strategies the caregiver has tried, and the caregiver's thoughts as to what he or she would prefer as an outcome.

Touring and observing each room also provides an opportunity for the occupational therapist and caregiver to engage in a prolonged dialogue as the basis for developing a working relationship. It helps the caregiver to convey his or her thinking processes and in turn enables the therapist to share his or her professional insights. This dialogue while touring and observing each room may appear to the caregiver to be an informal conversation. However, it is a structured process in which the therapist's knowledge of environmental attributes informs the types of questions, probes, and observations used in an effort to obtain an understanding of the demands and supports of each room in relation to the activities performed and the care recipient's capabilities.

There is one important caveat about a home tour: Some caregivers may feel reluctant or embarrassed about having a stranger examine their home without prior knowledge and permission. This is particularly the case for a caregiver, who may already be stressed by the health professional's visit or who is unable to maintain the home as he or she would prefer. The occupational therapist can alleviate any discomfort by informing the caregiver when setting up the contact that he or she would like to observe a few key rooms and why such observations are important. Additionally, it is important to assure the caregiver that the observations are being made to help the therapist understand ways to help the caregiver and that there is no need for the caregiver to clean or rearrange anything. In fact, it is best that the caregiver leave the home the way it usually is so the occupational therapist can obtain a realistic understanding of the environment. Once the caregiver has given permission for the tour, the therapist should be careful to not open doors, drawers, cabinets, or closets without first inquiring if it is acceptable; if the therapist wants to know where a particular object is kept, he or she should ask the caregiver to show him or her where it is kept.

Most importantly, the occupational therapist must work to ease the experience for the caregiver by making sure that he or she makes the purpose of the observations clear and avoids any hint of judgment. It also helps to reason out loud, such as by saying "I wonder if you have room in one of these drawers for his shaving items to be kept all together" and waiting for the caregiver to either open the drawer or reply "No, there is no room." Additionally, touring and observing a home can help clarify the way each member of the family uses space and thus how a suggested modification may affect others in the home; this is especially important if there are children living in the home. Thus, observing relevant rooms is an important approach, but the occupational therapist needs to handle it sensitively. In our research, we have found that very few caregivers refuse such observations, and many find a home tour to be helpful and an opportunity to share ways they have rearranged their homes to accommodate caregiving.

In evaluating use of space in the home, the occupational therapist should consider several aspects. Of utmost importance is the level of clutter in the home and whether it affects the ability of the care recipient or caregiver to navigate the home. Clutter, or excessive number of objects for diverse tasks, is a common problem in households that can contribute to disorientation and agitation. A common area of clutter is the kitchen or dining room table, which may be used to sort mail, bills, or read newspapers in addition to serving as a place to eat. However, these diverse objects may be confusing to the person with dementia, and he or she may have difficulty determining what to do at that setting. In Figure 9.1, the caregiver worked at home as an importer of baskets and jewelry, and the excessive clutter was a source of agitation to his father, who had difficulty navigating the area and eating in that room.

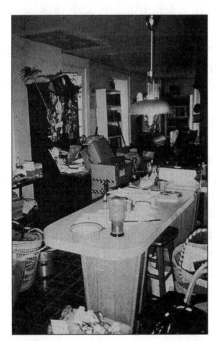

FIGURE 9.1. Areas of clutter may confuse the care recipient.

Another consideration is whether objects for a common purpose are clustered together to form a control center. A control center (see Figure 9.2) involves placing objects necessary for a particular task or common purpose in a central area for ease of use by the caregiver or care recipient. A control center may contain the medications needed for the day, or objects that will occupy a person near his or her favorite chair (e.g., newspaper, remote control, glass of water, reading glasses).

Another consideration in observing how space is used is whether objects of interest and meaning to the care recipient are easily accessible. For example, placing an activity

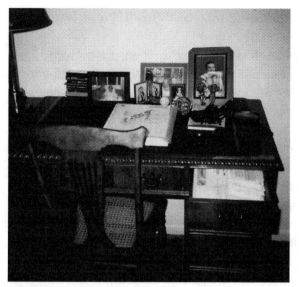

FIGURE 9.2. Control center.

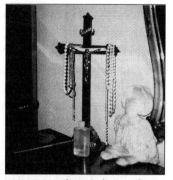

FIGURE 9.3. Placing religious objects in view of the care recipient can enhance quality of life.

board, favorite magazines, or meaningful religious objects (as in Figure 9.3) in full view of the care recipient can enhance quality of life and offer meaningful stimulation.

EVALUATION OF CAPABILITIES, CONCERNS, AND ENVIRONMENTAL FEATURES

The second principle is to evaluate individual capabilities, family concerns, and home environmental features. This principle lies at the heart of ESP and its competence–environmental press conceptual framework (discussed in Chapter 5). Appendix A provides several tools that can help occupational therapists evaluate the person, family, and environmental contexts independent of the others. Occupational therapists may find these tools helpful to identify the principal concerns of caregivers; the types of safety issues and home adaptations present; the caregiver's management style; and the care recipient's functional, behavioral, and cognitive profile. However, their usefulness is limited by the fact that they do not capture transactional processes; hence, it is up to the therapist, through clinical reasoning, to put it all together. For example, a therapist may obtain a preliminary understanding of a caregiver's concerns through the Caregiver Assessment of Management Problems, but the relationship of the caregiver's concerns to the care recipient's actual capacities or contextual attributes will not necessarily become apparent. The therapist must make those connections through clinical reasoning as he or she collects information. In our research, the presentation of cases helped occupational therapists synthesize the clinical information they had gathered and obtain feedback from colleagues as to appropriate treatment approaches. In the real world, such sharing may be difficult, but it is advantageous and recommended.

How do occupational therapists develop a comprehensive picture of the transactions among person, family, and context? Many experienced occupational therapists have their own visual or written techniques for documenting their clinical reasoning. We recommend the use of two techniques: field notes and force field analysis.

The recording of field notes in an ongoing log is a very common approach. Field notes can simply consist of the who, what, when, and where of each home visit; the therapist details his or her perceptions of the session, the care problems, and the caregiver's and care recipient's abilities and contrasts these perceptions with the caregiver's own story. Field notes can serve as a self-reflective tool; the therapist can ask himself or herself the following:

- What do I see happening in this household?
- Why do I see things differently than the caregiver sees them?
- What is the readiness level of this caregiver to adopt certain helpful strategies?
- Is this caregiver depressed, and could that be contributing to stress in the household?
- What would make things better for this caregiver?

Force field analysis is another simple and important clinical reasoning tool. Based on the work of social psychologist Kurt Lewin (1951), the force field is a visual map of factors that support and restrain function or a particular behavior that is the target of the intervention. The purpose of this approach is to identify supporting forces that can be strengthened and restraining forces that can be eliminated to improve function. This approach begins with the family and occupational therapist identifying target problem areas and a specific obtainable goal as part of the assessment and problem-solving processes. The therapist evaluates the capabilities of the person with dementia through direct observation and cognitive status tests such as the Mini Mental Status Examination (Folstein, Folstein, & McHugh, 1975) and then evaluates the attributes of the environment using the HEAP. The therapist and caregiver plot all factors in both the care recipient and the home environment as either restraining forces (i.e., factors that limit goal achievement) or supporting forces (i.e., factors that sustain or promote goal achievement).

Case Example 9.1 illustrates the use of force field analysis in devising a solution to the R family's concerns about Mr. R's difficulty gathering his clothing in the morning. Figure 9.4 is the force field diagram representing the supporting and restraining forces in Mr. R's ability to gather his clothing.

The map of supporting and restraining factors obtained using the force field technique helps the occupational therapist visualize potential solutions. In the case example, one possibility would be to reproduce the context- and person-based factors that were in place when Mr. R was able to function at his optimal

---

CASE EXAMPLE 9.1. Mr. R

Mr. R, a person with mild-stage dementia, has retired and is suddenly unable to gather clothing to dress himself in the morning. His wife, Mrs. R, wants her husband to be able to independently gather his clothing. This seems to be a reasonable goal, based on what can typically be expected of individuals with mild-stage dementia. "Independently gather clothing" is established as the goal, based on the concerns and priorities expressed by the family. Using a force field analysis, the occupational therapist and caregiver identify the restraining factors— those context- and person-based factors that limit Mr. R's capability to achieve this goal. The therapist and caregiver problem solve together and identify the following restraining forces:

- Mr. R is unable to remember where his clothing is kept (person-based factor).
- Mr. R becomes upset when he cannot perform a "simple" activity, and his anxiety reduces his performance (person-based factor).
- The family recently purchased new bedroom furniture, and Mr. R cannot remember where his clothing is kept (context-based attribute).
- Mrs. R developed a new arrangement for closets and drawers (context-based attribute).
- Mrs. R purchased new clothing to reflect Mr. R's retired status (context-based attribute).
- Mr. R is arising later than he did before retirement (context-based attribute).

The supporting forces identified are as follows:

- Mr. R is motivated to dress himself (person-based factor).
- Mr. R is physically capable of safely gathering clothing (person-based factor).
- The bedroom is familiar, having remained structurally unchanged for 25 years (context-based factor).
- The new bedroom furniture is quite similar to the set Mr. and Mrs. R used formerly (context-based factor).

---

level. However, the family has invested money and time in new furniture and is unlikely to bring back the old furniture. The therapist considered the following in the search for ways to reduce the effect of the restraining forces on Mr. R's performance:

- Start with the restraining forces that are easiest to address. For example, the occupational therapist may suggest that two context-based solutions (returning to preretirement wake-up time and returning to the original arrangement of closets and drawers) and one person-based solution (reducing the care recipient's anxiety through deep breathing) as a good beginning. If the results are not satisfying, the occupational therapist may confer with the caregiver about addressing other factors that are more difficult to implement (such as returning to the old bedroom furniture).

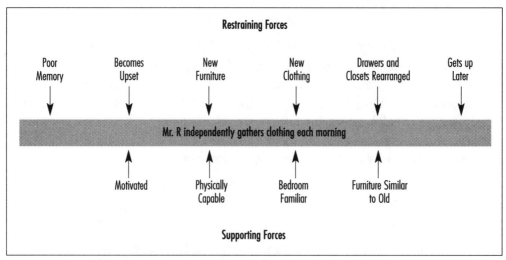

FIGURE 9.4. Force field analysis: Restraining or supporting forces.

- Consider whether any of the supporting forces can be strengthened. For instance, Mrs. R can reinforce her husband's motivation to dress himself by providing him with a goal for getting dressed, such as going to a museum or for a walk.
- Determine the relative strength of the forces on the problem, and tackle them from strongest to weakest. The occupational therapist determined through observation of Mr. R and discussion with Mrs. R that the arrangement of drawers and closets was a strong factor, because the husband seemed to search for his clothing.

Force field analysis is beneficial because it provides a map of the constellation of factors that work interdependently to shape an individual's functional performance. The occupational therapist can weigh each factor as a basis for determining what to modify first. Furthermore, the therapist can update the force field diagram as he or she obtains additional information. Some caregivers may benefit from viewing this visual portrayal and using it as a management tool.

INVOLVEMENT IN EVALUATION AND DECISION MAKING

The third principle is to involve family members and, if possible, the person with dementia in the evaluation and decision-making processes. The collaborative process discussed in previous chapters by necessity requires family involvement. Furthermore, the person with dementia can help shape the intervention goals and methods by expressing his or her opinions and concerns, if able. Alternatively, the caregiver can focus decisions on what he or she knows about the care recipient's preferences and interests and previous roles and habits. In fact, few occupational therapists would opt to exclude the family and client from these important aspects of evaluation and treatment, yet involving them efficiently and effectively is difficult and the methods for doing so often unclear. Four strategies necessary to achieve a high level of family involvement include allowing adequate time for the caregiver to provide input and tell his or her story, engaging in clear communication about the purpose of the intervention and the identification of goals, remaining flexible about recommendations, and providing choices.

Adequate Time

Most caregiver interactions with health professionals, including occupational therapists, tend to be based on a prescriptive, medical-model approach. This experience may be particularly typical for older cohorts, who may have spent decades interacting with medical professionals as authority figures. Thus, families may not be clear as to the focus and purpose of ESP and may need time and guidance to learn how to maximize this opportunity to address the problems and concerns of utmost interest to them. The shift from a medical or prescriptive approach to a collaborative model can feel different for both occupational therapists who have not worked from this framework and for caregivers.

It is thus important for the occupational therapist to give the collaborative process time to unfold. Some families will be immediately comfortable discussing their most pressing and intimate concerns, whereas others may not be able to raise critical issues until trust and rapport have been well established. Nevertheless, as discussed in Chapter 7, our research suggests that occupational therapists can establish a strong collaborative therapeutic relationship relatively quickly—by the second intervention contact. Using the techniques discussed in previous chapters—such as approaching the caregiver from a collaborative framework and treating him or her as a lay practitioner whose expertise and story of caregiving are important—facilitates the development of an effective therapeutic relationship.

Clear Communication

ESP is based on the premise that families are active partners in identifying problem areas and deriving solutions in conjunction with occupational therapists. Thus, it is important that therapists communicate clearly the intervention approach and help family members provide input in the assessment, treatment planning, and evaluation stages. As described in Chapter 8, in each contact the therapist begins by providing the caregiver with a road map, or overview, of the purpose of the contact and what they will accomplish. After outlining the contact's purpose, the therapist checks in with the caregiver to make sure he or she understands and agrees to what they have outlined; adjustments to the road map are made based on caregiver input and agreement. Likewise, each contact ends with the therapist taking a few minutes to obtain closure by reviewing the major points covered, the treatment goals jointly established, and the strategies recommended. These simple yet highly effective therapeutic tools (introductory road map and wrap-up) reinforce therapeutic messages and serve to organize and optimize communication between caregiver and therapist.

The occupational therapist can further facilitate clear communication by the way he or she names and frames the issues and derives decisions. Case Example 9.2 illustrates the complexities of communicating clearly in decision making about the treatment process.

Flexibility Regarding Recommendations

In ESP, it is important to convey that the strategies the therapist proposes represent a point of departure for discussion and that the caregiver can accept, modify, or reject the strategies proposed. The therapist also needs to explain that any one strategy may need to be modified either by the occupational therapist or the caregiver to fit the particular situation and resolve the target problem. A caregiver's modification of a recommendation demonstrates that the caregiver understands the strategy's purpose and has learned how to increase its potential effectiveness for his or her particular context. Because the ultimate goal of ESP is to build problem-solving skills in caregivers and to enable use of the environment

---

CASE EXAMPLE 9.2. Mrs. B

Mrs. B wanted to make sure her husband received adequate nutrition, yet she also recognized the need for her own respite. The occupational therapist suggested sending Mr. B to a local day care center that serves hot meals at lunchtime. The caregiver initially rejected this suggestion, and the therapist began to explore the reasons why. In response to the therapist's probing questions, Mrs. B revealed that she was concerned that the staff would not take the time needed to feed her husband. In addition, she believed that only she could provide proper care for him, so she opted to continue to keep him at home.

In discussing this issue further, the occupational therapist proposed some alternative approaches, such as having Mr. B attend adult day care on a limited basis. In thinking about this, Mrs. B decided to try adult day care for 3 days each week to give her some respite. Additionally, the therapist and Mrs. B came up with another solution to address her concern with his eating. They derived a strategy by which Mrs. B would send her husband to day care with homemade soup in a container. That way, Mrs. B would know how much he ate, and even if he did not consume all of the soup she would be assured that the partially eaten meal would be nutritious. Providing Mr. B with hot soup also was an important and symbolic care gesture. It provided Mrs. B with a way to continue to provide Mr. B with the best personal care she could and represented an offering of love, nurturance, and continuity in their relationship.

as a management tool, caregiver modification of a strategy is one important indicator of the success of the therapeutic process. For this reason, the Treatment Receipt and Enactment tool (Tool A.7 in Appendix A) and the Therapeutic Engagement Index (see Chapter 7) include items that refer to the caregiver's sense of ownership of the intervention process.

Provision of Choices

Most caregivers are overwhelmed and fatigued and may have little energy for making decisions and actively participating in a therapeutic process that involves active problem solving and behavioral change. Caregivers also may be reluctant to engage if they are used to a medical, prescriptive approach in which a health professional prescribes or dictates a set of directives for the caregiver to follow. Alternatively, some caregivers may have difficulty focusing on the intervention or may be distracted by other issues that cannot be addressed in the intervention, such as financial, legal, or marital matters. Finally, caregivers may be overwhelmed by having to consider more than one possible solution to a care issue, and they may need guidance in narrowing their choices.

With such caregivers, it is helpful for the occupational therapist to be more directive in the therapeutic process and to offer no more than two choices of strategy to reduce the press of the intervention on the caregiver. By reducing the caregiver's decision to a few choices, provided with a brief explanation of their relative pros and cons, the therapist helps to simplify the decision-making process while empowering the caregiver to take ownership of a decision. Additionally, if a caregiver is overwhelmed, providing a basic choice allows him or her to remain involved in the decision-making process without adding further burden or pressure to an already stressful situation.

One clue that the intervention may be overwhelming for a caregiver is if he or she agrees to have the occupational therapist visit but does not practice or use recommended strategies and shows little to no progress from session to session. Our research has shown that this may be the case for caregivers who are clinically depressed (Gitlin, 2001; Gitlin, Corcoran, Winter, Boyce, & Marcus, 1999). In this case, it is very important for the therapist to first refer the caregiver to a health professional to be treated for depression. Second, it is important for the therapist to avoid placing any additional burden on the caregiver. Although a therapist may be able to identify many strategies that could be helpful to the caregiver, it is best to introduce just one strategy that would be easy for the caregiver to implement and for which the caregiver would have some immediate success (e.g., "Take three deep breaths before you wake your mother up to try to dress her"). The therapist must be careful not to bombard the caregiver with too many strategy recommendations and to proceed slowly in each session.

INCREMENTAL CHANGES

The fourth principle is to introduce small, incremental changes to the home environment. This principle is important for several reasons. First, changing the physical and social aspects of a household may have unexpected negative effects. For example, in one household the caregiver and occupational therapist created a quiet, soothing room for the caregiver's husband by decluttering and removing unnecessary objects (e.g., stacks of newspapers, pictures, chairs, tables). The caregiver would bring her husband to sit in the room to listen to quiet music and look out the window, which overlooked a beautiful garden and bird feeders. However, the back door to the garden was located in that room; decluttering the room made this door much more noticeable to the caregiver's husband, and he tried to exit. Thus, whereas decluttering initially had a positive effect (e.g., decreased agitation, engagement in a pleasant activity), it also had an unintended negative effect (elopement attempts). The caregiver and therapist problem solved and developed a way to camouflage the door with a poster that her husband enjoyed looking at. Another way the elopement problem could have been handled is by placing a "stop" sign on the door, as shown in Figure 9.5.

Second, objects and their placement in a home typically have deeply held meanings. Thus, small changes may be more acceptable to a family and easier to tolerate. For example, Figure 9.6 shows a wall where family photos are displayed in the home of a caregiver who participated in the ESP study. This was a meaningful area in the home that the caregiver wanted the care recipient to access, despite the fact that the care recipient was experiencing balance problems. The solution was to keep the area as is but to add a hand rail so the care recipient could stand and enjoy the photographs. It is important to remember, however, that reactions can be highly individualized so a positive change for one family member may cause distress for others. Proceeding with suggestions slowly and carefully provides opportunities for the occupational therapist to observe and reflect on potential reaction of each family member to the suggested modification.

Third, families may be able to tolerate only a few changes in the environment. Our research has shown that, whereas occupational

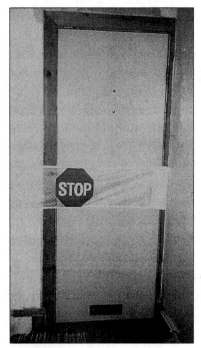

FIGURE 9.5. Use of a stop sign to deal with elopement problems.

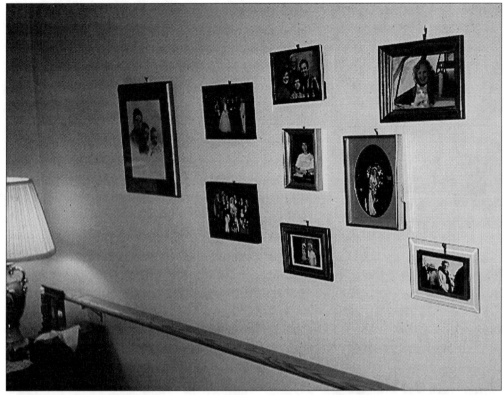

FIGURE 9.6. A display of family photos is a meaningful area for many care recipients.

therapists generated an average of 16 strategy recommendations per caregiver-identified problem area, caregivers chose to implement an average of 4 of these strategies. Family caregivers may have a limit as to how much change is tolerable (Corcoran & Gitlin, 2001). Thus, it is important to choose only strategies that are key to the success of achieving an identified treatment goal. For example, caregiver communication strategies are critical to any problem area; the therapist should introduce them early on because they can also be generalized easily to other care problems.

Finally, the occupational therapist should introduce modifications in the home in an incremental fashion to reflect the level of competence of the person with dementia. A modification is rather temporary in that it addresses an immediate problem and is designed to reflect the capabilities of the care recipient at one point in time. However, as the disease progresses and the person declines in ability, the modification may need additional refinement. For example, a care recipient is having difficulty recognizing and distinguishing objects used for grooming (e.g., toothbrush, toothpaste, floss). An initial strategy might be to label the objects (see Figure 9.7) or post a picture as to how the care recipient should use

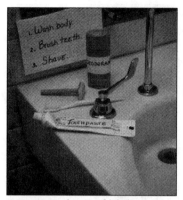

FIGURE 9.7. The use of labels to distinguish items for grooming.

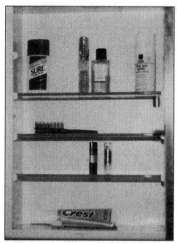

FIGURE 9.8. Grouping items used for each grooming task is one strategy to help care recipients recognize objects.

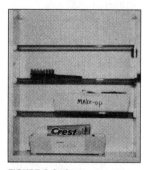

FIGURE 9.9. Care recipients may be aided by grouping objects in labeled containers.

each object. However, with decline, the caregiver may need to change this strategy by grouping objects for a particular task on one shelf (see Figure 9.8) or in a container with a label (e.g., all objects for brushing one's teeth in container labeled "Teeth" that is in the care recipient's visual field; see Figure 9.9). When the disease has progressed further, the caregiver may have to remove all grooming objects from the sink area and hand one object at a time to the care recipient while providing verbal cueing.

USE OF VALIDATING STATEMENTS

The fifth principle is to use validating statements while reevaluating with the caregiver what works and what does not work. An important aspect of ESP is empowering the caregiver by validating his or her efforts and recognizing him or her as a skilled provider. Caregivers ultimately want to do the right thing and provide the best care possible. Thus, caregivers need validation that they are doing a great job. They rarely receive any feedback, are left on their own to determine what to try and how to provide care, and may never be complimented on the job they are doing. Thus, validation of what the caregiver does and why it is working is critical for skill building and empowerment and serves as a powerful therapeutic tool.

Likewise, caregivers need to feel empowered to reject recommendations that they are offered and to speak freely to the therapist as to what they believe will or will not work and to choose what they are willing to try. Validating statements include recognition of what the caregiver has attempted or achieved; examples include "You are putting so much energy, thought, and effort into caring for your wife," "That was a difficult strategy to use, but you stuck with it," and "If it doesn't work, then we will try something else—it is important for you to try different strategies to find the right one. This is a trial-and-error approach; there is no one right way." The following simple guidelines can help the therapist maintain an accepting therapeutic tone while providing suggestions for change:

- Show the caregiver what he or she should do, as opposed to what he or she should not do. For example, instead of telling the caregiver not to raise his voice with his wife, suggest instead that he keep his voice very quiet and accepting. The therapist must provide a concrete alternative approach.
- Avoid the word *you*, if possible, by focusing on the strategy itself and not how the caregiver implemented it. For example, rather than "It looks like you weren't able to change his resistance to your care by using the bath bench," the therapist can say, "Using the bath bench didn't work as well as we'd hoped, did it?"
- Always point out to the caregiver what worked well first, and then indicate what needs more work to be effective.
- Ask the caregiver to talk about how he or she thought the strategy worked. This provides an opportunity for you to agree with the analysis and to help specify the aspects of the strategy that need to be changed.
- Offer to provide whatever is needed to improve how the strategy is implemented, such as information or practice. Demonstrate that the effectiveness of the strategy depends on you, the occupational therapist, doing your job well and that you are willing to work harder to ensure success.

USE OF ROLE-PLAY AND DEMONSTRATION

The sixth principle is to use role-play or demonstration to instruct the caregiver in the use of new strategies. Role-play and demonstration are a visual approach to learning; seeing and doing are a useful way to build skills. Additionally, the skills required of caregivers in ESP may not be simple to learn or implement. By virtue of its nature, ESP demands that the caregiver modify his or her environment; interact in a calm and supportive manner with the person who has dementia; and respond quickly and effectively to unpredictable actions, some of which may be annoying or dangerous. Therefore, essential to ESP is engaging the caregiver in an active therapeutic process by using role-playing or demonstrations to provide ample practice opportunities and to solidify new skills and their integration into daily caregiving.

In a role-play, the caregiver and occupational therapist assume the roles of anyone who is involved in the strategy being practiced. The caregiver can play the part of the care recipient if the purpose of the role-play is to understand more about the perspective of the person with dementia during implementation of the strategy. Alternatively, the caregiver can play his or her own part in the role-play, and the therapist can provide opportunities to respond to a range of possible actions and reactions by the care recipient. The latter role assignment is especially useful if the strategy being practiced requires the caregiver to maintain a calm and reassuring attitude.

In a demonstration, the occupational therapist works with the care recipient while the caregiver observes, thereby providing an opportunity for the caregiver to watch someone else model the strategy. Demonstration is beneficial when the therapist wishes to increase the caregiver's engagement in modifying or critiquing the strategy, because it provides a positive mechanism for eliciting the caregiver's comments and suggested changes. Recent research shows that interventions that engage the caregiver in the active use of strategies are more effective than those that are more didactic or that rely on print and educational approaches only (Belle et al., 2003; Chee, Hauck, Dennis, & Gitlin, 2004).

READJUSTMENT OF ENVIRONMENTAL STRATEGIES

The seventh principle is to readjust environmental strategies based on family feedback as to what works best. At the beginning of each session, it is important to review with the caregiver what strategies he or she tried and each strategy's outcome or effectiveness. In discussing each strategy, the occupational therapist should review its purpose, examine its effect on the care recipient's behavior or function, and determine whether it increased or decreased the caregiver's burden of care. For example, whereas a toileting schedule may decrease bladder accidents, it may increase caregiver burden because it requires the caregiver to bring the care recipient to the bathroom every 2 hours.

Role-play can be helpful in determining which aspects of a strategy may need adjustment. Careful and detailed interviewing regarding the who, what, when, and where of the strategy also may yield important information. Encouraging caregivers to keep notes, a diary, or a behavior log to help evaluate the effectiveness of a strategy can be helpful; some caregivers may find such documentation burdensome, however. No matter how the information is collected, the occupational therapist should continue with the collaborative techniques he or she initiated by engaging the family in reasoning about how well the strategy is meeting treatment goals and how to modify it. The therapist should reason aloud to share his or her perspective and to encourage the same by the caregiver. Together, they can then decide on the next steps.

PROVISION OF INFORMATION ABOUT THE DISEASE

The eighth and final principle is to provide the family with information about the disease and skills to implement other environmental strategies in the future. The ultimate goal of ESP is to build skills for addressing current and future issues associated with family caregiving in the home. Over the course of the disease, symptoms emerge and disappear, and function slowly dissipates. The family's burden of care changes from vigilance in the early stages to advocacy in the later stages. At present, few mechanisms are in place for supporting ongoing involvement by occupational therapy in a family's care decisions over time, so it is imperative that the caregiver be able to apply the skills to emerging or worsening care issues. Additionally, as part of the final contact, the occupational therapist should provide families with community, online, material, and print resources as appropriate (see Appendix C).

CONCLUSION

In this chapter, we have presented eight principles that underlie the conduct of ESP and that help ensure individuation of the treatment and skill-building processes. First, families need information about the disease process and about the ways different aspects of the home environment may affect their caregiving efforts and the behavior of their family member. Second, it is important to evaluate both the care recipient's and the caregiver's capabilities and perceived needs and to examine the environmental context in which a care problem occurs; inclusion of the family member in the decision-making process as to which strategy to use is to be encouraged. Use of role-play, demonstration, or simulations that actively engage the caregiver in demonstrating a new technique and allow ample opportunity for practice help reinforce the acceptance and use of strategies. Strategies may need to be adjusted or refined, so it is important that therapists obtain feedback from families as to what worked best and why after a brief trial period.

Finally, dementia is progressive and irreversible; families need to adopt different strategies over the course of the disease. People with dementia may have increasing difficulty navigating the physical environment and processing and interpreting cues. Therefore, teaching families how to problem solve and use their environment to address newly emerging care challenges also is an important component of this approach.

REFERENCES

Belle, S., Czaja, S. J., Schulz, R., Burgio, L., Gitlin, L. N., Jones, R., et al. (2003). Combining diverse interventions using a new taxonomy to combine the uncombinable: Integrating results across diverse caregiving interventions. *Psychology and Aging, 18,* 396–405.

Chee, Y., Hauck, W., Dennis, M., & Gitlin, L. N. (2004, November). *Predictors of adherence to in-home caregiver interventions for managing dementia.* Paper presented at the Gerontological Society of America Meetings, Washington DC.

Corcoran, M. A., & Gitlin, L. N. (2001). Family acceptance and use of environmental strategies provided in an occupational therapy intervention. *Occupational and Physical Therapy in Geriatrics, 19*(1), 1–20.

Folstein, M. F., Folstein, S. E., & McHugh, P. R. (1975). Mini-mental state: A practical method for grading the cognitive state of patients for the clinician. *Journal of Psychiatric Research, 12,* 189–198.

Gitlin, L. N. (2001). Effectiveness of home environmental interventions for individuals with dementia and family caregivers. *Home Health Care Consultant, 8,* 22–26.

Gitlin, L. N., Corcoran, M., Winter, L., Boyce, A., & Marcus, S. (1999). Predicting participation and adherence to a home environmental intervention among family caregivers of dementia patients. *Family Relations, 48,* 363–372.

Lewin, K. (1951). *Field theory in social science.* New York: Harper.

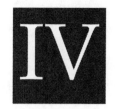

Practicalities of Implementing the Home Environmental Skill-Building Program

10

Involving Other Formal Care Providers:

Tracey Vause Earland, MS, OTR/L
Laura N. Gitlin, PhD

The Home Environmental Skill-Building Program in Diverse Care Settings

How did I find the resources? I went [to the Alzheimer's Association and] found the caregivers' seminars very helpful, to [generate] ideas. . . . But no, did I get stuff from the doctors? No. In fact, I did a one-page summary of the resources I found and gave it to my doctor for their office . . . and they were real glad to have it.

—Corcoran, *Styles Study* # NIA R29-AG13019 10411#1: 227–233

I think in the Washington [DC] area you may have more available sources then you would in other parts of the country. [But] it was surprising to me when I went to the support group in Alexandria [VA], those people had been participating in that [group] for months, or maybe a year or two, and how little they seemed to know. They had gone to a neurologist; some were complaining the neurologist didn't answer their calls or didn't respond, at least they thought they should, and so on, but it's everybody's problem in knowing what to do.

—Corcoran, *Styles Study* # NIA R29-AG13019 10381#1: 478–485

The vast majority of older adults in the United States have a strong desire to remain in their homes and communities as long as possible—to "age in place" (Gitlin, 2003). The home remains the primary care setting for more than 4 million Americans who have been diagnosed with dementia. However, many families must seek formal assistance to help keep their loved ones at home. National health care trends suggest that community-based settings, home care agency interventions, special-care (dementia) units, and assisted-living facilities will increasingly serve as care delivery networks for people with dementia (Spitzer, 1998; Wahl & Gitlin, 2003).

Thus far, this book has illustrated the Home Environmental Skill-Building Program (ESP) as an occupational therapy service in the home to help family caregivers manage complex dementia-related behaviors and functional dependence. Nevertheless, many of the approaches, principles, and strategies of ESP that occupational therapists use with family caregivers in the home setting are applicable to and successful in other care delivery environments.

In this chapter, we discuss the basic principles and intervention strategies of ESP that are transferable to other settings. Figure 10.1 portrays the numerous clinical arenas in which formal care providers can use ESP principles; these arenas include nursing homes or special-care units, adult day care centers, and assisted-living facilities, which are the settings we focus on in this chapter. The principles of ESP can inform inservice programs for home health agencies, caregiver support groups, and health providers and administrators, as well as guide targeted interventions for residents or program participants. The basic principles of ESP offer care providers who are in environments other than the home with essential tools to manage difficult behaviors and functional dependence.

Use of ESP in other care settings can potentially decrease the level and type of assistance that may be required for a person with dementia and hence reduce the burden of care on formal care providers. As illustrated in the quotes at the start of this chapter, perhaps one of the most important roles an occupational therapist can play is to educate other health professionals about the disease and its impact on caregivers and help them identify when it is appropriate to refer a family to an occupational therapist for ESP intervention.

ESP IN NURSING HOMES AND SPECIAL-CARE UNITS

More than 80% of nursing home residents have a diagnosis of dementia, behavior disorder, psychosis, or major clinical depression, alone or in combination (Burns et al., 1993). There is growing research evidence suggesting that modifying the physical and social environment within long-term-care facilities can reduce behavioral disturbances and improve the lives of residents with dementia (Calkins, 1989; Gitlin, Liebman, & Winter, 2003). Adapting the physical environment (e.g., smaller unit size, way-finding strategies, use of adaptive equipment) and the social environment (e.g., caregiver approach, communication strategies)

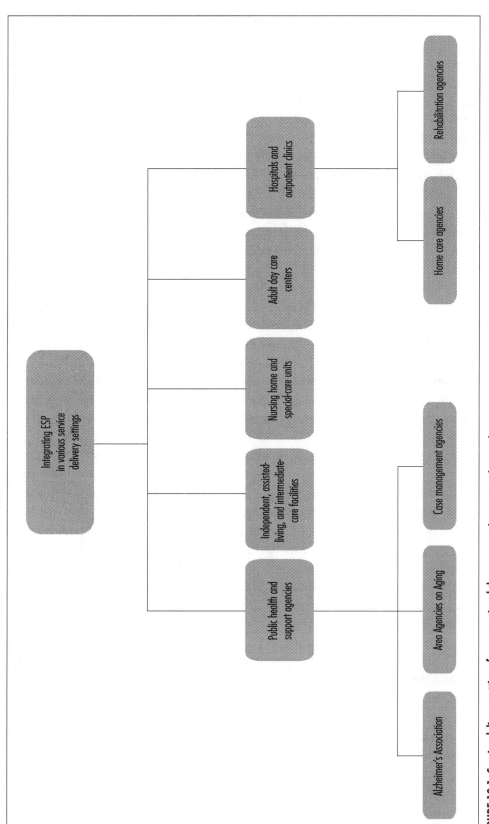

FIGURE 10.1. Service delivery settings for occupational therapy caregiver supportive services.

to support an individual's preserved cognitive abilities has been associated with less decline in activities of daily living (ADL) performance and improved social participation (Gitlin, Corcoran, Winter, Boyce, & Hauck, 2001; Rogers et al., 1999; Rovner, Steele, Shmuely, & Folstein, 1996; Wells, Dawson, Sidani, Craig, & Pringle, 2000).

How, then, can ESP be applied to the nursing home environment? The occupational therapist has two important roles: providing education and skills training and intervening with residents with targeted problem behaviors. First, occupational therapists are in an important position to provide consultative support to formal care providers such as nursing assistants, aides, recreational therapists, and administrators. This support includes specific education about the role of the environment in promoting or inhibiting meaningful and appropriate occupation. Core concepts of ESP—understanding the environment as multilayered, the need for the best person–task–environment fit, the role of culture emergent in shaping daily care, and collaborative techniques in work with caregivers—are all applicable to the nursing home setting.

However, educating staff is only one step in managing disruptive behaviors. Skills training, collaborative problem solving, feedback, and reinforcement all contribute to empowering the care provider. For example, skills training in detecting early-warning signs for catastrophic reactions (e.g., wringing hands, refusal to make eye contact, increased volume, restlessness) can help the care provider formulate effective strategies to prevent or de-escalate potentially difficult situations. Occupational therapists can help formal providers understand dementia-related behaviors and their effect on occupation. Together, the care provider and the occupational therapist can design routines that facilitate engagement in occupation and support participation in the environment (Corcoran, 2001). For example, identifying a sturdy piece of furniture in the day room with a name or picture label will cue the resident to sit down in his or her personal seat during activity sessions. Establishing a structured oral care routine in a well-lit environment increases the individual's sense of control and decreases the need for physical assistance from the aide.

Occupational therapists also can be called into the nursing home environment to work with residents whose behavior or functional dependency is difficult to manage. After evaluating the environment and resident capabilities, occupational therapists can introduce strategies to decrease troublesome behavior and instruct the staff in how to individualize such strategies to fit the unique person–environment system within the nursing home context. As in the home, the evaluation process is important; an environmental modification for one person may not work for another with similar deficits because of the person's individual capabilities or the particular interaction of the person and the environment. Case Example 10.1 shows how ESP modifications to both the physical and social environments of care led to greater gains for a resident with dementia and her care providers.

ESP IN ADULT DAY CENTERS

Although nursing home placement was previously one of the few options available in dementia care, today there are other potential solutions for families. Adult day centers offer a full-day program for people with cognitive impairments and provide health and human services in a secure, engaging environment for part of the day. Having a family member attend adult day programs offers caregivers respite from daily care responsibilities and can help postpone a long-term residential placement.

The National Institute on Adult Daycare (NIAD) defines *adult day care* "as a community-based group program designed to meet the needs of functionally impaired adults through an individual plan of care" (Conyers, 1996, p. 452). These centers have become the fastest growing component of community-based long-term care; the national Alzheimer's Association has actively encouraged their use.

Occupational therapy can serve as a valuable resource to adult day care center staff in numerous ways. Adult day care centers are designed to maintain the person's present level of functioning as long as possible while receiving health services in a community-based setting (Conyers, 1996). Thus, occupational therapy plays a vital role by using occupation to improve the individual's well-being and enable him or her to retain meaningful life skills. Occupational therapists can help care providers understand dementia-related behaviors and, based on the culture or philosophy of the center, can help plan acceptable activities for the participants and staff.

In the adult day care setting, the occupational therapist can use principles of ESP to conduct a comprehensive evaluation that includes assessment of
- The individual's functional performance,
- Safety and daily routines,

CASE EXAMPLE 10.1. Mrs. J

Mrs. J was able to dress herself daily by selecting a dress from one of the three hanging in her closet and putting on undergarments, stockings, and shoes that a nursing aide laid out for her in the morning. However, the nursing staff noted a sharp decline in Mrs. J's self-care one week, and they could not identify why. Consultation with an occupational therapist revealed that a new nursing assistant laid out Mrs. J's clothing with slight differences that caused Mrs. J great confusion. Training of the new nursing assistant resulted in a return to Mrs. J's previous level of assistance and functioning.

- The center's physical and social environment and potential environmental modifications to maximize performance,
- Residents' sense of mastery and control of the environment, and
- The daily routines at home and in the center to inform strategies to promote continuity across settings (Osorio, 1993).

The occupational therapist may serve as a consultant and design a structured program for center staff to implement. An ESP intervention might consist of staff education, recommendations for physical adaptations, skill-building workshops for staff and family caregivers, and follow-up sessions to obtain feedback from staff as to what works and what does not work. Examples of recommended environmental strategies include installing adequate lighting at the activity table, reducing the number of objects or choices in a given leisure activity, reducing stimuli (e.g., by turning off radios and televisions in the dayroom), and creating a memory board to remind care recipients of basic information.

Moreover, the occupational therapist can play an important role in developing and implementing caregiver training programs for both family members and center staff. Workshop or training topics of particular importance include the following:

- The disease process,
- Environmental triggers to disruptive behavior,
- Safety considerations in the adult day center environment,
- Ways to improve collaboration and communication with family caregivers,
- Ways to simplify tasks (e.g., task breakdown and cueing strategies), and
- Self-protection techniques for the formal caregiver.

People with dementia often have difficulty in making the transition from the home to the center and back again. Thus, helping families and staff to communicate effectively with each other and to establish similar routines in the home and the center are of particular benefit for the person with dementia. Adult day centers are often underused by families, often because of resistance to attend on the part of the person with dementia. Occupational therapists can play a critical role in helping families set up a schedule and approach that minimize morning upset and resistance to adult day care attendance.

Community-based programs, including adult day centers, are undergoing great growth and expansion as families search for acceptable alternatives to long-term-care placement. Caregivers of individuals with dementia seek caring, engaging, and protective settings that promote health and well-being for their loved ones and that provide support and resources for the family. An ESP works with families and adult day care staff to offer important tools in the management of dementia-related behaviors and promotion of meaningful occupation within this setting. Case Example 10.2 illustrates the effective use of communication techniques, activity engagement, and task simplification resulting in reduced recipient upset and caregiver burden.

CASE EXAMPLE 10.2. Mrs. S

Mrs. S was initially reluctant to have her husband attend an adult day center, because he never really liked group activities and had not participated in community programs before the onset of his disease. However, she was in desperate need of time off from the oversight she provided him 24 hours a day, 7 days a week. The occupational therapist working with Mrs. S helped her understand that Mr. S might enjoy the adult day center because it would offer opportunities for stimulation and engagement in meaningful activities. Additionally, the therapist helped Mrs. S realize that Mr. S would not view the adult day setting now in the same way he would have viewed it before the onset of dementia. Encouraging Mrs. S to understand this change was the first hurdle.

Once Mrs. S had made the decision to enroll Mr. S in a day care setting and had arranged for his transportation, she found that the three mornings he attended were almost impossible to bear. Mr. S would become very anxious and start pacing the living room, repeatedly asking Mrs. S where she was going and what was happening. He appeared so distressed and angry that Mrs. S was overwhelmed and felt guilty for the rest of the day, believing that she had made the wrong decision.

After a few days, the center staff reported that Mr. S was smiling, ate well, and enjoyed working on a craft project and listening to music. Nevertheless, the mornings were still difficult, and sometimes he became angry and agitated after returning home. The therapist worked with Mrs. S to help her acknowledge the benefits of day care for her husband and to develop approaches for establishing a morning and late-afternoon routine to address these new behaviors.

First, Mrs. S observed in the day center for a short period and saw firsthand that her husband settled down quickly and was absorbed positively in a simple card game. Second, the occupational therapist helped Mrs. S communicate differently with Mr. S in the morning. Instead of telling her husband as soon as he woke up that he was going to the center, Mrs. S learned how to simplify his dressing and breakfast routines to ensure that he would be on time for his transportation to the center. Additionally, she learned how to introduce a simple activity to divert his attention (e.g., photos to look at, a favorite magazine) as they waited for the van to arrive. When his ride came, Mrs. S told her husband that he was going to play cards now and that she would see him soon. On some days, she gave him his favorite magazine to take with him, if that seemed appropriate.

Thus, by simplifying morning routines and keeping them consistent and predictable, and by simplifying communication by not informing Mr. S of his departure until it was time to go, she eased the transition to the center. Likewise, Mrs. S was prepared for Mr. S's return in the afternoon by ensuring a calm environment, having a small snack ready, and giving him his favorite magazine to look at on his return.

ESP IN ASSISTED-LIVING FACILITIES

Within the past decade, a new senior housing and care option for individuals in the early stages of dementia has emerged. Assisted-living facilities specializing in early-stage dementia care are congregate housing environments that offer individualized health and personal care assistance in a homelike setting. Assisted living is appropriate for people who do not need nursing home care but who may benefit from 24-hour supervision and minimal physical and cognitive assistance (as required), food preparation, and other supports.

Despite the specialized focus of some assisted-living facilities on dementia care, the physical environment may not always match the cognitive abilities of residents; staff often need training and assistance in managing complex dementia-related behaviors. Furthermore, because state standards and regulations vary, family members often need assistance in determining what services a facility provides and whether the appropriate level of care is available. Some assisted-living facilities expect the resident to be independent and ambulatory, other facilities provide assistance only with showering and homemaking tasks, and others require the resident to be totally physically independent in performing daily self-care activities. Many assisted-living programs are currently modifying their high functioning admission criteria and providing additional care to moderately impaired individuals.

There are three points of entry for occupational therapy into assisted-living facilities. First, care providers (e.g., nursing assistants) in assisted-living environments may require educational support and training to address troublesome behaviors associated with dementia. Occupational therapists can provide ESP to staff to give them tools and management strategies to enhance residents' functional performance and decrease the overall burden of care. Based on the needs of the care providers, the occupational therapist can develop customized training sessions using ESP. Direct intervention may include developing new routines for people with dementia based on their cognitive level; identifying needed modifications and simple environmental changes that will promote safety and functional performance; and recommending adaptive equipment such as bathroom safety aids (e.g., grab bars), bedrail assists, a talking clock, and so on to increase residents' independence level. A critical component of occupational therapy intervention in such facilities is the one-on-one formal provider training in the task simplification techniques, cueing strategies, and problem solving that are necessary to best support residents' ability to function.

A second way in which occupational therapists can import ESP principles into assisted-living settings is to offer workshops or training programs similar to those provided in the nursing home and adult day environments. Relevant activities include training in systematic problem-solving approaches to managing troublesome behaviors and instruction in simple environmental modifications for specific problems such as wandering or agitation. Such workshops should also address the care providers' own stress levels and offer training in stress reduction techniques and self-protection strategies against physical or aggressive behaviors (see Table 10.1 for a sample of the workshops being offered through a collaboration between the Department of Occupational Therapy and the Center for Applied Research on Aging and Health at the Jefferson College of Health Professions, Thomas Jefferson University, Philadelphia). Again, ESP offers occupational therapists a practical framework for teaching formal care providers effective strategies for minimizing disruptive behaviors in their settings.

TABLE 10.1. Outline of Educational Workshop Ideas for Family Members and Formal Care Providers

Workshop Title	Objectives
Workshop A (Introductory Level): A Closer Look at Alzheimer's Disease and Related Disorders	By the end of this session, participants will be able to • Define the terms *dementia* and *Alzheimer's disease* • Understand the potential causes and symptoms of Alzheimer's disease • Recognize the stages of dementia • Identify the current medical treatments used to help symptoms • Understand disruptive behaviors—Why do they occur? • Understand the impact of the physical and social environment on behavior and function.
Workshop B: Useful Communication Strategies to Minimize Behavior Difficulties and Enhance Participation	By the end of this session, participants will be able to • Describe components of communication—verbal, nonverbal, positive, and negative communication • Identify effective verbal communication strategies to address behavior problems or facilitate function • Explore other methods of communicating without using words to engage people with dementia.
Workshop C: Environmental Adaptations for People With Dementia: An Innovative Approach to Enhance Function, Safety, and Comfort in the Home	By the end of this session, participants will be able to • Discuss caregiving challenges in the home environment (potential hazards and unsafe behaviors) • Define *home environment* • Understand the environmental influences on dementia-related behaviors • Identify basic principles in changing the home environment • Ise the ABC process to managing troublesome behaviors • Describe environmental modifications for specific problem behaviors (e.g., wandering, agitation) and activities.
Workshop D: Taking Care of the Caregiver or Care Provider	By the end of this session, participants will be able to • Acknowledge the complex, multitask role of caregiving • Understand the symptoms of stress and the contributing factors • Identify strategies to manage and prevent unhealthy stress response • Demonstrate how to prevent aggressive behavior and protect onself from injury.
Workshop E: Engaging People With Dementia in Meaningful Activities	By the end of this session, participants will be able to • Understand preserved capabilities of people with dementia • Identify assessment approaches to evaluate capabilities • Understand ways to set up activities for people at different levels of cognitive functioning • Demonstrate how to establish an activity program.

Note. This list contains sample education programs offered by the Center for Applied Research on Aging and Health, Thomas Jefferson University, Philadelphia.

A third approach is to work with administrators and health professionals who seek a better understanding of how and when to request an occupational therapy evaluation for a resident with dementia or who seek the added value of the ESP model in improving the care they provide. Many health providers are not aware of the specialized services occupational therapists can provide to this population, which include evaluation of an individual's preserved capabilities and functional performance, establishment of a self-care routine program, and determination of the amount or type of assistance required to successfully and safely complete ADL. Table 10.2 offers a brief screening tool we currently use to advocate for a referral to occupational therapy services as part of the Farber Family Clinical Services offered at Thomas Jefferson University, Philadelphia.

REFERRAL TO OTHER HEALTH PROFESSIONALS

Occupational therapists working in community-based settings, as well as in the home, often identify other health care needs of people with dementia. In many cases, referral to a physical therapist, social worker, or physician is warranted.

Physical Therapy

An underused referral is to physical therapy. If the person with dementia is experiencing new or progressive mobility problems (e.g., increased incidence of falls, trunk or lower back pain, ambulation problems), a physical therapist evaluation may be highly advised. Table 10.3 provides five screening questions used in ESP to determine the need for physical therapy for a caregiver or care recipient (Cornman-Levy, Gitlin, Corcoran, & Schinfeld, 2001).

TABLE 10.2. Screening Indicators to Determine Need for Occupational Therapy Referral

Carefully review each statement and check off each statement that applies to the person with dementia or the caregiver. One or more check marks indicate the need for an occupational therapy referral.

The person has had a recent decline in daily function (e.g., self-care performance, mobility).	❏
The person has new safety issues limiting daily function (e.g., change in balance, increased confusion).	❏
The person has experienced one or more falls in the living environment.	❏
The person has resisted assistance with bathing, eating, toileting, transferring, or other self-care activity.	❏
The person has difficulty participating in a daily self-care routine.	❏
The person has difficulty navigating the living environment because of confusion and disorientation.	❏
The person wanders, rummages excessively, or becomes extremely upset or agitated easily, limiting his or her ability to participate in daily activities safely.	❏
The person exhibits self-destructive behaviors (e.g., not eating, pulling at skin, cutting self).	❏
The person is cared for by a family caregiver who is overwhelmed or upset or who reports difficulties in managing disruptive behaviors or functional dependence.	❏

Note. Developed by Vause-Earland & Gitlin, the Center for Applied Research on Aging and Health, Thomas Jefferson University. All rights reserved.

TABLE 10.3. Screening Indicators to Determine Need for Physical Therapy Referral

Carefully review each statement and check off accordingly. One or more check marks indicate the need for a physical therapy referral for the caregiver or the person with dementia.

The caregiver has experienced back or neck pain within the past 3 months while physically helping or transferring the person with dementia.	❏
The caregiver is concerned about hurting his or her back while physically helping or transferring the person with dementia.	❏
Either the caregiver or the person with dementia has musculoskeletal problems or balance problems that represent a risk while the caregiver is physically helping or transferring the person with dementia.	❏
Either the caregiver or the person with dementia has had a fall or near fall in the past 6 months.	❏
Musculoskeletal aches or pains in the caregiver or person with dementia	❏
Other:	❏

Note. Reprinted from Cornman-Levy, D., Gitlin, L. N., Corcoran, M., & Schinfeld, S. (2001). Caregiver aches and pains: The role of physical therapy in helping families provide daily care. *Alzheimer's Care Quarterly, 2,* 47–55. © 2001. Reprinted with permission from Lippincott Williams & Wilkins.

Health professionals also can use physical therapy consultation to minimize the physical burden of caregiving experienced by family caregivers and staff in assisted-living facilities. Through verbal instruction, demonstration and modeling, written material, and an individualized exercise program, the physical therapist can help care providers avoid musculoskeletal injuries and improve general strength and balance. This, in turn, promotes the safety and mobility of the person with dementia. Case Example 10.3 describes intervention by an occupational therapist and a physical therapist with Mrs. G, who was experiencing recent mobility-related difficulties.

Social Work

A social worker's knowledge of resources and available services in the community can be essential in assisting both family caregivers and formal care providers. If family members disagree over the course of treatment or type of care to be provided, a social worker can provide counsel and assist the family with resolving differences.

Physicians

Referral to a physician can be critical, particularly in the management of problem behaviors. New onset of a disruptive behavior or sudden increased confusion may indicate a need for a physician referral sooner than the scheduled routine checkup. Underlying medical conditions such as infection, dehydration, constipation, or drug interactions can cause sudden changes in mental status or behavior and require the attention of a nurse or physician. If a family member or formal care provider notices grimacing, an increase in moaning or crying, or

---

CASE EXAMPLE 10.3. Mrs. G

Mrs. G is a 78-year-old resident at an assisted-living facility. She is in the early stages of Alzheimer's disease. Within the past few weeks, Mrs. G has experienced three falls. The staff recently noticed her unsteadiness, especially when she walks down the hall to the dining area. In the morning, Mrs. G has difficulty rising up from the bed. She gets "stuck" in a sitting position and is unable to stand independently. Last week, when the care provider attempted to assist Mrs. G out of bed, she strained her back in the process. Mrs. G refuses to use her cane, stating, "I don't need that thing anymore!"

Decreased functional mobility, recent falls, resistance to care, and initiation difficulties prompted a physical therapy evaluation. The physical therapist evaluated Mrs. G's cognitive and physical capacity. She noted lower body weakness, balance and motor planning difficulties, and decreased ability to scan the environment. Physical therapy intervention included ambulation training (using a rolling walker with a brightly colored walker bag attached for visual cueing), an exercise program for lower extremity strengthening, and balance activities. Caregiver training was pivotal to achieving positive functional outcomes. The physical therapist focused on transfer and guarding techniques and on effective communication approaches to elicit safe mobility.

The occupational therapist instructed care providers to use specific verbal prompts to help Mrs. G out of bed. They learned to speak slowly and to allow Mrs. G additional processing time to complete an action. Mrs. G now uses a bedrail assist to reduce the physical effort needed to transfer out of bed.

A simple visual cue (brightly colored, personalized walker bag) attached to Mrs. G's walker reminded her to use it and to carry her personal items with her throughout the day. Mrs. G now exhibits safe, independent mobility as she performs her daily occupations within this setting.

---

mobility changes, any of which may indicate pain, he or she should contact the appropriate medical personnel. Furthermore, referral to a physician is in order if the person with dementia is depressed, suicidal, or extremely physically aggressive or has psychotic delusions. Finally, referral to a physician may be required to arrange hospice care.

ADDITIONAL CONSIDERATIONS WHEN WORKING WITH FORMAL CARE PROVIDERS

Occupational therapists have many important opportunities to consult, coach, and instruct formal care providers on environmental adaptations in all types of care facilities. The following underlying principles used in work with caregivers in the home are applicable to work with health care providers in community-based settings:

- Use of a collaborative approach;
- Cultural sensitivity;
- Assessment of the demands of the physical and social environment;
- Introduction of small, incremental changes to the environment;
- Reinforcement and validation of the care provider's actions; and
- Readjustment of or follow-up on recommended strategies based on the care provider's feedback.

Collaboration is the cornerstone and foundation for work with caregivers both in the home and in other health care settings. Regardless of setting or health profession, the occupational therapist must create a climate of trust and respect in which knowledge is shared to resolve difficult management problems (Gitlin, Corcoran, & Leinmiller-Eckhardt, 1995). It is important to involve the care provider actively in identifying the problems he or she considers most pressing. Communication pathways must be honest, clear, and free of jargon. The occupational therapist must recognize and respect the knowledge and skills that the care provider brings to the working relationship.

Assessing the cultural environment in the community-based setting helps the occupational therapist understand the care provider's roles and actions. Appreciating what is important and valued by staff will enhance collaborative efforts. Insight into the setting's philosophy of dementia care, expectations, and role demands is essential for an effective partnership with the caregiver. The occupational therapist must be realistic and flexible and be able to tailor the intervention to fit the dynamics of the culture.

An important dimension of the cultural environment is the work demands placed on staff. Integrating environmental strategies may be difficult in some settings because of resource and time constraints. New skills place demands for behavioral change that may prove overwhelming to busy formal care providers (Shaw, Kearney, Vause Earland, & Eckhardt, 2003). Understanding the work culture and then providing reasonable, achievable treatment goals and strategies that the care provider can easily implement may enhance their utility and eliminate some of the stress encountered by care providers. Once a strategy has proved successful, the care provider acquires trust, ownership, and a sense of mastery and may more easily accept other recommendations that are more difficult or challenging to implement.

Another principle to consider when coaching care providers on dementia management is validating effective caregiving. Care providers have in-depth knowledge about the daily behaviors of care recipients and what may or may not work in providing care. The occupational therapist can use this information in understanding the care recipient's capabilities and limitations. The nursing assistant, for example, has important insights into the preferred routines, goals, and values of the care recipient or his or her family. Acknowledging care providers' expertise and validating their ideas and strategies promote ongoing collaborative problem solving that benefits both the care provider and the person with dementia.

Finally, the occupational therapist should always follow up on or monitor the effectiveness of recommended strategies. Based on the care provider's feedback, strategies for dementia-related behaviors may require modification. A change in a care recipient's performance in areas of occupation or performance skills could result in the need for additional caregiving training.

The caregiving role, whether in the home or in a community-based setting, can be a difficult and stressful position to fulfill. The health and well-being of a person with dementia is contingent on the well-being of the care provider (Ortigara, 2000). Frontline care providers within institutional settings are often undervalued and may have limited input in the decision-making process. It is essential that the occupational therapist who is serving in the role of ESP consultant in various treatment settings nurture and support the well-being of care providers by arranging meaningful educational experiences; providing coaching and skill training; and promoting ongoing communication for feedback, reinforcement, and validation.

FUNDING CONSIDERATIONS

Although Chapter 12 tackles this issue more carefully, it is important to recognize funding issues for occupational therapy in institutional contexts. In accordance with the Centers for Medicare and Medicaid Services (CMS, 2004) regulation manual, skilled occupational therapy is a reimbursable service if prescribed by a physician who indicates a decline in function, safety issues limiting function, or risk for medical complications (falls, broken bones, dehydration) or medical noncompliance. Coverage for occupational therapy services cannot be denied to persons with dementia solely on the basis of diagnosis (CMS, 2001). In a facility that is eligible to obtain Medicare B coverage for residential care, such as nursing homes, occupational therapists can develop a contractual arrangement to provide resident-based functional maintenance training, and the nursing home can be reimbursed. However, this may not be the case in other facilities, such as adult day care centers and assisted-living facilities. In these environments, occupational therapists can provide consultation services to help develop programs based on ESP principles, provide care-centered consultation, and train staff members. A contract, signed by both the facility and the occupational therapist, should clearly define the purpose of the consultation, expectations, procedures, and fee structure (McCormack, Jaffe, & Goodman-Lavey, 2003). Using client-focused, educational, behavioral, or program development models, occupational therapists can successfully contribute to the delivery of ESP services in various settings in the role of consultant.

CONCLUSION

People with Alzheimer's disease and related disorders experience increased difficulties completing routine daily tasks and exhibit a variety of disruptive behaviors such as wandering, resistance to care, and verbal or physical aggression. These behaviors interfere with daily function and safety in community-based living environments and prove challenging to often stressed formal care providers.

Helping health and human services providers manage dementia-related behaviors and functional dependency can improve both quality of life for the person with dementia and, perhaps, work conditions for the care provider.

Regardless of type of setting, the occupational therapist brings an important and unique perspective to the dementia management team. The occupational therapist is skilled in methodically evaluating care recipients' preserved capabilities and occupational performance, assessing the environmental contingencies (social and physical) that affect function, and respecting the cultural environment that shapes the delivery of care in that particular facility. Occupational therapists are proficient at evaluating the best functional fit between the person with dementia and his or her environment. Through educational workshops for care providers, occupational therapists introduce approaches to developing individualized management strategies that prevent or reduce behavioral disturbances common in dementia and care settings. One-on-one training in problem solving, communication, cueing, and task simplification techniques can help support care recipients' ability to function in their living environment and empower care providers with skills to address stressful behaviors. ESP can thus serve as a practice model for providing care and training intervention to people with dementia in a variety of community-based settings.

REFERENCES

Burns, B. J., Wagner, H. R., Taube, J. E., Magaziner, J., Permitt, T., & Landerman L. R. (1993). Mental health service use by the elderly in nursing homes. *American Medical Journal of Public Health, 83,* 331–337.

Calkins, M. P. (1989). *Design for dementia.* Owings Mills, MD: National Health.

Centers for Medicare and Medicaid Services. (2001). *Medical review of services for patients with dementia* (Program Memorandum, CMS Publication 60AB). Retrieved June 21, 2004, from http://www.cms.hhs.gov/manuals/102_policy/bp102.c15.pdf.

Centers for Medicare and Medicaid Services. (2004). Retrieved June 21, 2004, from http://www.cms.hhs.gov/manuals/102-policy/bp102.c15.pdf

Conyers, K. (1996). Adult day care. In K. O. Larson, R. G. Sterns-Ratchford, L. Pedretti, & J. Crabtree (Eds.), *ROTE: The role of occupational therapy with the elderly. A self-paced clinical course* (pp. 451–482). Bethesda, MD: American Occupational Therapy Association.

Corcoran, M. (2001). *Occupational therapy practice guidelines for adults with Alzheimer's disease.* Bethesda, MD: American Occupational Therapy Association.

Cornman-Levy, D., Gitlin, L. N., Corcoran, M., & Schinfeld, S. (2001). Caregiver aches and pains: The role of physical therapy in helping families provide daily care. *Alzheimer's Care Quarterly, 2,* 47–55.

Gitlin, L. N. (2003). Conducting research on home environments: Lessons learned and new directions. *Gerontologist, 43,* 628–637.

Gitlin, L. N., Corcoran, M., & Leinmiller-Eckhardt, S. (1995). Understanding the family perspective: An ethnographic framework for providing occupational therapy in the home. *American Journal of Occupational Therapy, 49*(6), 802–809.

Gitlin, L. N., Corcoran, M., Winter, L., Boyce, A., & Hauck, W. (2001). A randomized controlled trial of a home intervention: Effect on efficacy and upset in caregivers and on daily function of persons with dementia. *Gerontologist, 41,* 4–14.

Gitlin, L. N., Liebman, J., & Winter, L. (2003). Are environmental interventions effective in the management of Alzheimer's disease and related disorders? A synthesis of the evidence. *Alzheimer Care Quarterly, 4,* 85–107.

McCormack, G., Jaffe, E., & Goodman-Lavey, M. (2003). *The occupational therapy manager* (4th ed.). Bethesda, MD: American Occupational Therapy Association.

Ortigara, A. (2000). The heart of education and training: Person-centered care. *Alzheimer's Care Quarterly, 1,* 73–74.

Osorio, L. P. (1993). Adult day care. In H. L. Hopkins & H. D. Smith (Eds.), *Willard and Spackman's occupational therapy* (pp. 812–815). Philadelphia: Lippincott.

Rogers, J. C., Holm, M. B., & Burgio, L. D., Granieri, E., Hsu, C., Hardin, J. M., & McDowell, B. J. (1999). Improving morning care routines of nursing home residents with dementia. *Journal of the American Geriatric Society, 47,* 1049–1057.

Rovner, B. W., Steele, C. D., Shmuely, Y., & Folstein, M. (1996). A randomized trial of dementia care in nursing homes. *Journal of the American Geriatric Society, 44,* 7–11.

Shaw, G., Kearney, P., Vause Earland, T., & Eckhardt, S. (2003). Managing dementia-related behaviors. *Home and Community Health Special Interest Section Quarterly, 10*(1), 1–3.

Spitzer, A. (1998). Nursing in the health care system of the postmodern world: Crossroads, paradoxes, and complexity. *Journal of Advanced Nursing, 28*(1), 164–171.

Wahl, H.-W., & Gitlin, L. N. (2003). Future developments in living environments for older people in the U.S. and Germany: Potential and constraints. In K. W. Schaie, H.-W. Wahl, H. Mollenkopf, & F. Oswald (Eds.), *Aging independently: Living arrangements and mobility* (pp. 281–301). New York: Springer.

Wells, D. L., Dawson, P., Sidani, S., Craig, D.,& Pringle, D. (2000). Effects of an ability-focused program of morning care on residents who have dementia and on caregivers. *Journal of the American Geriatric Society, 48,* 442–449.

Common Challenges and Effective Strategies in Working With Family Caregivers

Susan Toth-Cohen, PhD, OTR/L
Laura N. Gitlin, PhD

With this anxiety going on, it's very difficult [for caregivers] to be open to new ideas and try out and collaborate. They're the ones that need [the occupational therapist to say], "OK, you're going to do A, B, and C."

—Toth-Cohen, Text Unit 23, Interview 2, Participant 3

There are many challenges in providing services to families and people with dementia in their homes. These challenges result, in large part, from the complexities of the disease process, the intensity of the relationship between caregiver and care recipient, and the fact that the caregiver is providing care in a highly personalized context (e.g., the home) rather than in the standard, prescriptive setting of a clinic. Thus, delivering the Home Environmental Skill-Building Program (ESP) is a thoughtful process requiring ongoing reflection and self-evaluation. In this chapter, we discuss some of the most common challenges that occupational therapists confront in implementing ESP and the approaches we have found to be effective in handling those challenges (see Table 11.1).

CHALLENGES IN IMPLEMENTING THE HOME ENVIRONMENTAL SKILL-BUILDING PROGRAM

The challenges we discuss in this chapter are not unlike those that occupational therapists encounter in other practice arenas and with other clinical populations. For example, making a positive therapeutic connection with a client can be challenging in any practice context and with any individual. However, when working with families in the context of the home and dealing with the particularly complex issues of dementia, therapeutic practice takes on a different dimension and level of involvedness (Gitlin, Corcoran, & Leinmiller-Eckhardt, 1995). Additionally, there are challenges that are unique to this population and to the delivery of ESP, such as shifting the focus of treatment from the person with dementia to the family member while simultaneously integrating the care recipient into the treatment process when possible and appropriate.

Finally, there is the added complexity of the intervention or treatment process itself. ESP is a behaviorally demanding intervention requiring caregivers to accept the significance of a dementia diagnosis and to change their long-held and habitual approaches to communicating, caring, and reacting. Thus, some caregivers are ready and able to accept, use, and integrate ESP strategies at the first session, whereas others require additional time, effort, and practice with a limited set of strategies. The particular response of any one caregiver to the intervention may be shaped by multiple factors, including cultural values and beliefs, the availability of social and material resources, the age and health status of caregivers, the degree to which the caregiver understands the diagnosis and accepts the caregiving role, and the level of cognitive disability of the person with dementia. We discuss in this section four issues that present as the most pressing challenges to occupational therapists in delivering ESP: developing rapport, using open-ended and probing questions, adopting the caregiver's language, and providing validation.

TABLE 11.1. Summary of Common Challenges in Working With Caregivers and Recommended Strategies

Challenge	Recommended Strategies
Developing rapport	Use open-ended questions. Use the caregiver's language. Validate the caregiver's strategies.
Ensuring optimal fit between intervention and family	Examine one's own values and beliefs in relation to those of the caregiver. Understand the caregiver's priorities. Re-evaluate the intervention approach.
Meeting the needs of both caregiver and person with dementia	Educate the caregiver about dementia. Provide environmental adaptations. Identify activities that are meaningful for the person with dementia.
Enabling caregivers to obtain resources	Educate oneself about local, state, and national resources to present to the caregiver. Discuss or write a list of caregiving tasks with the caregiver, and determine which tasks the caregiver might consider assigning to others. Role-play help-seeking strategies with the caregiver.
Assisting the overwhelmed caregiver	Educate the caregiver about dementia. Validate the caregiver's existing strategies. Involve and collaborate with family members and other supportive people.
Assisting the depressed caregiver	Identify resources that may help the caregiver. Encourage the caregiver to discuss possible treatment for depression with his or her family physician. Educate the caregiver about appropriate resources. Help the caregiver identify tasks he or she can allow others to perform. Role-play with the caregiver ways of asking for help. Work on one problem area and strategy at a time so as not to overwhelm the caregiver. Provide validation by pointing out things the caregiver does well. Introduce an easy strategy for which the caregiver can see immediate positive results.
Assisting the master caregiver	Explore quality-of-life issues; consider strategies to engage the care recipient in occupations linked to previous interests and roles. Validate the caregiver's existing strategies.

Developing Rapport

A classic challenge in working with caregivers in their homes is developing rapport (Toth-Cohen et al., 2001). As discussed in previous chapters, building rapport is critical to the delivery of ESP and an essential ingredient of a collaborative therapeutic relationship. Rapport building typically occurs gradually and builds over each treatment session. That is, rapport building is not a one-time event or single behavioral action on the part of the occupational therapist but is rather an approach that infuses all therapeutic interactions. It requires the therapist to purposely and strategically relate to the caregiver in a way that demonstrates and promotes respect, trust, and sensitivity to the cultural dimensions of the household. A primary objective of rapport building is to enable caregivers and occupational therapists to work productively together to identify the "real" issues that concern the caregiver and the best approaches for managing them. Establishing rapport is central, in that without a climate of trust and comfort, caregivers may not disclose their most intimate concerns. To effectively build rapport, the therapist conceptualizes the caregiver as a lay practitioner with expert knowledge about the caregiving situation (Hasselkus, 1988), as discussed in Chapter 4.

Using Open-Ended and Probing Questions

Using questions and prompts such as "Tell me about a typical day" and "What is it like for you since you began taking care of your mother?" encourages caregivers to talk about current concerns and to describe what daily life is like for them. Another benefit of open-ended questioning is that caregivers' responses often reveal the underlying values and beliefs that guide their decision making with regard to the care they are giving and that serve as a window into which strategies might work and which might not. This dialogue provides the occupational therapist with a more in-depth and nuanced understanding of the care situation and what matters most in the household.

Adopting the Caregiver's Language

Using the caregiver's own language and word choice to describe care activities and disease processes is important for several reasons. First, it provides implicit feedback to caregivers that what they are describing or explaining makes sense and that the occupational therapist has appropriately heard and understood what he or she is saying. Using the same words or phrases as the caregiver demonstrates empathy and ensures that the therapist is "on the same page" as the caregiver. Second, it validates that the way the caregiver conceptualizes the issue is acceptable and helps to "demedicalize" the situation, keeping the discussion within the scope of the family's everyday life.

Providing Validation

Corroborating a caregiver's actions is very important. Statements such as "That's a great way to handle the problem" or "That's exactly what I would have recommended" demonstrate respect and support for the caregiver's efforts. Furthermore, validation is a great teaching moment. It is an opportunity to explain why the strategies or actions of the caregiver are effective so that the caregiver can apply them to other situations.

OTHER CHALLENGES

Ensuring Optimal Fit

Another challenge in delivering ESP is optimizing the acceptability of strategies. Acceptable strategies are customized to fit the particular needs, beliefs, and values of the caregiver and care recipient. Because ESP strategies are intimate—that is, they often involve changes to self-care and personal practices—the occupational therapist must develop and introduce recommendations carefully to maximize acceptance and integration into the household structure.

Ensuring an optimal fit among strategy, caregiver need, and household structure can be difficult, particularly when the value system of the therapist differs from or conflicts considerably with the family's value system. The culture of the occupational therapy profession places high value on doing, occupying, and being independent. For example, the occupational therapist may seek opportunities to recommend strategies that optimize the participation of the person with dementia in his or her own self-care; in contrast, the caregiver may prefer the family member to be a passive recipient of care. Although the therapist may view the situation in terms of the caregiver promoting excess disability, the caregiver may prefer this approach for a variety of important reasons that the therapist needs to understand and respect. For example, the caregiver's approach may be easier and save time to accomplish other necessary tasks, or the care recipient may have always depended on the caregiver to carry out that particular task, so that continued dependency is consistent with their lives before the onset of dementia.

When the values and beliefs of the occupational therapist clash with those of the caregiver, it may interfere with the development of effective strategies. It is important for therapists to reflect on and examine their own values and beliefs and their influence on strategy development. Reflective, helpful questions include the following:

- What are the main issues here?
- How does the caregiver think about this?
- Why do I think differently?
- Are my personal values different from or interfering with my ability to understand the caregiver's perspective or to be objective about these issues?

Thus, an important strategy for ensuring optimal fit between the intervention and the family is for the occupational therapist to be vigilant about the ways in which his or her personal values and beliefs interface with those of the caregiver and family.

Identifying Caregiver Concerns

Basic to ESP is the initial identification of the caregiver's concerns and subsequent prioritization of those concerns in a treatment plan. However, identifying caregiver concerns and prioritizing them is not necessarily easy or clear cut. An important strategy is the use of open-ended questions that elicit the caregiver's story and help to identify the caregiver's explicit and implicit concerns. Follow-up probes to explore facets of the story and to clarify what is most important to the caregiver and why are part of the process of need identification. For example, a probe such as "Tell me more about why it is important for your husband to bathe every day" may reveal that the caregiver wishes to reclaim part of her life with her spouse as it was before the dementia, in which this self-care practice was part of his daily routines and habits—what he used to do and be like. In addition to open-ended questions and probes, use of the Caregiver Assessment of Management Problems can help identify the priorities of the caregiver and guide the approach to intervention (see Tool A.1 in Appendix A).

Integrating the Perspectives of Caregiver and Care Recipient

Most occupational therapists are accustomed to working with a patient with a particular diagnosis. However, rarely are occupational therapists referred for a person specifically because of a dementia diagnosis. Although occupational therapists treat people with dementia, the referral is usually for an acute problem that is potentially compounded by cognitive impairment. Work with a family member in the home to address issues related to dementia is thus quite different from typical practice. Although the main focus of ESP is skill training for the caregiver, the purpose of such training is to enhance the quality of life of both the caregiver and the person with dementia. This dual focus can be challenging. Even if treatment sessions include only the caregiver, the therapist must gain an understanding of the abilities, needs, and previous habits, likes, and dislikes of the person with dementia in developing appropriate strategies.

In the mild to early moderate stages of the disease it may be possible and appropriate for the occupational therapist to include the person with dementia in discussions about daily life and ways to make task performance easier. This inclusion supports the dignity of the person with dementia by establishing him or her as someone who can contribute to the family (Hellen, 2000). Having the person with dementia participate in a treatment contact also may serve as an important opportunity to model for the caregiver effective communication strategies and approaches and to enable the caregiver to maintain a positive connection and sense of partnership; loss of a close relationship is an important source of caregiver stress (Pearlin, Mullan, Semple, & Skaff, 1990). The person with dementia also benefits from participating in decisions about his or her care, because it provides an opportunity to exercise some control over daily life (Alzheimer's Association, 2002).

In the later stages of the disease, the occupational therapist may be able to engage the person with dementia by acknowledging his or her presence, briefly explaining the purpose of the visit, and engaging him or her in a brief conversation. When the therapist lets the care recipient know who he or she is and why he or she is in the home (e.g., "Hello, Mrs. S, how are you today? I am here to help your daughter"), the anxiety that the care recipient may feel over a stranger in the home can be eased.

Another important way to involve a care recipient is to introduce an activity that is meaningful and engaging. This activity may enable a caregiver to see what his or her loved one can actually do and his or her preserved capabilities. In turn, the care recipient may find enjoyment in performing simple activities, which have been shown to decrease agitation and enhance well-being in people with dementia (Chung, 2004).

Enabling Caregivers to Obtain Resources

Many caregivers, especially those who are overwhelmed or depressed, lack basic knowledge about the role and scope of services such as respite and adult day care and about how to obtain such services (Toth-Cohen et al., 2001). Thus, it is important in the course of ESP to help caregivers understand these service opportunities and their availability in the community. In some cases, it is helpful to model for the caregiver by making an initial contact with a service provider or role-playing with a caregiver the kinds of questions to ask. For example, some caregivers may need skill development in effective interaction with formal services and providers, including what questions to ask, how to ascertain the quality of a particular service, and how to arrange for service provision.

A related challenge is helping caregivers feel comfortable with accepting help from others. Caregivers may be reluctant to accept help, even from close family members, for several reasons. The caregiver may believe that he or she is the only one who knows best or can meet the needs of the person with dementia or that he or she is a good caregiver only if he or she is on duty 24 hours a day, 7 days a week. The caregiver may believe that having another helper—whether a formal care provider or another family member—may contribute to agitation or distress in the person with dementia.

To approach the issue of a caregiver's reluctance to receive help, it may be helpful for the occupational therapist to discuss or write down a list of caregiving tasks and to review each one with the caregiver to determine if he or she might consider asking for help with any of them. Even if the therapist identifies only one task, such as a family member picking up groceries during his or her regular shopping trip, the caregiver may benefit from having one less demand on his or her time and energy.

Caregivers may need help in identifying the type of assistance they may benefit from and how best to coordinate others who become involved in caregiving tasks. Additionally, the occupational therapist should problem solve with the caregiver about how to introduce a new person in the home to assist in daily care so that the care recipient experiences minimum upset.

Another potential obstacle to obtaining help is that caregivers may have difficulty asking for it. For example, caregivers may express annoyance that other family members do not participate in daily care chores, but they may be too embarrassed or fearful to ask for the help they want. Additionally, caregivers may think that they have asked for help, but they may not have asked for help in a way that others understand. Role-play of different situations and opportunities to practice are powerful ways of modeling and help caregivers gain important skills and experience in managing daily care needs and clearly delineate the types of activities and tasks for which they can seek help. Assertiveness techniques and communication skills are other critical tools.

CAREGIVER RESPONSES

Caregivers vary considerably in their emotional response to and level of expertise in the caregiving role. Three types of caregiver are encountered frequently in ESP intervention—the overwhelmed caregiver, the depressed caregiver, and the master caregiver.

The Overwhelmed Caregiver

Caregivers may feel overwhelmed at different points in the trajectory of caregiving. In delivering ESP, it is important for the occupational therapist to be aware of the caregiver's unique needs and to adjust his or her approach accordingly. Feeling overwhelmed is a customary response when the diagnosis of dementia is initially obtained and the role of caregiver is initiated. In the early stages of the disease, families may have difficulty understanding or accepting the diagnosis and its implications for home safety and continued employment. For caregivers of people in the early stages of dementia, the occupational therapist must be careful to address potential safety risks while presenting suggestions in a way that supports the caregiver's confidence and fits his or her values and beliefs.

For example, a caregiver may believe that it is very important for his father with dementia to continue to walk freely in the community. The occupational therapist, however, may find cause for concern that the care recipient will wander and become lost. In this case, the therapist might discuss the safety concerns with the caregiver while simultaneously acknowledging the caregiver's desire not to restrict his father's activities. The therapist might also explore the strategies of setting up a network of neighbors to watch out for his father and obtaining a personal identification bracelet for his father to wear. Education about Alzheimer's disease and related disorders might also be beneficial; the therapist can explain that wandering behaviors typically become more problematic as the disease progresses.

Caregivers often need time to understand the meaning of the diagnosis and the immediate and long-term effects of dementia on their family, so it may initially be difficult for them to realize how best to use the expertise of the occupational therapist and the potential benefits of the ESP intervention. The occupational therapist should be prepared to present information about dementia in different ways and to repeat this information frequently to allow caregivers to fully process and understand the magnitude of the disease process.

Additionally, occupational therapists must consider how caregiver factors such as gender, level of education, and previous roles influence a caregiver's ability to address a problem behavior (see Chapter 4). For example, older wives may find it difficult to be assertive in assuming responsibility for finances, such as balancing the checkbook or managing investments. Conversely, men may find it difficult to discuss their wives' incontinence issues or to assume responsibility for tasks that their wives had previously performed, such as preparing meals or doing housework and laundry.

At the moderate and late stages of dementia, care recipients' increasing cognitive decline, behavioral problems, and functional impairments (e.g., incontinence) may cause caregivers to experience feelings of burden and a sense of captivity in the caregiving role (Aneshensel, Pearlin, Mullan, Zarit, & Whitlatch, 1995). During these stages, caregivers may consider nursing home placement, a decision that usually produces major stress and feelings of guilt or inadequacy.

The Depressed Caregiver

As many as half of caregivers of people with dementia show signs of clinical depression (Alzheimer's Association, 2003). Depression is especially prevalent at the moderate stage of the disease process (Schulz, Visintainer, & Williamson, 1990). Caregivers with clinical depression may have difficulty fully participating in ESP, which requires behavioral activation. Clinically depressed caregivers may become easily overwhelmed by the intervention and have difficulty following through with recommendations (Gitlin, Corcoran, Winter, Boyce, & Marcus, 1999).

It is normal for caregivers to feel a sense of profound loss and sadness in response to the changes they witness on a daily basis in their loved one with dementia. However, feelings of loss and grief are different from clinical depression. Signs of clinical depression include suicidal ideation, feelings of worthlessness, self-reproach, excessive guilt, difficulty in thinking or concentrating, and loss of interest or pleasure in usual activities (Alzheimer's Association, 2003). Experiencing these and other symptoms, such as weight change, disturbed sleep, or agitation, over a period of at least 2 weeks may indicate that the caregiver is clinically depressed and could benefit from psychotropic treatment.

Sometimes caregivers do not recognize that they are clinically depressed. They may believe that their symptoms are a natural part of the caregiving process.

It is important for occupational therapists to recognize the signs of depression and to refer caregivers for treatment. An introduction to the topic such as the following can be very helpful: "Mr. Jones, you appear very distressed, and while deep sadness is, of course, normal in light of your wife's condition, you are experiencing more pain than others in your situation. You may benefit from talking to your doctor about your feelings, and there may be some medication or other treatments that can be helpful to you."

Caregivers who are depressed tend to welcome the occupational therapist into the home, but contacts may feel as if they are not going anywhere or are circular, or as if there is no movement forward. Caregivers who deny the severity of a situation, who minimize difficulties ("It is not that bad"), or who seem to agree to everything but refuse to try a strategy may in fact be depressed. In these cases, it is best to simplify the intervention approach and work on one very small area of concern or problem. Introducing a strategy that can enable the caregiver to experience immediate success is another effective approach. Providing one strategy and working with the caregiver to incorporate it into daily routines may gradually move the treatment process along successfully.

The Master Caregiver

The caregiver who appears completely masterful also presents challenges. The occupational therapist may question whether assistance is necessary and, if so, how best to help a highly skilled caregiver. It is important to remember that, although master caregivers have an impressive repertoire of skills, there are still many possibilities for improving quality of life both for them and for their loved ones with dementia.

For example, even caregivers who provide high-quality care and address the physical needs of the person with dementia may not recognize or understand how best to involve the person in a meaningful activity or occupation. Engaging in occupations that are appropriate for their current stage of dementia can contribute care recipients' quality of life and provide a pleasant event (or perhaps some free time) for their caregivers.

If an occupational therapist is unable to identify a specific strategy that is helpful or appropriate, master caregivers may still benefit from having the therapist name and frame their management techniques, why they are effective, and how they work. This validates the caregivers' approaches and confirms that their efforts are worthwhile and effective. Additionally, the therapist can ask master caregivers to describe the strategies they have found to be most effective to help build the therapist's repertoire of strategies and enable the master caregiver to contribute to the larger society in a meaningful and productive way.

CONCLUSION

This chapter discusses some of the most common challenges that occupational therapists confront when working in the home with a family caregiver. These challenges include the need to develop rapport; ensure optimal fit between intervention strategies and family values, structure, and needs; involve people with dementia; and enable caregivers to obtain resources. Caregivers who are overwhelmed or clinically depressed or who display extreme proficiency in caregiving present specific and additional challenges. The occupational therapist's ability to meet these challenges effectively will improve the caregiver's response to treatment. Becoming aware of these challenges and knowledgeable about the specific measures that can be used to overcome them enables occupational therapists to provide effective, customized intervention in ESP.

REFERENCES

Alzheimer's Association. (2002). *Fact sheet: Feelings.* Retrieved October 15, 2004, from http://www.alz.org/Resources/FactSheets/FSfeelings.pdf.

Alzheimer's Association (2003). *Depression.* Retrieved June 20, 2003 from http://www.alz.org/hc/counseling/depression.htm.

Aneshensel, C. S., Pearlin, L. I., Mullan, J. T., Zarit, S. H., & Whitlatch, C. J. (1995). *Profiles in caregiving: The unexpected career.* San Diego, CA: Academic Press.

Chung, J. C. C. (2004). Activity participation and well-being of people with dementia in long-term-care settings. *Occupational Therapy Journal of Research: Occupation, Participation and Health, 24,* 22–31.

Gitlin, L. N., Corcoran, M. C., & Leinmiller-Eckhardt, S. (1995). Understanding the family perspective: An ethnographic framework for providing occupational therapy in the home. *American Journal of Occupational Therapy, 49,* 802–809.

Gitlin, L. N., Corcoran, M., Winter, L., Boyce, A., & Marcus, S. (1999). Predicting participation and adherence to a home environmental intervention among family caregivers of persons with dementia. *Family Relations, 48,* 363–372.

Hasselkus, B. R. (1988). Meaning in family caregiving: Perspectives on caregiver/professional relationships. *Gerontologist, 28,* 686–691.

Hellen, C. R. (2000). Being, doing, belonging: Upholding the sense of self with meaningful activities. *Alzheimer's Care Quarterly, 1,* 35–49.

Pearlin, L. I., Mullan, J. T., Semple, S. S., & Skaff, M. M. (1990). Caregiving and the stress process: An overview of concepts and their measures. *Gerontologist, 30,* 583–591.

Schulz, R., Visintainer, P., & Williamson, G. M. (1990). Psychiatric and physical morbidity effects of caregiving. *Journal of Gerontology, 45,* 181–191.

Toth-Cohen, S., Gitlin, L. N., Corcoran, M. A., Eckhardt, S., Johns, P., & Lipsitt, R. (2001). Providing services to family caregivers at home: Challenges and recommendations for health and human services professions. *Alzheimer's Care Quarterly, 2,* 23–32.

Documentation and Reimbursement for the Home Environmental Skill-Building Intervention

Laura N. Gitlin, PhD
Geri Shaw, OTR/L
Tracey Vause Earland, MS, OTR/L

12

The development and evaluation of the Home Environmental Skill-Building Program (ESP) were supported by federal grant monies, which offset costs associated with the purchase and installation of assistive devices, training in the protocols, supervisory and quality monitoring, and intervention contacts and telephone calls. Nevertheless, ESP can be integrated into existing practice arenas (see Chapter 10) and reimbursed by third-party payers under various mechanisms, including Medicare. In this chapter, we consider different approaches for integrating ESP into current clinical structures, strategies for obtaining reimbursement, and appropriate treatment documentation to support the role of occupational therapy in dementia care.

OVERVIEW OF MEDICARE GUIDELINES

The Centers for Medicare and Medicaid Services (CMS) publishes Medicare manuals describing the provision of services and billing procedures for each treatment setting. Exhibit 12.1 provides the relevant excerpts from these manuals that justify the role of occupational therapy in the care of dementia patients.

Under Medicare guidelines, skilled services include but are not limited to the following:
- Evaluation of the patient
- Determination of measurable goals with the patient and patient's caregiver and other professionals
- Analysis and modification of functional tasks
- Instruction in the tasks for the patient and the caregiver.

Occupational therapists may document any period of practice required by the patient and the patient's caregiver to learn the steps of the task, as well as time required to verify the task's effectiveness in improving function and to check for safety.

A *New York Times* article published in 2002 highlighted a new policy by which Medicare can no longer deny reimbursement for the costs of mental health services, home health care, and hospice care just because an individual has Alzheimer's disease. This article cited a memorandum by CMS dated September 25, 2001, instructing contractors not to install edits that result in the automatic denial of services based solely on the *International Classification of Diseases* (9th edition; ICD-9) codes for dementia:

> A claim submitted with *only* a diagnosis of Alzheimer's Disease (ICD-9 code 331.0) may entitle a beneficiary to (occupational therapy) evaluation and management visits if the contractor (occupational therapist) determines that these therapies are reasonable and necessary when reviewed in the context of a beneficiary's overall medical condition. (Pear, 2002)

The development of this chapter was supported in part by funds from the Farber Family Foundation.

EXHIBIT 12.1. Excerpts From CMS on Reimbursement for Dementia Services

Services must be prescribed by a physician and furnished under a physician-approved plan of care developed by a physician or an occupational therapist. Services must be reasonable and necessary for the treatment of the individual's illness or injury. Occupational therapy is considered reasonable and necessary when it is expected that the therapy will result in significant improvement in the patient's level of function within a reasonable amount of time. (*Medicare Benefit Policy Manual* [CMS Pub.100-2, Chapter 7, 40.2])

Services of skilled therapists for the purpose of teaching the patient, family, or caregivers, necessary techniques, exercises, or precautions are covered to the extent that they are reasonable and necessary to treat illness or injury. For the cognitively impaired patient, refusal to perform an activity can escalate into aggressive, destructive, or verbally abusive behavior if pressed by the therapist or caregiver to perform. In these cases, a reduction in these behaviors will be considered significant; however, these behaviors must be documented, including the skilled OT provided to reduce the abnormal behavior. (U.S. Department of Health and Human Services, *Medicare: Health Insurance for the Aged, Home Health Agency Manual,* Chapter 4, Section 452, p. 49.7)

Medicare contractors recommend that occupational therapy service providers enter the primary diagnosis or condition as well as a secondary condition that reflects the "medical necessity" of the billed service. For example, if a patient shows resistance toward eating or displays motor-planning difficulties during self-feeding, the provider would enter ICD-9 code 783.3 (feeding difficulties and mismanagement) as the secondary diagnosis to support the medical necessity of the occupational therapy service.

DOCUMENTATION AND MEDICARE GUIDELINES FOR OCCUPATIONAL THERAPY

The basic premise of documentation for reimbursement is that it must reflect the language and parameters of the Medicare guidelines. As with all documentation, reports must include patient identification, medical and social history, assessments, treatment plan, and discharge planning. The treatment plan should specify measurable goals, the interventions necessary to achieve the goals, and the frequency and duration of occupational therapy treatment. The occupational therapist's assessment should establish the reason for the referral (e.g., decline in functional activities, decrease in safety, escalating behavior disturbances).

Documentation should indicate what level of assistance is needed for sequencing, safety, and continuation of the task targeted for intervention:

- *Standby assistance* is the need for supervision by one person for the individual to perform new procedures or activities that the occupational therapist adapted to increase safety and effective performance.
- *Minimum assistance* is necessary to correct repeated mistakes, to check for established safety procedures, or to solve problems posed by unexpected hazards.

- *Moderate assistance* indicates that the occupational therapist or caregiver needs to be in the immediate environment for the patient to complete a functional activity.
- *Maximum assistance* involves the need for visual demonstrations or one-on-one tactile stimulation, such as hand-over-hand guiding, to elicit the activity.

Occupational therapists should document any modifications made to facilitate the specific activity, such as changes to the environment, use of equipment, and caregiver training. Caregiver training must take place with the patient present and before the patient is discharged from therapy. Table 12.1 provides examples of treatment goal statements (Corcoran, 2000).

REIMBURSABLE SERVICE MODELS

Older adults form the fastest growing segment of the North American population. Nevertheless, legislation in support of health care, including the delivery of occupational therapy services, to older adults is still inadequate and lags behind the statistics. Within the Medicare system, the extent to which occupational therapy services are allowable and the level of reimbursement vary by setting. The occupational therapist must thus consider four critical reimbursement-related factors: (1) cost and payer source, (2) expected occupational performance outcome, (3) any service limitations that may apply, and (4) documentation requirements (e.g., demonstration that functional progress and improved safety resulted from skilled intervention).

There are several service provider structures for Medicare reimbursement. Medicare coverage guidelines, as determined by fiscal intermediaries and their respective local coverage determination (LCD; formerly referred to as a *local*

TABLE 12.1. Examples of Treatment Goals

Daily Living Activity	Sample Goal
Grooming	Individual will wash face and brush teeth following setup and minimal verbal cues from caregiver.
Dressing	Individual will dress self after caregiver sets up clothes in proper order for dressing.
Eating	Individual will demonstrate increased attention to meals following environmental changes made by caregiver, such as decluttering the table.
Meal preparation	Individual will get lunch from refrigerator using visual reminders.
Household task	Individual will fold laundry following setup by caregiver. Individual will sweep kitchen floor with minimal verbal cueing by caregiver.
Leisure activity	Individual will sew quilt pieces together following setup by caregiver. Individual will practice golf putting once a week with relative.

medical review policy), apply to all service provider settings. Each service setting or payer system determines the criteria for payment, but it is critical for providers of a "designated health service" (e.g., occupational therapy) to understand how the Medicare intermediary interprets Medicare guidelines and to determine how the facility's fiscal intermediary believes occupational therapy services should be coded and billed. The occupational therapist also must have a clear understanding of the documentation requirements for each billing entity in the various practice settings in order to prevent claim denials.

Table 12.2 provides a brief description of the pros and cons of the various provider models for Medicare reimbursement. Occupational therapists can provide Medicare-covered services for people with Alzheimer's disease or related dementia disorders in settings such as hospitals, skilled-nursing facilities, rehabilitation hospitals, home health agencies, outpatient therapy clinics, a physician's office, and an occupational therapy private practice. Home health agencies primarily serve Medicare A clients under a different billing system. Given that ESP was designed for implementation primarily within the home environment, the service provider models outlined in Table 12.2 focus on systems that deliver home-based intervention primarily covered by Medicare Part B. Table 12.3 lists referral sources and their payment mechanisms.

Private Practice

A growing number of occupational therapists have chosen the entrepreneurial path and established a private practice. These occupational therapists can either bill Medicare directly for services rendered or contract with a Medicare-certified facility that submits claims to Medicare. There are more than 1,500 occupational therapists enrolled with Medicare as private practitioners (McCormack, Jaffe, & Goodman-Lavey, 2003; CMS, 2004a). To bill Medicare directly, the occupational therapist must apply for a Medicare provider number by completing the provider application form through his or her local intermediary or on CMS's Web site. The applicant's Medicare carrier issues a provider identification number to the occupational therapist for Medicare Part B reimbursement that identifies on the Medicare claim form who provides the service.

There are several advantages to private practice. Occupational therapists in private practice can perform services anywhere (e.g., private home, office, adult day care center, assisted-living facility), have flexibility in scheduling, and are self-directed. However, starting a private practice involves financial and professional risks. Start-up capital is required for expenditures associated with the new practice prior to generating revenue. In addition, the occupational therapist is responsible for adhering to all state rules and regulations, tax structures, and licensure compliance guidelines. If the occupational therapist in private practice hires additional employees, the therapist can use his or her provider number only

TABLE 12.2. Pros and Cons of Service Provider Models for Medicare or Medicaid Reimbursement

Model	Pros	Cons
Occupational therapy private practice	Occupational therapist can provide services anywhere under Part B. A physician's prescription is required, but not direct supervision. Scheduling is flexible. Work is self-directed. Therapist determines business standards and makes decisions.	Occupational therapist assumes all financial and professional risks. Therapist bears full responsibility for compliance with state rules, regulations, and taxes.
Physician's office	An immediate referral source is available. Services can be given in a timely fashion. Physician's office bills Medicare for services.	Services must be performed in the "same building" as physician. Physician must supervise home intervention.
Outpatient therapy providers	Provider site is responsible for compliance with certification and regulations. Provider site bills Medicare. Services can be performed in clinic or client's home. Referrals can be received from different physicians.	Travel expense to and from home is not reimbursable. Service delivery in clinic is more cost effective than home intervention.
Home health agency (Medicare A)	Provides a "home setting" treatment environment. Agency is responsible for regulation compliance. Agency bills Medicare. Agency is a good referral source. Prospective payment system fosters interdisciplinary teamwork.	Occupational therapy intervention requires physical therapy, nursing, or speech therapy to "open case" and refer. Under Medicare A prospective payment system, clients must qualify as "homebound."

for occupational therapy services and is responsible for employee benefits and withholding taxes (unless the employees are independent contractors who provide their own insurance and tax management).

Physician's Office

Another service provider type is the physician's office; the physician employs the occupational therapist to provide services in his or her office or in a physician-directed clinic. Occupational therapy services are covered under Medicare Part B as incidental to a physician's services (McCormack, Jaffe, & Goodman-Lavey, 2003). The physician's group provider number is documented on the Medicare claim form. Occupational therapy must be "under arrangement for services" and must abide by the "fair market" standards.

There are a few advantages to this provider type. The physician's office provides the occupational therapist with an immediate referral source, and the therapist can implement services with little delay. The physician's office is responsible

TABLE 12.3. Referral Sources and Payment Mechanisms for Occupational Therapy Services

Referral Source	Payment Mechanism
Inpatient (e.g., geropsychiatry rehabilitation hospital)	Medicare Part A: Occupational therapy services must wait until the care recipient returns home, unless home care is coordinated with the hospital.
Outpatient (physician's office)	Medicare Part B: A prescription is needed from the physician for occupational therapy services. There is a 30-day treatment period from the date of prescription; then a new prescription is needed. Treatment may be provided in the home or an outpatient setting. Documentation must focus on goals for the care recipient and on maintenance for the caregiver through training. Treatment must focus on function, safety, and medication. There is no restriction on the number of service days (length of service must be "reasonable and necessary"). A 60-day service window is allowed if the patient is already receiving home care.
Private pay	Occupational therapists should set payment schedules in line with Medicare reimbursement rates.
Assisted-living facility, nursing home, or home care	For assisted-living facility residents, Medicare can be billed for occupational therapy services. For nursing home residents not in a Medicaid room, the occupational therapist is a consultant, and the nursing home can bill Medicare for his or her services.

for administering occupational therapy billing. With regard to implementing ESP, the occupational therapist is limited to providing services in the office (or "same building") of the physician. Thus, occupational therapy can occur in the home only if the physician is present as well. According to Medicare regulations, the physician must physically supervise an in-home session (CMS, 2004b).

Outpatient Therapy Providers or Ambulatory Clinics

Outpatient therapy providers or ambulatory clinics constitute yet another option for providing ESP intervention under Medicare B. The Medicare-certified provider provides occupational therapy services to a beneficiary in the home or outpatient facility. The institutional provider can accept referrals from different physicians. The provider bills Medicare directly, and payment for all outpatient therapy services is made under the Medicare physician fee schedule (McCormack et al., 2003). Few institutional providers offer home-based intervention, primarily because of the cost of providing such intervention (e.g., travel expenses are not reimbursable). Operationally, service efficiency may be compromised when treatment is provided in the individual's home rather than in the clinic.

Home Health Agency System

Home health agencies (HHAs) provide Medicare A services under the prospective payment system (PPS), "a method of paying for predefined group of health services for a specific illness or injury over a specific duration of time" (e.g., per episode, per day; McCormack et al., 2003, p. 386). Intermittent skilled-nursing care, physical therapy, or speech pathology "opens" the case for the client and allows occupational therapy services to be provided in the home. Clients receiving Medicare A home health services must qualify as "homebound."

With the PPS, Medicare pays a single rate for each 60 days of service, determined by the information entered in the Medicare form, Outcome & Assessment Information Set. The HHA oversees all reimbursement and payment issues. This provider type offers a good referral source and provides the optimal environment (the home) to conduct occupational therapy services and ESP. Another benefit of HHA and the PPS is that they foster interdisciplinary teamwork for the good of the client (Boerkoel, 2004).

CONCLUSION

Occupational therapists must be aware of the specific coverage and payment policies affecting the settings in which they work. There are pros and cons within each Medicare provider type. Occupational therapy intervention incorporating ESP can be reimbursed through these models of service delivery if the clinician is mindful of billing policies and documentation regulations.

REFERENCES

Boerkoel, D. (2004). Thriving within PPS. *OT Practice, 9*(20), 9–12.

Centers for Medicare and Medicaid Services. (2004a). Accessed June 24, 2004, from http://www.cms.hhs.gov/manuals/102_policy/bp102.c15.pdf.

Centers for Medicare and Medicaid Services. (2004b). Accessed June 24, 2004, from http://cms.hhs.gov/providers/enrollment/providers/agency.asp.

Corcoran, M. (2000). *Occupational therapy practice guidelines for adults with Alzheimer's disease* (Practice Guidelines Series). Bethesda, MD: American Occupational Therapy Association.

McCormack, G., Jaffe, E., & Goodman-Lavey, M. (2003). *The occupational therapy manager* (4th ed.). Bethesda, MD: American Occupational Therapy Association.

Medicare Benefit Policy Manual. CMS Pub.100-2.

National Center for Health Statistics. (2000). *International Classification of Diseases, Ninth Revision, Clinical Modification (ICD-9-CM).* Salt Lake City: Medicode.

Pear, Roberto. (2002, March 31). In a first, Medicare coverage is authorized for Alzheimer's. *The New York Times.*

U.S. Department of Health and Human Services. *Medicare: Health Insurance for the Aged, Home Health Agency Manual.* Washington, DC: Author.

Appendixes

A

Assessment Tools

TOOL A.1. Caregiver Assessment of Management Problems at Baseline and During Treatment (CAMP 1)

Caregiver's name　_____

Occupational therapist's name　_____

Management Area	1. *Ask caregiver:* On a typical day, how difficult is it for you to help with or handle this area? 1 = not at all difficult 2 = a little difficult 3 = moderately difficult 4 = very difficult 5 = extremely difficult	2. *Ask caregiver:* How important is it for you to learn new strategies to handle this area? 1 = not at all important 2 = a little important 3 = moderately important 4 = very important 5 = extremely important	3. *Ask caregiver:* How effective are you in handling problems in this area? 1 = not at all effective 2 = a little effective 3 = moderately effective 4 = very effective 5 = extremely effective		Comments
	CG Rating	CG Rating	Rating		
			CG	OT	
1. Bathing					
2. Dressing					
3. Eating					
4. Toileting and incontinence					
5. Wandering					
6. Catastrophic reactions					
7. Mobility					
8. Safety					
9. Leisure and instrumental activities of daily living					
10. Personal hygiene					
11. Communication					
12. Caregiver-centered concerns					
13. Other					

TOOL A.2. Caregiver Assessment of Management Problems Following Intervention (CAMP 2)

Caregiver's name _____

Occupational therapist's name _____

Management Area	1. Was management area addressed in contacts 1 to 6?		2. *Ask caregiver:* On a typical day, how difficult is it for you to help with or handle this area? 1 = not at all difficult 2 = a little difficult 3 = moderately difficult 4 = very difficult 5 = extremely difficult	3. For each management area addressed, ask the caregiver about the outcome: Have things in this area become 1 = much better 2 = somewhat better 3 = stayed the same 4 = somewhat worse 5 = much worse?		Comments
	Yes	**No**	**CG Rating**	**Rating**		
				CG	**OT**	
1. Bathing	1	0				
2. Dressing	1	0				
3. Eating	1	0				
4. Toileting and incontinence	1	0				
5. Wandering	1	0				
6. Catastrophic reactions	1	0				
7. Mobility	1	0				
8. Safety	1	0				
9. Leisure and instrumental activities of daily living	1	0				
10. Personal hygiene	1	0				
11. Communication	1	0				
12. Caregiver-centered concerns	1	0				
13. Other	1	0				

TOOL A.3. Task Management Strategy Index

Caregiver's name _____

Occupational therapist's name _____

Ask caregiver (or observe if strategy is used):	Check if used	Comments
Do you introduce an activity that uses the same motion over and over, such as sweeping, raking, dusting?		
Do you give short instructions (two or three words)?		
Do you use pictures or labels to identify objects in rooms?		
Do you keep talking to your family member when he or she is doing something so that he or she knows what to do?		
Do you place items in the order in which your family member needs to use them?		
Do you provide rest breaks or quiet time for your family member?		
Do you place your hand over your family member's hand to guide him or her through an activity?		
Do you take your family member's arm to get him or her to go somewhere with you?		
Do you keep things that your family member likes to use, look at, or touch within easy reach?		
Do you put items that your family member needs in a place where he or she will notice them?		
Do you show your family member what to do by demonstrating the activity?		
Do you put away items that aren't needed for what your family member is doing?		
Do you use pictures to help your family member remember what to do?		
Do you use bright color or signs to help your family member notice an item?		
Do you use clothing that is easy for your family member to put on or take off?		
Do you have your family member do simple chores such as folding laundry, making beds, or drying dishes?		
Do you try to ignore your family member's mistakes?		
Do you plan a routine for your family member and try to stick to it?		
Do you use an intercom or other monitoring device to supervise your family member when he or she is in another room?		

TOOL A.4. Home Environmental Assessment Protocol (HEAP) Assessment

ENTRANCE TO HOME

Date _____ (verify with CG) _____

Time of Day $\leq$1 morning—noon $\leq$2 12:01 pm—3 pm $\leq$3 3:01—sunset $\leq$4 Dark

1a. Number of entrances to home: _____

1b. Number of entrances used by CR: _____

1c. Can main entrance used by CR be evaluated?
  1 Yes
  2 No

1d. If no, why?
  1 Refused
  2 Other (specify _____)

	Yes	No	N/A	Comments
I. POTENTIAL HAZARDS				
A. Exterior				
1. Are external steps uneven, steep, loose, cracked, sloping or slippery?				
2. Is there a securely attached banister or handrail that covers all steps?				
3. Is lighting to entrance adequate? *Probe: Is lighting to entrance in working order?*				
B. Interior				
4. Is a lock or dead bolt present on interior of door?				
5. Is door threshold >1 inch?				
II. ADAPTATIONS				
A. Exterior				
1. Is there a ramp, stair glide, or elevator to entrance?				
B. Exterior or Interior				
1. Any other visual cues or adaptations? *Probe: Have you changed anything in the entrance to make it easier for yourself or CR? (specify)*				
2. Any other safety hazards? (specify)				

Note: CG = caregiver, CR = care recipient. When you see CR, use care recipient's name.

(Continued)

213

TOOL A.4. Home Environmental Assessment Protocol (HEAP) Assessment *(Continued)*

LIVING ROOM

1. Is there a living room/den?

   ☐ 1 Yes
   ☐ 2 No

2. Does CR ever enter or use the living room/den?

   ☐ 1 Yes
   ☐ 2 No

3a. Can living room/den be observed?

   ☐ 1 Yes
   ☐ 2 No

3b. If no why

   ☐ 1 CG refused
   ☐ 2 CR in room
   ☐ 3 Living room converted to bedroom
   ☐ 4 Other (specify) _____

4. Is living room used as living room/bedroom combination?

   ☐ 1 Yes
   ☐ 2 No

	Yes	No	N/A	Comments
I. POTENTIAL HAZARDS				
A. Tripping/Falling				
1. Observe condition of floor				
a) If linoleum or tile, is floor slippery?				
b) If carpeting, is it frayed, torn, or are there folds?				
c) If tiled, is it broken?				
d) If throw rugs, not secured?				
2. Is door threshold > 1 inch?				
3. Are objects on floor in pathways?				
4. Are electrical/phone cords on floor in pathways?				
5. Is furniture that CR uses stable? *PROBE: Where does CR usually sit? Does CR use other furniture to get up and down from this chair/sofa?* If that furniture is unstable, then code = 1 (no).				
6. Is lighting adequate? TIME OF DAY _____				

B. Electrical

7. Are cords, switches, outlets, in good repair?
   PROBE: Do you frequently blow fuses or circuit breakers? (If this occurs, code = 1)

8. Are electrical cords in dangerous positions?

C. Accessible Objects

9. Are dangerous objects accessible to <u>CR?</u>
   PROBE: Do you keep scissors or other sharp objects in this room? IF YES, where do you keep them in this room?

10. Are medications accessible to <u>CR?</u>
    PROBE: Do you keep any medications (prescriptions and over-the-counter types) in this room? IF YES, where do you keep them?

D. Other

11. Any other safety hazards with regard to falling, access to dangerous items or electrical shock?
    Specify: _____

II. ADAPTATIONS

1. Are there any structural renovations?
   PROBE: Have you made any major alterations or renovations in this room to make things easier for yourself or <u>CR</u>? This includes any change, floors, walls, ceiling, wiring, and/or plumbing. Specify: _____

2. Has any door leading to or in living room been modified? If no doors, code = 8
   PROBE: Have you done anything to doors in living room?
   a) Has door been removed?
   b) Have locks or chains been installed, removed, or placed in unusual manner?
   c) Was doorway made wider?
   d) Is there a pressure gate or other barrier to room?
   e) Other

Note: CG = caregiver, CR = care recipient. When you see <u>CR</u> use care recipient's name.

215

LIVING ROOM *(Continued)*

	Yes	No	N/A	Comments
3. *PROBE: Have you removed any objects in response to CR's problems?* (e.g., throw rugs, plants, fireplace equipment, framed pictures, magazine holders, matches, etc.) *Specify:* _____ _____				
4. Have objects or furniture been added, modified, or rearranged? *PROBE: Have you added, modified, or rearranged any furniture or objects in response to CR's problems or to make caregiving easier for you?* _____ _____ _____				
5. *PROBE: Are there devices or special equipment in this room that CR uses or you use to help CR for:* a) leisure activities? b) seating? c) monitoring or communicating? d) toileting? e) other (specify)? _____ _____				
6. Is there a Control Center set up for CR's use?				
III. VISUAL CUES				
1. Are any objects labeled (television, knitting) with drawings, signs, or written information?				
2. Is there a picture, label, or arrow pointing to bathroom?				

3. Is there a drawing, picture, or short instruction list for living room tasks or daily schedule?

4. Is there use of colors or color contrast to highlight an object?

5. Are objects kept together or in containers by task for caregiving activities or for CR's use?
   PROBE: Can you show me where you keep items that CR uses in this room or that you use to care for CR?

6. Any other visual cues, adaptations, or observations? Specify:

IV. COMFORT

1. PROBE: Have you purposely placed items that are comforting, or provide meaning to CR in this room (e.g., photos, doll, stuffed animal, touch stone)?

For LR/BR combination only:

2. Is the bedroom quiet?

3. Is there a sense of privacy?

Note: CG = caregiver, CR = care recipient. When you see CR, use care recipient's name.

(Continued)

TOOL A.4. Home Environmental Assessment Protocol (HEAP) Assessment *(Continued)*

KITCHEN AREA

1. Does CR use or enter kitchen area?
   - ☐ 1 Yes
   - ☐ 2 No (go to next room)

2a. Can kitchen area be observed?
   - ☐ 1 Yes
   - ☐ 2 No

2b. If no, why?
   - ☐ 1 CG refused
   - ☐ 2 CR in room
   - ☐ 3 Other (specify) _____

	Yes	No	N/A	Comments
I. POTENTIAL HAZARDS				
A. Tripping/Falling				
1. Observe condition of floor: a) If linoleum or tile, is floor slippery? b) If carpeting, is it frayed, torn, or are there folds? c) If tiled, is it broken? d) If throw rugs, are they loose?				
2. Is door threshold >1 inch?				
3. Are objects on floor in pathways?				
4. Are electrical/phone cords on floor in pathways?				
5. Is furniture that CR uses stable? *PROBE: Where does CR usually sit? Does CR use other furniture to get up and down from this chair/sofa?* If that furniture is unstable, then code = 1 (no).				
6. Is lighting adequate? TIME OF DAY _____				

218

B. Electrical

7. Are cords, switches, outlets, in good repair?
   PROBE: Do you frequently blow fuses or circuit breakers? (If this occurs, code = 1)

8. Are electrical cords in dangerous positions?

C. Accessible Objects

9. Are dangerous objects accessible to <u>CR</u>?
   PROBE: Please show me where you keep cleaning fluids, detergents, and sharp knives in this room.

10. Are medications accessible to <u>CR</u>?
    PROBE: Do you keep any medications (prescriptions and over-the-counter types) in this room?
    IF YES, where do you keep them?

D. Other

11. Any other safety hazards with regard to falling, access to dangerous items, or electrical shock?
    (specify)

_____

_____

II. ADAPTATIONS

1. Are there any structural renovations?
   PROBE: Have you made any major alterations or renovations in this room to make things easier for yourself or <u>CR</u>? This includes any changes to floors, walls, ceiling, cabinets, wiring, and/or plumbing.
   If YES: Specify

_____

_____

2. Has any door leading to or in kitchen been modified in response to <u>CR</u>'s problems?
   PROBE: Have you done anything to the kitchen door?
   a) Has door been removed?
   b) Have locks or chains been installed, removed, or placed in unusual manner?
   c) Was doorway made wider?
   d) Is there a pressure gate or other barrier to room?
   e) Other?

Note: CG = caregiver, CR = care recipient. When you see <u>CR</u>, use care recipient's name.

(Continued)

219

KITCHEN AREA *(Continued)*

	Yes	No	N/A	Comments
3. *PROBE: Have you removed any items/objects in response to <u>CR's</u> problems? Specify:*				
4. Have objects or furniture been added, modified, or rearranged? *PROBE: Have you added, modified, or rearranged any furniture or objects in response to <u>CR's</u> problems or to make caregiving easier for you? If YES: Specify*				
5. *PROBE: Are there devices or special equipment in this room that CG uses to help <u>CR</u> for:* a) feeding and meal preparation? b) monitoring and communication? c) seating? d) other (specify)?				
6. Is there a safety latch or childproof lock on the inside or outside of any cabinet door or drawer? *PROBE: Do you use safety latches, childproof locks or other types of locks on the inside of cabinet doors or drawer?*				
7. Any adaptations to oven? *PROBE: Have you changed or modified your oven in response to <u>CR's</u> problems?*				

III. VISUAL CUES

1. Are any objects labeled (sink, refrigerator, bowls, food) with drawings, signs, or written information?

2. Is there a picture, label, or arrow pointing to bathroom?

3. Is there a drawing, picture, or short instruction list for kitchen tasks or daily schedule?

4. Is there use of color or color contrast to highlight an object?

5. Are objects kept together or in containers by task for caregiving activities or for CR's use?
   PROBE: *Can you show me where you keep items that CR uses in this room or that you use to care for CR?*

6. Does CR have own chair at table or is there a place at table labeled with CR's name?

7. Are there any other visual cues, adaptations, or other observations?

   _____

   _____

	< 25%	26–50%	51–75%	76–100%

IV. OBSERVATION ONLY

	< 25%	26–50%	51–75%	76–100%
1. To what extent are counter surfaces covered with objects?				
2. To what extent are eating surfaces covered with objects?				

Note: CG = caregiver, CR = care recipient. When you see CR, use care recipient's name.

(Continued)

221

TOOL A.4. Home Environmental Assessment Protocol (HEAP) Assessment *(Continued)*

DINING AREA

1. Does CR use or enter dining area?

   ☐ 1 Yes
   ☐ 2 No (go to next room)

2a. Can dining area be observed?

   ☐ 1 Yes
   ☐ 2 No

2b. If no, why?

   ☐ 1 CG refused
   ☐ 2 CR in room
   ☐ 3 Other (specify) _____

	Yes	No	N/A	Comments
I. POTENTIAL HAZARDS				
A. Tripping/Falling				
1. Observe condition of floor:				
a) If linoleum or tile, is floor slippery?				
b) If carpeting, is it frayed, torn, or are there folds?				
c) If tiled, is it broken?				
d) If throw rugs, are they loose?				
2. Is door threshold >1 inch?				
3. Are objects on floor in pathways?				
4. Are electrical/phone cords on floor in pathways?				
5. Is furniture that CR uses stable? *PROBE: Where does CR usually sit? Does CR use other furniture to get up and down from this chair/sofa?* If that furniture is unstable, then code = 1 (no).				
6. Is lighting adequate? TIME OF DAY _____				

222

B. Electrical

7. Are cords, switches, outlets, in good repair?
   PROBE: Do you frequently blow fuses or circuit breakers? (If this occurs, code = 1)

8. Are electrical cords in dangerous positions?

C. Accessible Objects

9. Are dangerous objects accessible to <u>CR</u>?
   PROBE: Please show me where you keep cleaning fluids, detergents, and sharp knives in this room.

10. Are medications accessible to <u>CR</u>?
    PROBE: Do you keep any medications (prescriptions and over-the-counter types) in this room?
    IF YES, where do you keep them?

D. Other

11. Any other safety hazards with regard to falling, access to dangerous items, or electrical shock?
    (specify)

II. ADAPTATIONS

1. Are there any structural renovations?
   PROBE: Have you made any major alterations or renovations in this room to make things easier for yourself or <u>CR</u>? This includes any change to floors, walls, ceiling, cabinets, wiring, and/or plumbing.
   IF YES: Specify

2. Has any door leading to or in dining room been modified in response to <u>CR</u>'s problems?
   PROBE: Have you done anything to the dining door?
   a) Has door been removed?
   b) Have locks or chains been installed, removed, or placed in unusual manner?
   c) Was doorway made wider?
   d) Is there a pressure gate or other barrier to room?
   e) Other?

Note: CG = caregiver, CR = care recipient. When you see <u>CR</u>, use care recipient's name.

(Continued)

223

DINING AREA *(Continued)*

	Yes	No	N/A	Comments
3. PROBE: Have you removed any items/objects in response to <u>CR's</u> problems? Specify:				
4. Have objects or furniture been added, modified, or rearranged? PROBE: Have you added, modified, or rearranged, any furniture or objects in response to <u>CR's</u> problems or to make caregiving easier for you? Specify:				
5. PROBE: Are there devices or special equipment in this room that CG uses to help <u>CR</u> for: a) feeding and meal preparation? b) monitoring and communication? c) seating? d) other (specify)?				
6. Is there a safety latch or childproof lock on the inside or outside of any cabinet door or drawer? PROBE: Do you use safety latches, childproof locks, or other types of locks on the inside of cabinet doors or drawer?				
7. Any adaptations to oven? PROBE: Have you changed or modified your oven in response to <u>CR's</u> problems?				

III. VISUAL CUES

				<25%	26–50%	51–75%	76–100%
1. Are any objects labeled (sink, refrigerator, bowls, food) with drawings, signs, or written information?							
2. Is there a picture, label, or arrow pointing to bathroom?							
3. Is there a drawing, picture, or short instruction list for kitchen tasks or daily schedule?							
4. Is there use of color or color contrast to highlight an object?							
5. Are objects kept together or in containers by task for caregiving activities or for CR's use? PROBE: Can you show me where you keep items that CR uses in this room or that you use to care for CR?							
6. Does CR have own chair at table or is there a place at table labeled with CR's name?							
7. Are there any other visual cues, adaptations, or other observations?							

IV. OBSERVATION ONLY

	<25%	26–50%	51–75%	76–100%
1. To what extent are counter surfaces covered with objects?				
2. To what extent are eating surfaces covered with objects?				

Note: CG = caregiver, CR = care recipient. When you see CR, use care recipient's name.

(Continued)

225

TOOL A.4. Home Environmental Assessment Protocol (HEAP) Assessment *(Continued)*

STAIRS

1. How many flights of stairs (staircases) in the interior
   of home? _____ (If "0" go to next room/area)

2. How many staircases are used by CR?

3a. Can staircases used by CR be evaluated?

   ☐ 1 Yes
   ☐ 2 No

3b. If no, why?

   ☐ 1 CG refused
   ☐ 2 Other (specify) _____

	Yes	No	N/A	Comments
I. POTENTIAL HAZARDS				
A. Tripping/Falling				
1. Observe condition of floor:				
a) If linoleum or tile, is floor slippery?				
b) If carpeting, is it frayed, torn, folds, or not secured?				
c) If tiled, is it broken?				
2. Are stairs uneven, steep, loose, cracked, sloping, or slippery?				
3. Are objects on stairs?				
4. Is there a securely attached banister or handrail present that covers *all* steps?				
5. Is there adequate lighting of staircase?				
6. Any other specific hazards? (specify)				
II. ADAPTATIONS				
1. Are steps edges outlined or is there use of color or color constrast?				
2. Are stairs closed off or are there pressure gates at either end of staircase?				
3. Are there any other visual cues, adaptations, or observations? (specify)				

HALLWAYS

1. Number of hallways in home: _____

2. Number of hallways in home used by <u>CR</u>: _____

3a. Can hallways used by <u>CR</u> be evaluated?

      ☐ 1   Yes
      ☐ 2   No

3b. If no, why?

      ☐ 1   CG refused
      ☐ 2   Other (specify) _____

	Yes	No	N/A	Comments
I. POTENTIAL HAZARDS				
A. Tripping/Falling				
1. Observe condition of floor				
a) If linoleum or tile, is floor slippery?				
b) If carpeting, is it frayed, torn, or are there folds?				
c) If tiled, is it broken?				
d) If throw rugs, are they loose?				
2. Is door threshold >1 inch?				
3. Are objects on floor in pathways?				
4. Are electrical/phone cords on floor in pathways?				
5. Is lighting adequate? _____ TIME OF DAY				
B. Electrical				
6. Are cords, switches, outlets, in good repair?				
7. Are electrical cords in dangerous positions?				

Note: CG = caregiver, CR = care recipient. When you see <u>CR</u>, use care recipient's name.

(Continued)

227

TOOL A.4. Home Environmental Assessment Protocol (HEAP) Assessment *(Continued)*

HALLWAYS *(Continued)*

	Yes	No	N/A	Comments
C. Other				
8. Any other safety hazards? (specify) _____				
II. ADAPTATIONS				
1. Are there any structural renovations? *PROBE: Have you made any major alterations or renovations in this room to make things easier for yourself or CR? This includes any changes to floors, walls, ceiling, cabinets, wiring, and/or plumbing.* (specify) _____				
2. Has any door in hallway been modified? *PROBE: Have you done anything to the door(s) in hallway?* a) *Has door been removed?* b) *Have locks or chains been installed, removed, or placed in unusual manner?* c) *Was doorway made wider?* d) *Is there a pressure gate or other barrier to room?* e) *Other?*				
3. *PROBE: Have you removed any objects in response to CR's problems? (e.g., throw rugs) Specify:* _____				

228

4. Have objects or furniture been added, modified, or rearranged?
   PROBE: Have you added, modified, or rearranged any furniture or objects in response to CR's problems or to make caregiving easier for you? If yes, specify.

_____

III. VISUAL CUES

1. Are any objects labeled (door, closet) with drawings, signs, or written information?

2. Is there a picture, label, or arrow pointing to bathroom?

3. Is there use of colors or color contrast to highlight an object?

4. Are there any other visual cues, adaptations, or other observations? (specify)

_____

Note: CG = caregiver, CR = care recipient. When you see CR, use care recipient's name.

(Continued)

229

TOOL A.4. Home Environmental Assessment Protocol (HEAP) Assessment *(Continued)*

BATHROOM

1a. How many bathrooms do you have in your (house/apartment) that CR either enters or uses? _____

1b. If CR does not use bathroom, ask CG: *Where do you bathe CR?* If not bathed in bathroom, ask:

1c. Are there any special devices/equipment you use for bathing CR (including washing hair)? If YES, specify:

_____

_____

2a. *If CR enters bathroom: Please show me the bathroom CR uses most often.* (If more than one bathroom and used with same frequency, choose bathroom where CR is bathed.)

2b. Can bathroom be observed?

   [1] Yes

   [2] No

2c. If no, why?

   [1] CG refused

   [2] CR in room

   [3] Other (specify) _____

	Yes	No	N/A	Comments
I. POTENTIAL HAZARDS				
A. Tripping/Falling				
1. Observe condition of floor				
a) If linoleum or tile, is floor slippery?				
b) If carpeting, is it frayed, torn, or are there folds?				
c) If tiled, is it broken?				
d) If throw rugs, are they loose?				
2. Is door threshold >1 inch?				
3. Are objects on floor in pathways?				
4. Are electrical/phone cords on floor in pathways?				
5. Is lighting adequate? Time of Day _____				
6. Is there a nightlight or is bathroom light on at night? *PROBE: Do you use a nightlight or leave the bathroom light on for CR?*				

230

B. Electrical

7. Are cords, switches, outlets, in good repair?
   PROBE: Do you frequently blow fuses or circuit breakers? (If this occurs, code = 1)

8. Are electrical cords in dangerous positions?

C. Accessible Objects

9. Are dangerous objects accessible to CR?
   PROBE: Do you keep cleaning fluids, detergents, or sharp objects in this room?

10. Are medications accessible to CR?
    PROBE: Do you keep any medications (prescriptions and over-the-counter types) in this room?
    IF YES, Where do you keep them?

D. Other

11. Any other safety hazards with regard to falling, access to dangerous items or electrical shock?
    Specify: _____
    _____

II. ADAPTATIONS

1. Are there any structural renovations?
   PROBE: Have you made any major alterations or renovations in this room to make things easier for yourself or CR? This includes any change to tubs/shower, sink, floors, walls, ceiling, wiring, and/or plumbing?
   _____
   _____

2. Has any door in bathroom been modified?
   PROBE: Have you done anything to the bathroom door?
   a) Has door been removed?
   b) Have locks or chairs been installed, removed, or placed in unusual manner?
   c) Was doorway made wider?
   d) Is there a pressure gate or other barrier to room?
   e) Other?

Note: CG = caregiver, CR = care recipient. When you see CR, use care recipient's name.

(Continued)

231

TOOL A.4. Home Environmental Assessment Protocol (HEAP) Assessment *(Continued)*

BATHROOM *(Continued)*

	Yes	No	N/A	Comments
3. Is there a safety latch or childproof lock on the inside or outside of any cabinet door or drawer? *PROBE: Do you use safety latches, childproof locks, or other types of locks on the inside or outside of cabinet doors or drawer?*				
4. Have any receptacles been removed from the bathroom? *PROBE: Have you removed the laundry basket, waste basket, and/or magazine holder in response to CR's problems?*				
5. Are there grab bars: a) in tub/shower? b) at toilet? c) at sink?				
6. Is there a raised toilet seat or adjusted seat height in use by CR?				
7. Is there a tub bench, hand held shower, or other devices used for bathing CR?				
8. Are there adaptive grooming devices?				
9. Is there a bathmat or non-skid abrasive strips (in good repair) in bathtub/shower?				
10. Is the hot water temperature adjusted? *PROBE: Have you adjusted the temperature on the hot water heater?*				
11. *PROBE: Have you removed any objects in response to CR's problems (e.g., laundry basket, waste basket, magazine holder, razors, cleaning fluids, etc.) Specify:*				

12. *PROBE: Are there other assistive devices or changes you have done in response to* <u>CR</u>'s *problem that we have not talked about?*
Have you rearranged or added any objects?

III. VISUAL CUES

	< 25%	26–50%	51–75%	76–100%
1. Are any objects labeled (door, sink, toilet, bathtub, towels) with drawings, signs, or written information?				
2. Is there a drawing, picture, or short instruction list for a bathroom task or daily schedule?				
3. Is there use of color or color contrast to highlight an object (e.g., colored toilet seat)?				
4. Are objects kept together or in containers by task? *PROBE: Can you show me where you keep items that* <u>CR</u> *uses or that you use to care for* <u>CR</u>?				
5. Are there any other visual cues, adaptations, or other observations? (specify)				

IV. OBSERVATION ONLY

	< 25%	26–50%	51–75%	76–100%
1. To what extent is sink area covered with objects?				
2. To what extent is toilet top covered with objects?				

Note: CG = caregiver, <u>CR</u> = care recipient. When you see <u>CR</u>, use care recipient's name.

(Continued)

233

TOOL A.4. Home Environmental Assessment Protocol (HEAP) Assessment (Continued)

BEDROOM

1a. Please show me the bedroom or sleeping area that <u>CR</u> uses.

1b. Can bedroom be evaluated?
- ☐ 1 Yes
- ☐ 2 No

1c. If no, why?
- ☐ 1 CG refused
- ☐ 2 <u>CR</u> in room
- ☐ 3 Other (specify _____)

2b. Is bedroom an area that has been converted?
- ☐ 1 Yes
- ☐ 2 No

	Yes	No	N/A	Comments
I. POTENTIAL HAZARDS				
A. Tripping/Falling				
1. Observe condition of floor				
a) If linoleum or tile, is floor slippery?				
b) If carpeting, is it frayed, torn, or are there folds?				
c) If tiled, is it broken?				
d) If throw rugs, are they loose?				
2. Is door threshold >1 inch?				
3. Are objects on floor in pathways?				
4. Are electrical/phone cords on floor in pathways?				
5. Is furniture that <u>CR</u> uses stable? *PROBE: Where does <u>CR</u> usually sit? Does <u>CR</u> use other furniture to get up and down from this chair/bed?* If that furniture is unstable, then code = 1 (no).				
6. Is lighting adequate? TIME OF DAY _____				
7. Is there a nightlight or light by bed?				
8. Is there a lighted path from bedroom to bathroom/commode area? *PROBE: Do you keep a light on at night for the bathroom/commode area?*				

B. Electrical

9. Are cords, switches, and outlets, in good repair?
   PROBE: Do you frequently blow fuses or circuit breakers? (If this occurs code = 1)

10. Are electrical cords or phone cords in dangerous positions?

C. Accessible Objects

11. Are dangerous items accessible to <u>CR</u>?
    PROBE: Do you keep matches, scissors, razors, or other sharp objects in this room? IF YES, Where do you keep them in this room?

12. Are medications accessible to <u>CR</u>?
    PROBE: Do you keep any medications (prescriptions and over-the-counter types) in this room? IF YES, Where do you keep them?

D. Other

13. Any other safety hazards with regard to falling, access to dangerous items, or electrical shock?
    Specify:

II. ADAPTATIONS

1. Are there any structural renovations?
   PROBE: Have you made any major alterations or renovations in this room to make things easier for yourself or <u>CR</u>? This includes any changes to tubs/shower, sink, floors, walls, ceiling, wiring, and/or plumbing. Specify:

2. Has any door in bedroom been modified?
   PROBE: Have you done anything to the bedroom door?
   a) Has door been removed?
   b) Have locks or chains been installed, removed, or placed in unusual manner?
   c) Was doorway made wider?
   d) Is there a pressure gate or other barrier to room?
   e) Other

Note: CG = caregiver, CR = care recipient. When you see <u>CR</u>, use care recipient's name.

(Continued)

235

TOOL A.4. Home Environmental Assessment Protocol (HEAP) Assessment *(Continued)*

BEDROOM *(Continued)*

	Yes	No	N/A	Comments
3. *PROBE: Have you removed any items or objects in response to CR's problems?* *(e.g., receptacles – laundry basket, waste basket, magazine holder?)*				
4. Have objects or furniture been added, modified, or rearranged? *PROBE: Have you rearranged or added any furniture or objects in response to CR's problems?* *Specify:*				
5. *PROBE: Are there devices or special equipment CR uses or you use to help CR in this room for:* a) Dressing? b) Seating? c) Monitoring or communicating? d) Toileting/commode? e) Other				
6. Is there a Control Center set up for CR's use?				
III. VISUAL CUES				
1. Are any objects labeled (socks, closet) with drawings, signs, or written information?				
2. Is there a picture, label or arrow pointing to bathroom?				

3. Is there a drawing, picture, or short instruction list for bedroom tasks or daily schedule?				
4. Is there use of colors or color contrast to highlight an object?				
5. Are personal care items kept together and/or in containers by task for caregiving or for CR's use? *PROBE: Can you show me where you keep items that CR uses in this room or that you use to care for CR?*				
6. Is there a picture or name of CR on door?				
7. Is there a mirror present and visible?				
8. Any other visual cues, adaptations, or observations? (specify) _____ _____				
	< 25%	26–50%	51–75%	76–100%

IV. OBSERVATION ONLY

1. To what extent are is sink area covered with objects?				

V. COMFORT

1. *PROBE: Have you purposely placed items that are comforting, or provide meaning to CR in this room (e.g., photos, doll, stuffed animal, touch stone)?*				
2. Is the bedroom quiet?				
3. Is there a sense of privacy?				

Note: CG = caregiver, CR = care recipient. When you see CR, use care recipient's name.

(Continued)

237

TOOL A.4. Home Environmental Assessment Protocol (HEAP) Assessment *(Continued)*

	Yes	No	N/A	Comments
I. HOME MODIFICATION SERVICES				
1. Have adaptations, modifications, or assistive devices been observed? If yes ask CG: *Were changes made in response to:* ___ 1 OT suggestion ___ 2 PT suggestion ___ 3 education materials ___ 4 PCA or other Home modification program ___ 5 client thought of it ___ 6 Other (specify): _____ (Check all that apply)				
II. ASSISTIVE DEVICES				

1a. Does <u>CR</u> use a mobility device?
    a. cane (straight/quad)
    b. walker
    c. wheelchair
 1b. If wheelchair used, is it adapted?				

2. Does <u>CR</u> use any devices for hearing?				
3. Does <u>CR</u> use any devices for vision (magnifying glass, glasses)?				
III. STEP STOOL				
1a. Does <u>CR</u> use a step stool or other furniture to reach high storage areas anywhere in your house? 1b. If yes; observe step stool for its safety. IF safe, code = 0. If not safe, code = 1				
IV. FIRE SAFETY				
1a. Are there smoke detectors in the house? anywhere in your house? 1b. If yes, ask; How many smoke detectors are in working order? _____				

	Yes	No	N/A	Comments
V. UNMET NEEDS				
1. ASK CG *Does CR have any (physical) difficulty getting into or out of the house or any rooms?* IF YES: specify:				
2. ASK CG *Do you have any problems or issues in any room of your home that we have not discussed?* IF YES: specify:				
3. ASK CG *Do you need any special equipment to help CR that you do not have? IF YES: specify:*				
V. RECORD HOUSING TYPE Housing especially for elderly Single family ranch Single family 2+ stories Twin home Row home Apartment in house with 1 or more apartments Apartment in apartment building Other (specify)				

239

TOOL A.5. Caregiver Readiness

Caregiver name _____ Date _____

Readiness score (circle one)   1   2   3   4

Does the caregiver know or acknowledge that the family member has dementia?

No

1. Precontemplation
"Everything is OK."
"He or she is just old."
"He or she has always been like this."
"He or she is being manipulative."
The caregiver hears but does not listen.

Currently trying

2. Contemplation
The caregiver hears but does not listen.
The caregiver is not sure if the intervention will work.
"Nothing will work."
"I've tried it all."

Yes

Does the caregiver indicate willingness to try different strategies, such as behavioral or environmental changes, to help make caregiving easier?

Trying

3. Preparation
The caregiver tries to understand.
The caregiver reads about the diagnosis.
"Maybe, but I hope it is something else."

Yes

4. Action and Maintenance
The caregiver participates actively.
The caregiver asks questions.
The caregiver tries his or her own ideas.

TOOL A.6. Strategies List and Integration Status

Caregiver Name _____

Management Area _____

Care Recipient Name _____

Describe Strategy	Suggested by whom? 1 = occupational therapist 2 = caregiver 3 = both	During Which Contact?	Integrated by Contact 6? 1 = integrated 2 = not integrated 3 = pending	How long in use? (weeks)	Reason not implemented 1 = too difficult 2 = not effective 3 = made problem worse 4 = unacceptable 5 = not enough time 6 = didn't understand 7 = made new problem 8 = other	Comments

TOOL A.7. Treatment Receipt and Enactment

Caregiver name _____

Occupational therapist name _____

Management area _____

Overall, in the process of addressing this management area, did the caregiver		
Treatment Receipt	Yes	No
1. Indicate that using these strategies was too much to think about?	1	2
2. Seem confused or mistaken about the nature of the problem?	1	2
3. Seem reluctant to participate in development of management strategies for this problem area?	1	2
4. Resist implementing agreed-on strategies?	1	2
5. Offer ideas about the nature of the problem to be solved?	2	1
6. Indicate that he or she feels less upset with the care recipient's behavior?	2	1
7. Indicate that desired outcomes were met?	2	1
8. Indicate that the strategies had no effect or made matters worse?	1	2
Treatment Enactment	Yes	No
1. Indicate that he or she has new or refined insight into the specific management area?	2	1
2. Convey that he or she preferred the old way of handling this management issue?	1	2
3. Demonstrate understanding of new management strategies?	2	1
4. Modify strategies to fit his or her own needs better?	2	1
5. Express feeling confident about being able to solve this management issue or implement specific strategies?	2	1
6. Suggest new strategies that involve environmental modifications?	2	1
7. Express satisfaction with how strategies worked?	2	1
8. Express hopefulness or enthusiasm about strategies or plans?	2	1

Examples of Environmental Strategies for Targeted Management Areas

This list of examples of general strategies can help occupational therapists generate potential strategies to share with caregivers. This list is not all-inclusive, and occupational therapists may need to modify these strategies to fit the culture and circumstances of a particular household and consult other resources. Also, numerous strategies are relevant to more than one problem area and thus are listed in multiple places.

TOPICS COVERED

- Toileting and Incontinence
- Dressing
- Bathing
- Eating
- Personal Hygiene
- Communication
- Mobility
- Safety
- Leisure and Instrumental Activities of Daily Living
- Wandering
- Catastrophic Reactions
- Caregiver-Centered Concerns

TOILETING AND INCONTINENCE

Object Layer

Use and Manipulation of Common Objects

- Limit use of absorbent pads, diapers, and condom catheters, except at night if enuresis is a problem. If these are used, an incontinence spray or cream may be indicated to prevent skin irritation.
- Provide clothing that the care recipient can manipulate easily (e.g., clothing with an elastic waist or hook-and-loop fasteners).
- Remove any confusing objects from around or on the toilet or commode, including washcloths, clothing, reading material, or telephone. These objects can confuse the care recipient about the intended purpose of the toilet or commode.
- Place visual cues to help the care recipient know where to toilet. Visual cues should be simple and straightforward, such as a picture or photograph of the toilet, and the caregiver should place them in a prominent position. Painting the bathroom door a bright, eye-catching color will attract attention to the room and prompt the care recipient to toilet. If preferred, the caregiver may have success with closing all doors except the bathroom door to attract the care recipient's attention to that room and discourage urination in other rooms. Large arrows pointing the way to the bathroom from the living room or bedroom also can steer the care recipient toward the toilet.
- Modify the bathroom. Removing or covering all containers in the bathroom (e.g., sink, wastebasket, laundry hamper) can eliminate confusion about where to toilet. Hanging a drawing over the toilet of a man or woman using the toilet will further reduce confusion. Use of a colored, padded toilet seat can call attention to the toilet. In some cases, removing the toilet seat lid completely may be preferable. Caregivers may also consider using a nightlight in the evening and at night or even keeping the bathroom light on at all times to compensate for the reduced visual acuity that usually accompanies aging.
- Place objects within the triangle of efficiency (nose, right elbow, left elbow) to accommodate reach limitations associated with aging.
- Keep all stairways and passageways free of objects.
- Arrange stable furniture, if possible, so that the care recipient can use it as a support when moving toward the bathroom.
- Keep available objects or activities to distract the care recipient if she or he is engaging in intolerable behavior while toileting.
- Eliminate as much clutter and extraneous objects from the bathroom as possible.

Assistive Devices and Home Alterations

- Install window coverings to eliminate glare in the bathroom and in passageways leading to the bathroom.
- Because depth perception is likely to be impaired as a normal aspect of aging, consider the following techniques for stairways and passageways leading to the bathroom:
  - Paint a narrow strip at the edge of each step.
  - Paint the wall in the stairway leading to the bathroom a contrasting color from the steps to accentuate the stair rise.
  - Add lighting to the bathroom and passageways leading to the bathroom.
  - Secure handrails, broken steps, and loose carpeting in the bathroom and on stairs and in passageways leading to the bathroom.
  - Paint the door to the bathroom a bright, eye-catching color.
- Install equipment as needed for bathroom transfers (e.g., grab bars) and for safe mobility in passageways leading to the bathroom (e.g., banisters, stair glides).
- Order and install equipment for toileting (e.g., raised toilet seat).
- Install safety gates where indicated (e.g., at the top of stairs).
- Install an electronic monitor (such as those used to monitor infants) in the bathroom.
- Modify doorways for accessibility (e.g., wider openings, lower thresholds).
- Remove lock from bathroom.
- Install a screen or curtains to hide distracting items from view.
- Install bells or alarms on doors, cabinet doors, or drawers to alert the caregiver when the care recipient opens them.

Task Layer

- Consider establishing a routine for voiding every 2 hours. The routine favored by the caregiver may be revealed through his or her analysis of information from a bladder record, which records voiding patterns and frequency of incontinence. Once these natural tendencies are identified, the caregiver can develop a bathroom schedule that accounts for these factors and coincides with the caregiver's personal needs. For instance, if the caregiver notes that accidents usually occur at specified times, he or she can schedule toileting immediately before these times and then relax for a while afterward. It is important to avoid unnecessary changes in an established toileting routine.
- Eliminate ambiguity in communicating what behavior is desired. The caregiver should use simple, one-step instructions, such as "Take off your pants" instead of "Take off your pants and sit down." It is important that the caregiver give instructions in a stepwise manner, with subsequent instructions given

only after the care recipient has completed each request. The caregiver should give instructions in the form of a statement, instead of a question, unless the care recipient must make a choice. For instance, saying "We are going to the bathroom, now" instead of "Do you have to urinate?" will clarify intent and avoid provoking anxiety. When instructions are presented as a statement and not a question, the care recipient is less likely to refuse or feel anxious about responding correctly. The caregiver can enhance verbal communication with nonverbal cues, such as taking the care recipient's elbow and walking toward or pointing to the bathroom.

- Between planned times for toileting, or as a substitute for establishing a voiding routine, look for verbal or nonverbal cues that the care recipient needs to toilet. Although highly individualized, signs that a care recipient needs to void frequently include restlessness, anxious behavior, crying, wandering, and pressured speech.

- Speak to a physician or dietitian about implementing a high-fiber diet when fecal impaction is a factor in incontinence. If the physician recommends a fiber supplement, the caregiver should give it at the same time every day to establish a routine. Furthermore, reducing the intake of caffeine and alcohol eliminates these potential bladder irritants. A final possibility for dietary control is regulating fluid intake. A fluid intake routine designed to ensure adequate hydration (1,500–2,000 ml per day) can offset the negative effects of concentrated urine in the bladder. The caregiver may wish to expand this fluid intake routine to include reduction of fluids in the evening if enuresis is a problem.

- If preferred, or if a bathroom routine is unworkable, the next step is to physically help the care recipient to remove clothing and sit on the toilet. Usually, simple instructions that involve gentle demonstration and avoid verbal directions get the best results. In this way, the caregiver does not convey frustration and upset to the care recipient through voice intonations.

- Do not talk to the care recipient if he or she needs to concentrate on walking to the bathroom or transferring to the toilet. One-third of all falls occur because the person who fell was not paying sufficient attention while moving around (Hornbrook et al., 1994; Shaw et al., 2003).

- Allow adequate time for the care recipient to adjust to changes in light intensity when entering or leaving the bathroom. Provide a safe place to stand or sit until his or her eyes accommodate to the difference.

- Finally, if the care recipient appears to be unwell or not at his or her best, give extra assistance with toileting.

Social Groups

- In households where more than one caregiver is present, the primary caregiver should establish the bathroom routine and specifics of the management strategy. He or she should develop this routine in detail and formulate specific instructions to be conveyed to all caregivers. Smith and Newman (1991) described the use of a "Bowel and Bladder Program—Prompted Voiding Diary" to assist in instructing others in the bathroom routine. In this way, all caregivers approach toileting-related tasks in the same way.

- Use positive reinforcement as a powerful and effective tool to promote a degree of independence in toileting. For instance, if the care recipient gives the caregiver cues about the need to toilet, a good response is "Thanks for letting me know you have to go." Caregivers can use the same type of positive recognition to reinforce any level of participation in the act of toileting or to acknowledge a lower level of resistance. Smith and Newman (1991) termed this strategy "prompted voiding"; caregivers have found this to be effective with nursing home residents.
- Expand the family's support network to include paid or unpaid helpers to provide assistance with toileting.
- Make a schedule of daily helpers that indicates the scope of each helper's visit. If toileting is to be part of the helper's duties, the caregiver must clearly communicate the specifics of how to perform this task.
- Ask the physician or pharmacist about the possible side effects of medications on performance in this area.

Technical Supports

Physical Therapist
Indicators of the need for a physical therapist consultation include potential or actual problems related to unsafe transfers, poor balance, unsteadiness, debility, and low endurance; caregiver physical strain from helping the care receiver; and the occurrence of a toileting-related event that triggers a catastrophic reaction. The physical therapist should

- Evaluate and order ambulation equipment necessary for toileting.
- Teach the caregiver to transfer the care recipient safely to the toilet.
- Teach the caregiver back protection and back-strengthening techniques.
- Develop and monitor a program to improve the care recipient's mobility.

Social Worker
During the consultation, the social worker should

- Help the caregiver obtain information about dementia and incontinence and suggest contacting the local library and the Alzheimer's Association for materials about management of toileting and incontinence in people with dementia.
- Provide information about support groups and other community resource agencies that provide assistance, counseling, and respite.

- Provide information about the benefits of adult day care for respite from the daily pressures of providing personal assistance to a person with dementia. Give the caregiver specific information about adult day care in the area.
- Provide information about the benefits of partial respite gained by attending a senior citizen center with the care recipient. Give the caregiver specific information about senior citizen centers in the area.
- Help the caregiver obtain information from churches and religious organizations about volunteer or low-cost help for a range of services.

DRESSING

Object Layer

Use and Manipulation of Common Home Objects
- Limit choices about clothing styles and colors. The caregiver should purchase clothing items that can be mixed and matched in many ways. One suggestion is to choose a few basic colors and buy all solid trousers or shirts in those colors. The caregiver also can purchase blouses, sweaters, and shirts within the selected color scheme and either print or solid fabrics.
- Prepackage all clothing to be used for one morning. A package of clothing would include underwear, socks, and so forth, and the care recipient will not have to search for these items. An alternative to prepackaging clothing is to establish one place in the bedroom where the caregiver sets out all clothing needed for dressing.
- Set out clothing in the order in which the care recipient will don it.
- Remove all out-of-season, ill-fitting, or little-used clothing.
- Arrange closets and drawers so that like items are kept together.
- Post steps for dressing on a large poster in the bedroom. If reading is a problem, use pictures or drawings.
- Use clothing that is easy to don and doff. It is easy for the care recipient to handle hook-and-loop closures or pull-on clothing, for instance.
- Keep available objects or activities to distract the care recipient if she or he is engaging in intolerable behavior while dressing.
- Eliminate as much clutter and extraneous objects from the area as possible.

Assistive Devices and Home Alterations
- Install a countertop, shelving, or extra space to arrange items for dressing.
- Install a closet organizer for clothing.

- Install a mirror for visual feedback.
- Install adequate lighting in closets and around dressers.
- Install bells or alarms on doors, cabinet doors, or drawers to alert the caregiver when the care recipient opens them.
- Install a screen or curtains to hide distracting items from view.

Task Layer

- Hand items to the care recipient one at a time as they are to be donned.
- Use simple, clear, one-step directions, such as "Put your arm in the sleeve" or "Pull up your pants."
- Demonstrate for the care recipient what to do or use hand-over-hand guiding.
- Help with the task of dressing only as much as necessary. For instance, if the care recipient is unable to don a shirt, the caregiver should help only with this activity and should supervise the remainder of the dressing task.
- Establish a calm and accepting atmosphere while the care recipient is dressing.
- Avoid scolding, criticizing, or invading the personal space of the care recipient, especially if there are signs of agitation.
- Allow the care recipient to take as much time as needed for dressing, as feasible.
- Offer no more than two choices of clothing.

Social Groups

- Establish a social goal for dressing. For instance, the caregiver may tell the care recipient about a friend's upcoming visit and encourage him or her to dress in an attractive manner.
- Compliment the care recipient about how he or she looks and about the amount of effort he or she demonstrated.
- Ignore mistakes if they are of no significant consequence (e.g., clashing colors).
- The caregiver may find it beneficial to ask himself or herself "Is it really necessary for me to do the dressing? Can it be done later or by someone else?"
- Expand the family's support network to include paid and unpaid helpers to provide assistance with dressing.
- Make a schedule of daily helpers that indicates the scope of each helper's visit. If the helper is to assist with dressing, the caregiver must clearly communicate the specifics of how to perform this task.
- Ask the physician or pharmacist about the possible side effects of medications on performance in this area.

Technical Supports

Physical Therapist

Indicators of the need for a physical therapist consultation include potential or actual problems related to unsafe transfers, poor balance, unsteadiness, debility, and low endurance; caregiver physical strain from helping the care receiver; and the occurrence of a dressing-related event that triggers a catastrophic reaction. The physical therapist should

- Evaluate and order ambulation equipment necessary for dressing.
- Teach the caregiver to transfer the care recipient safely in the bedroom.
- Teach the caregiver back protection and back-strengthening techniques.
- Develop and monitor a program to improve the care recipient's mobility.

Social Worker

During the consultation, the social worker should

- Help the caregiver obtain information about dementia and dressing and suggest contacting the local library and the Alzheimer's Association for materials about management of dressing in people with dementia.
- Provide information about support groups and other community resource agencies that provide assistance, counseling, and respite.
- Provide information about the benefits of adult day care for respite from the daily pressures of providing personal assistance to a person with dementia. Give the caregiver specific information about adult day care in the area.
- Provide information about the benefits of partial respite gained by attending a senior citizen center with the care recipient. Give the caregiver specific information about senior citizen centers in the area.
- Help the caregiver obtain information from churches and religious organizations about volunteer or low-cost help for a range of services.

BATHING

Object Layer

Use and Manipulation of Common Home Objects

- Put a few drops of blue food coloring in the bathwater to strengthen its visual impact. The blue color also may make the water appear more inviting to the care recipient. Using just a few drops is not likely to leave any stain on the care recipient's skin.

- Check the water temperature with a thermometer. Be aware of the tendency for older people to perceive temperature differently due to normal aging changes. Pay attention to any complaints of the water being too hot or cold.
- Set the temperature on the hot water heater not to exceed 120° F.
- Warm the room sufficiently to increase the care recipient's willingness to remove clothing.
- Set out only what is needed for bathing, and make sure the items are arranged in the order they will be used.
- Use brightly colored items for bathing (e.g., soap, soap dish, towels) to provide greater visual emphasis.
- Post a bathing schedule and steps for bathing on a large poster in the bathroom. If reading is a problem, use pictures or drawings.
- Place objects within the triangle of efficiency to accommodate reach limitations associated with aging.
- Keep all passageways free of objects.
- Arrange stable furniture, if possible, so that the care recipient can use it as a support when moving toward the bathroom. Keep available objects or activities to distract the care recipient if he or she is engaging in intolerable behavior while bathing.
- Eliminate as much clutter and extraneous objects from the bathroom as possible.

Assistive Devices and Home Alterations
- Install window coverings to eliminate glare in the bathroom and in passageways leading to the bathroom.
- Because depth perception is likely to be impaired as a normal aspect of aging, consider the following techniques for stairways and passageways leading to the bathroom:
  - Paint a narrow strip at the edge of each step.
  - Paint the wall in the stairway leading to the bathroom a contrasting color from the steps to accentuate the stair rise.
  - Add lighting to the bathroom and the passageways leading to the bathroom.
  - Secure handrails, broken steps, and loose carpeting in the bathroom and on stairs and in passageways leading to the bathroom.
  - Paint the door to the bathroom a bright, eye-catching color.
- Install equipment as needed for bathroom transfers (e.g., grab bars) and for safe mobility in passageways leading to the bathroom (e.g., banisters, stair glides).
- Order and install equipment for bathing (e.g., shower chair, hand-held shower hose).

- Install safety gates where indicated (e.g., at the top of stairs).
- Install an electronic monitor (such as those used to monitor infants) in the bathroom.
- Modify doorways for accessibility (e.g., wider openings, lower thresholds).
- Change the lock on the bathroom door.
- Remove glass shower doors on bathtubs or otherwise alter bathing area for easier access.
- Install a screen or curtains to hide distracting items from view.
- Install bells or alarms on doors, cabinet doors, or drawers to alert the caregiver when the care recipient opens them.

Task Layer

- Consider alternative bathing schedules, such as a semiweekly tub bath and daily sponge baths.
- Hand bathing items to the care recipient one at a time as they are to be used.
- Use simple, clear, one-step directions, such as "Put soap on the washcloth" or "Lift your arm overhead."
- Demonstrate for the care recipient what to do or use hand-over-hand guiding.
- Help with the task of bathing only as much as necessary. For instance, if the care recipient is unable to wash his or her feet, the caregiver should help only with this activity and should supervise the remainder of the bathing task.
- Establish a calm and accepting atmosphere while the care recipient is bathing, especially when he or she is getting into and out of the tub or shower.
- Avoid scolding, criticizing, or invading the care recipient's personal space, especially if there are signs of agitation.
- Do not talk to the care recipient if he or she needs to concentrate on walking to the bathroom or getting into or out of the tub or shower. One-third of all falls occur because the person who fell was not paying sufficient attention while moving around (Hornbrook et al., 1994).
- Allow adequate time for the care recipient to adjust to changes in light intensity when entering or leaving the bathroom. Provide a safe place to stand or sit until his or her eyes accommodate to the difference.
- If the care recipient appears to be unwell or not at his or her best, avoid situations where falls might happen (e.g., bathtub, stairways, outdoors) and give extra assistance with bathing.

Social Groups

- Compliment the care recipient about how clean he or she is and the amount of effort he or she demonstrated.

- The caregiver may find it beneficial to ask himself or herself "Is it really necessary that I do the bathing or that the bathing is done in this way? Can it be done later or by someone else?"
- Expand the family's support network to include paid or unpaid helpers to provide assistance with bathing.
- Make a schedule of daily helpers that indicates the scope of each helper's visit. If bathing is to be part of the helper's duties, the caregiver must clearly communicate the specifics of how to perform this task.
- Ask the physician or pharmacist about the possible side effects of medications on performance in this area.

Technical Supports

Physical Therapist
Indicators of the need for a physical therapist consultation include potential or actual problems related to unsafe transfers, poor balance, unsteadiness, debility, and low endurance; caregiver physical strain from helping the care receiver; and the occurrence of a bathing-related event that triggers a catastrophic reaction. The physical therapist should
- Teach the caregiver back protection and back-strengthening techniques.
- Evaluate and order ambulation equipment necessary for self-care activities.
- Teach the caregiver to transfer the care recipient safely to the bathtub or shower.
- Develop and monitor a program to improve the care recipient's mobility.

Social Worker
During the consultation, the social worker should
- Help the caregiver obtain information about dementia and bathing and suggest contacting the local library and the Alzheimer's Association for materials about management of bathing in people with dementia.
- Provide information about support groups and other community resource agencies that provide assistance, counseling, and respite.
- Provide information about the benefits of adult day care for respite from the daily pressures of providing personal assistance to a person with dementia. Give the caregiver specific information about adult day care in the area.
- Provide information about the benefits of partial respite gained by attending a senior citizen center with the care recipient. Give the caregiver specific information about senior citizen centers in the area.
- Help the caregiver obtain information from churches and religious organizations about volunteer or low-cost help for a range of services.

EATING

Object Layer

Use and Manipulation of Common Home Objects
- Arrange utensils, dishware, and food in a consistent manner.
- Use a white plate to eliminate distractions from patterns on the dishware.
- Because perception of salty and sweet is reduced with age, use salt and sugar substitutes if allowed by the physician.
- Keep the table setting simple. Consider providing only one utensil.
- Use nonstick surfaces under the dishware, such as a placemat.
- Use a travel mug with a nonspill top or a cup with a top and straw if spilling is a problem.
- Ensure that there is an appetizing smell, if not from the food served, then from cinnamon or orange potpourri.
- Eliminate noxious odors (e.g., urine).
- Keep background noise low.
- Encourage the care recipient to use eyeglasses and dentures.
- Present courses or food items one at a time.
- Arrange food in an attractive manner on the plate and table.
- Offer chopped or soft foods if chewing is a problem. Moisten foods with gravy or sauce. Avoid foods with tough skins or that fall apart in the mouth (e.g., nuts, seeds) and dry, sticky foods (plain white bread, peanut butter).
- Cut food into small pieces if overstuffing is a problem.
- Place smaller portions on the plate if overeating is a problem.
- Have nutritious snacks available.
- Avoid using a bib. An alternative may be a shirt, smock, or apron (whatever article of clothing might normally be worn) to catch spills.
- If a wheelchair is used, transfer the care recipient to a regular chair when possible. If a wheelchair must be used at the table and the care recipient has good trunk support, remove the wheelchair's arms.
- Keep available objects or activities to distract the care recipient if she or he is engaging in intolerable behavior at mealtime.
- Eliminate as much clutter and extraneous objects from the eating area as possible.
- Remove knobs from the stove, and put away any sharp or dangerous items.

Assistive Devices and Home Alterations
- Install adequate lighting at the table and over countertops.
- Install safety gates where indicated (e.g., in doorway to kitchen).

- Install an electronic monitor (such as those used to monitor infants) in the kitchen or dining room.
- Modify doorways for accessibility (e.g., wider openings, lower thresholds).
- Install or change the lock on the kitchen door.
- Install locks on cabinet or appliance doors.
- Install a shutoff switch on electric or gas lines.
- Provide assistive devices (e.g., built-up utensils, scoop dishes).
- Provide a large, stable eating surface in an area where the family normally eats.
- Adjust the height of tables or chairs to position care recipient optimally.
- Install a screen or curtains to hide distracting items from view.
- Install bells or alarms on doors, cabinet doors, or drawers to alert the caregiver when the care recipient opens them.

Task Layer

- Position care recipient so that a 10- to 12-inch distance between plate and mouth can easily be maintained. Drinking liquids and eating semisolids may require an 8- to 10-inch distance.
- Allow and encourage finger feeding when the care recipient cannot use utensils efficiently.
- Turn off the television during mealtime if distraction is a problem.
- Do not rush the care recipient to finish eating.
- If the caregiver needs to feed the care recipient, he or she should use appropriate feeding techniques, including allowing sufficient time to swallow before another bite is introduced, not overloading the care recipient's mouth, encouraging the care recipient to hold the food or utensil and guiding his or her hand to the mouth, and not mixing food into a "hash." Light downward pressure on the chin may help prompt the care recipient to open his or her mouth.
- Engage in calm and pleasant social interaction.
- If overeating or undereating is a problem, offer smaller, nutritious meals more often during the day.
- If motor problems are present, explore positioning needs.
- Establish an eating routine and reinforce it with environmental cues (e.g., eat after some routine activity, post a daily schedule).
- When possible, encourage other family members (including the caregiver) to stay at the table and eat with the care recipient.

Social Groups

- If family members or friends who are not customarily present are asked to share in a meal, try to appoint one familiar person to attend primarily to the social interaction needs of the care recipient. If possible, keep the social group small (4 total, including the caregiver and care recipient).

- Explore how touch is generally used in the family. Refine touching to include hand-over-hand techniques, inhibitory touch to calm, or stimulating touch to refocus attention, and incorporate these normal patterns into the dining experience. Touch has been indicated to have a positive effect on nutritional intake (Mattes, 1987; Eaton, Mitchell-Bonair, & Friedmann, 1986).
- If the care recipient wears street clothes for lunch and dinner, socially acceptable behavior while eating may be encouraged.
- The caregiver may find it beneficial to ask himself or herself "Is it really necessary to prepare a meal? Can it be done more simply, later, or by someone else?"
- Expand the family's support network to include paid or unpaid helpers to provide assistance with mealtime.
- Make a schedule of daily helpers that indicates the scope of each helper's visit. If feeding is to be part of the helper's duties, the caregiver must clearly communicate the specifics of how to perform this task.
- Ask the physician or pharmacist about the possible side effects of medications on performance in this area.

Technical Supports

Physical Therapist
Indicators of the need for a physical therapist consultation include potential or actual problems related to unsafe transfers, poor balance, unsteadiness, debility, and low endurance; caregiver physical strain from helping the care receiver; and the occurrence of an eating-related event that triggers a catastrophic reaction. The physical therapist should

- Teach the caregiver to transfer the care recipient safely at the table.
- Teach the caregiver back protection and back-strengthening techniques.
- Develop and monitor a program to improve the care recipient's mobility.

Social Worker
During the consultation, the social worker should

- Help the caregiver obtain information about dementia and mealtime and suggest contacting the local library and the Alzheimer's Association for materials about management of eating for people with dementia.
- Provide information about support groups and other community resource agencies that provide assistance with meals, counseling, and respite.

- Provide information about the benefits of adult day care for respite from the daily pressures of providing personal assistance to a person with dementia. Give the caregiver specific information about adult day care in the area.
- Provide information about the benefits of partial respite and nutritional support gained by attending a senior citizen center with the care recipient. Give the caregiver specific information about senior citizen centers in the area.
- Help the caregiver obtain information from churches and religious organizations about volunteer or low-cost help for a range of services.

PERSONAL HYGIENE

Object Layer

Use and Manipulation of Common Home Objects
- Place all items for one specific grooming task in a marked container. Containers may be clear plastic or opaque, depending on distractibility. Containers should be marked with one of the following labels (arranged from simplest to most complex):
  - A picture of the care recipient performing the task for which the objects are needed,
  - A drawing or picture of another person performing the task,
  - A drawing of the objects, and
  - A label specifying the task or objects.
- Remove all objects that the care recipient does not use daily. Also remove from view all objects that belong to other family members.
- Put grooming items out in the sequence they will be needed, one task at a time.
- Only use products and product packaging that are familiar to the care recipient. For instance, pump-type containers of soap and toothpaste may be confusing to a person with memory problems.
- Purchase several identical personal care items so that familiar replacements are on hand. For instance, buy several toothbrushes or combs, all in one style and color, and use these to replace worn or lost items.
- Use labels or pictures to mark items as needed for certain tasks. For example, all shaving items may be marked "Shaving" and include a picture of a person shaving. If reading is a problem, a photograph of the care recipient shaving can be used.
- Provide physical assistance with all electrical appliances used in the bathroom, or arrange for the care recipient to use those appliances in another room. When necessary, remove all electrical appliances from the bathroom.

- Adjust the hot water heater to no higher than 120° F to avoid burns.
- If distractions are a problem, simplify the surroundings by removing items from the bathroom.
- Eliminate extraneous noise.
- Keep the bathroom comfortably warm.
- Keep available objects or activities to distract the care recipient if he or she is engaging in intolerable behavior during personal hygiene routines.
- Eliminate as much clutter and extraneous objects from the area as possible.

Assistive Devices and Home Alterations
- Install adequate lighting over the sink and countertops.
- Install window coverings to eliminate glare in the bathroom and in passageways leading to the bathroom.
- Because depth perception is likely to be impaired as a normal aspect of aging, consider the following techniques for stairways and passageways leading to the bathroom:
  - Paint a narrow strip at the edge of each step.
  - Paint the wall in the stairway leading to the bathroom a contrasting color from the steps to accentuate the stair rise.
  - Add lighting to the bathroom and passageways leading to the bathroom.
  - Secure handrails, broken steps, and loose carpeting in the bathroom and on stairs and in passageways leading to the bathroom.
  - Paint the door to the bathroom a bright, eye-catching color.
- Install equipment as needed for bathroom transfers (e.g., grab bars) and for safe mobility in passageways leading to the bathroom (e.g., banisters, stair glides).
- Order and install equipment for toileting (e.g., raised toilet seat).
- Install safety gates where indicated (e.g., at the top of stairs).
- Install an electronic monitor (such as those used to monitor infants) in the bathroom.
- Modify doorways for accessibility (e.g., wider openings, lower thresholds).
- Change the lock on the bathroom door.
- Install a screen or curtains to hide distracting items from view.
- Install bells or alarms on doors, cabinet doors, or drawers to alert the caregiver when the care recipient opens them.

Task Layer

- Post pictures or written directions to communicate the sequence of steps to be performed.
- Provide physical assistance in the form of hand-over-hand guiding for grooming tasks.

- Perform only those parts of tasks that the care recipient cannot perform, and allow the care recipient to participate at the level he or she is able to handle.
- Use short, one-step directions (e.g., "Turn toward me" or "Open your mouth").
- Engage in grooming tasks at the same time every day, and provide temporal cues if possible (e.g., always after breakfast).
- Do not ask the care recipient if he or she wants to brush teeth or shave. Tell him or her "We are going to brush your teeth now."
- Hand grooming items to the care recipient as they are needed. Name each item as it is presented.
- Allow the care recipient to take as much time as needed to complete the tasks.
- If the care recipient performs grooming tasks in an unusual but effective way, do not correct.

Social Groups

- Schedule the care recipient's grooming for periods of the day when other family members are not waiting for the bathroom. This will allow the care recipient to take the necessary amount of time for grooming.
- Establish a social goal for good grooming, such as saying "You look so clean and nice. Let's go for a walk and show you off."
- The caregiver may find it beneficial to ask himself or herself "Is this task really necessary? Can it be done later or by someone else?"
- Expand the family's support network to include paid or unpaid helpers to provide assistance with grooming.
- Make a schedule of daily helpers that indicates the scope of each helper's visit. If grooming is to be part of the helper's duties, the caregiver must clearly communicate the specifics of how to perform this task.
- Ask the physician or pharmacist about the possible side effects of medications on performance in this area.

Technical Supports

Physical Therapist

Indicators of the need for a physical therapist consultation include potential or actual problems related to poor balance, unsteadiness, debility, and low endurance; caregiver physical strain from helping the care receiver; and the occurrence of a self-care-related event that triggers a catastrophic reaction. The physical therapist should

- Teach the caregiver to transfer the care recipient safely.
- Teach the caregiver back protection and back-strengthening techniques.
- Develop and monitor a program to improve the care recipient's mobility.

Social Worker

During the consultation, the social worker should

- Help the caregiver obtain information about dementia and performance of personal hygiene tasks, such as grooming, and suggest contacting the local library and the Alzheimer's Association for materials about management of personal hygiene for people with dementia.
- Provide information about support groups and other community resource agencies that provide assistance with grooming and other self-care tasks, counseling, and respite.
- Provide information about the benefits of adult day care for respite from the daily pressures of providing personal assistance to a person with dementia. Give the caregiver specific information about adult day care in the area.
- Provide information about the benefits of partial respite gained by attending a senior citizen center with the care recipient. Give the caregiver specific information about senior citizen centers in the area.
- Help the caregiver obtain information from churches and religious organizations about volunteer or low-cost help for a range of services.

COMMUNICATION

Learning to communicate effectively with a person with dementia is very important and key to enhancing his or her ability to engage in everyday activities. The strategies listed here reflect ways to simplify verbal and nonverbal communication to enhance task performance.

- Use the most easily understood methods to convey information. Communication methods may be used in combination to augment each other and include, arranged from simplest to most complex,
  - Gentle and slow hand-over-hand guiding,
  - Physical demonstration of one step in a process,
  - A picture of the care recipient doing what is being communicated,
  - A drawing or picture of another person doing what is being communicated,
  - Simple and short one-step verbal directions, and
  - Written labels or instructions.
- Use nouns and names instead of pronouns ("Mary" or "Paul" instead of "she" or "he").
- Emphasize nonverbal communication. Some research has shown that the nonverbal communication of individuals with dementia is no different than that of individuals without dementia (Hoffman, 1990).
- Use facial expressions, universally understood hand signs (e.g., for "come here" and "stop"), and touch to convey information.

- Use positive affective nonverbal messages to elicit positive affective nonverbal responses. Likewise, negative affective nonverbal messages may elicit withdrawal and catastrophic reactions.
- Allow several minutes for the care recipient to respond to nonverbal and verbal messages.
- Keep verbal messages short and simple.
- Use "yes–no" or "either–or" questions when possible.
- If the care recipient is searching for a word, it is all right to provide it.
- Avoid interrupting the care recipient.
- If a hearing problem is present or if attention is distracted, gain the care recipient's attention with a touch. Once he or she is facing you, speak slowly, clearly, and simply in a slightly louder but lower-pitched voice.
- If the care recipient uses a hearing aid, check the batteries regularly. A hearing aid battery has a very short life span, as little as 2 weeks if used often. When disposing of hearing aid batteries, be careful to remove them from any areas where the care recipient may find and ingest them.
- Be vigilant in identifying and receiving the nonverbal messages the care recipient is sending.
- Do not pull or push to get the care recipient to do what you want him or her to do. Move up behind him or her and to one side, take his or her elbow, and gently walk with him or her while calmly stating where the two of you are going. If the care recipient resists, do not force him or her to comply.
- Use of humor can defuse a tense situation. However, the care recipient should not be the target of the humor, and sarcasm should be avoided.
- Use a portable tape recorder with headphones to provide a small respite from repetitive questioning or other verbal perseveration.
- Keep available objects or activities to distract the care recipient if she or he is engaging in intolerable behavior during communication efforts.
- Remove from view objects that stimulate upsetting topics.

Social Groups

- Keep a record of nonverbal communication techniques the care recipient uses to assist others who may wish to interact with him or her.
- Convey calm, accepting, reassuring attitudes and messages as much as possible. Although communication is impaired, the care recipient may actually be more acutely aware of emotional tones than previously.
- Make a schedule of daily helpers that indicates the scope of each helper's visit. The caregiver must provide specific instructions for communicating with the care recipient.

- Ask the physician or pharmacist about the possible side effects of medications on performance in this area.

Technical Supports

Social Worker

A social work consultation is indicated when difficulty communicating triggers catastrophic reactions. During the consultation, the social worker should

- Help the caregiver obtain information about dementia and communication and suggest contacting the local library and the Alzheimer's Association for materials about management of communication with people with dementia.
- Provide information about support groups and other community resource agencies that provide assistance and information about communication, counseling, and respite.
- Provide information about the benefits of adult day care for respite from the daily pressures of providing personal assistance to a person with dementia. Give the caregiver specific information about adult day care in the area.
- Provide information about the benefits of partial respite gained by attending a senior citizen center with the care recipient. Give the caregiver specific information about senior citizen centers in the area.
- Help the caregiver obtain information from churches and religious organizations about volunteer or low-cost help for a range of services.

MOBILITY

Object Layer

- Eliminate glare from all areas where the care recipient is transferring or ambulating.
- Remove items from the floor, stairways, and passageways.
- Place sturdy furniture strategically for use as an ambulation and transferring aid.
- Install window coverings to eliminate glare in key rooms and in passageways throughout the house.
- Because depth perception is likely to be impaired as a normal aspect of aging, consider the following techniques for stairways and passageways:
  - Paint a narrow strip at the edge of each step.
  - Paint the wall in the stairway a contrasting color from the steps to accentuate the stair rise.
  - Add lighting to the rooms and passageways where the care recipient must transfer or ambulate.

- Secure handrails, broken steps, and loose carpeting in key rooms, on stairs, and in passageways.
- Paint the doors to key rooms a bright, eye-catching color.
- Install a vertical strip of wallpaper or paint a vertical line as a visual cue to rise from a chair.

- Install equipment as needed for transfers (e.g., grab bars) and for safe mobility in key rooms and passageways (e.g., banisters, stair glides).
- Order and install equipment to eliminate the need to transfer or ambulate when these activities are unsafe (e.g., urinal, long-handled reacher, remote control, environmental control unit).
- Install safety gates where indicated (e.g., at the top of stairs).
- Install electronic monitors (such as those used to monitor infants) in key areas of the home.
- Modify doorways for accessibility (e.g., wider openings, lower thresholds).
- Consider installing a ramp for easier and safer access to the outdoors.

Task Layer

- When rising to stand, direct the care recipient's attention along a vertical line or to a place above his or her head to encourage back extension.
- Use one-word commands when the care recipient is transferring or ambulating (e.g., "turn," "pivot," "sit").
- Gently lean on the care recipient as appropriate to encourage weight shifting.
- Walk arm-in-arm with the care recipient; do not pull or push.
- Do not speak to the care recipient while he or she is walking or moving.
- Do not let the care recipient pull on you to stand. Instead, stand slightly to one side and help the care recipient push himself or herself to a standing position.
- Tighten your stomach muscles before moving care recipient to avoid back strain and sprain.
- When the care recipient is immobilized because of fear or uncertainty, entice him or her to move by pointing out a goal (e.g., "Let's go see those flowers on the table").
- When possible, eliminate the need to transfer or ambulate by arranging needed items close to the care recipient.
- Allow adequate time for the care recipient to adjust to changes in light intensity, such as when entering a dark building on a bright day. Provide a safe place to stand or sit until his or her eyes accommodate to the difference.
- If the care recipient appears to be unwell or not at his or her best, avoid ambulating and transferring or provide more assistance than typically is needed.

Social Groups

- Praise the care recipient for safe behaviors (e.g., watching where he or she is going, holding the handrail, paying attention).
- In households where more than one caregiver is present, the primary caregiver establishes routines and specifics of ambulation and transfers. He or she should develop this routine in detail and formulate specific instructions to be conveyed to all caregivers.
- Use positive reinforcement as a powerful and effective tool to promote a degree of independence in mobility.
- Expand the family's support network to include paid or unpaid helpers to provide assistance with transfers and ambulation.
- Make a schedule of daily helpers that indicates the scope of each helper's visit. If the helper is to assist with transfers and ambulation, the caregiver must clearly communicate the specifics of how to perform these tasks.
- Ask the physician or pharmacist about the possible side effects of medications on performance in this area.

Technical Supports

Physical Therapist

Indicators of the need for a physical therapist consultation include potential or actual problems related to poor balance, unsteadiness, debility, and low endurance; caregiver physical strain from helping the care receiver; and a mobility-related event that triggers a catastrophic reaction. The physical therapist should

- Teach the caregiver to transfer the care recipient safely (e.g., bed to chair, chair to stand).
- Teach the caregiver back protection and back-strengthening techniques.
- Develop and monitor a program to improve the care recipient's mobility.
- Assess for and provide equipment to improve mobility.

Social Worker

During the consultation, the social worker should

- Help the caregiver obtain information about dementia and mobility and suggest contacting the local library and Alzheimer's Association for materials about management of mobility for people with dementia.
- Provide information about support groups and other community resource agencies that provide assistance, equipment, counseling, and respite.
- Provide information about the benefits of adult day care for respite from the daily pressures of providing personal assistance to a person with dementia and as an outlet for practice with ambulation and transfers. Give the caregiver specific information about adult day care in the area.

- Help the caregiver obtain information from churches and religious organizations about volunteer or low-cost help and equipment for a range of services.

SAFETY

Object Layer

Use and Manipulation of Common Home Objects
- Use "hot" colors to increase the visibility of objects. Hot colors include yellows, oranges, and reds. Avoid "cool" colors, which include greens and blues.
- Use dark colors and increase the size of letters, forms, or pictures used to communicate information to the care recipient.
- Reduce glare by
  - Providing polarized sunglasses outdoors;
  - Eliminating highly polished surfaces, especially floors;
  - Placing a nonskid rug over bare floors under windows; and
  - Using light letters on a dark background for signs.
- In the bathroom, place objects within the triangle of efficiency to accommodate reach limitations associated with aging.
- Eliminate background noise that may interfere with the care recipient's ability to hear conversation.
- If the care recipient uses a hearing aid, check the batteries regularly. A hearing aid battery has a very short life span, as little as 2 weeks if used often. When disposing of hearing aid batteries, be careful to remove them from any areas where the care recipient may find and ingest them.
- Leave all toxic substances in the original container and lock them up.
- Arrange the furniture, if possible, so that the care recipient can use it as a support when moving about the house. Use nightlights and safety gates at the top of stairs.
- Leave the light on in the bathroom.
- Consider using an electronic monitor (such as those used to monitor infants) as much as possible to supervise the activities of the care recipient.
- Place locks or bells at the tops of doors to prevent the caregiver from walking outdoors unsupervised. Also, a "stop" sign on the front door may deter the care recipient from leaving.
- Remove knobs from the stove, and put away any sharp or dangerous items from the kitchen.

Assistive Devices and Home Alterations
- Because depth perception is likely to be impaired as a normal aspect of aging, consider the following techniques for stairways:

- - Paint a narrow strip at the edge of each step.
  - Paint the wall in the stairway a contrasting color from the steps to accentuate the stair rise.
  - Illuminate stairways at all times.
  - Secure handrails, broken steps, and loose carpeting in key rooms, on stairs, and in passageways.
  - Do not speak to the care recipient unnecessarily when going up or down steps. The care recipient may become distracted and fall.
  - Install a screen or other device to eliminate shadows on outside stairways. Where light and dark areas meet can be confused for a step.
  - Eliminate shadows from windows on indoor stairways with curtains or blinds.
  - Keep all stairways and passageways free of objects.
- Use bright but diffuse lighting to create overall illumination and eliminate pockets of light and shadow.
- Install window coverings to eliminate glare in key rooms and in passageways throughout the house.
- Add lighting to rooms or passageways where care recipient must transfer or ambulate.
- Install a vertical strip of wallpaper or paint a vertical line as a visual cue to rise from a chair.
- Paint doors to key rooms a bright, eye-catching color.
- Install equipment as needed for transfers (e.g., grab bars) and for safe mobility in key rooms and passageways (e.g., banisters, stair glides).
- Order and install equipment to eliminate the need to transfer or ambulate when these activities are unsafe (e.g., urinal, long-handled reacher, remote control, environmental control unit).
- Consider adaptive equipment for the bathroom to assist in bathing and toileting. Especially useful are raised toilet seats, grab bars, extended shower hoses, bath mats, and bath seats.
- Install safety gates where indicated (e.g., at the top of stairs).
- Modify doorways for accessibility (e.g., wider openings, lower thresholds).
- Install smoke and carbon monoxide detectors, and check the batteries regularly.
- Install adequate lighting at the table and over countertops.
- Install or change the locks on key doors.
- Install locks on cabinet or appliance doors.
- Install a shutoff switch on electric or gas lines.
- Adjust the height of tables or chairs to position care recipient optimally.
- Install a screen or curtains to hide distracting items from view.

- Install bells or alarms on doors, cabinet doors, or drawers to alert the caregiver when the care recipient opens them.

Task Layer

- Take the care recipient's arm when walking in unfamiliar, distracting, or uneven areas.
- Do not talk to the care recipient if he or she needs to concentrate on walking. One-third of all falls occur because the person who fell was not paying sufficient attention while moving around (Hornbrook et al., 1994).
- Allow adequate time for the care recipient to adjust to changes in light intensity, such as when entering a dark building on a bright day. Provide a safe place to stand or sit until his or her eyes accommodate to the difference.
- If the care recipient appears to be unwell or not at his or her best, avoid situations that present risk for falls (e.g., bathtub, stairways, outdoors).
- Develop and practice a fire evacuation plan.
- Place emergency numbers by the telephone and practice using them.
- Set the temperature on the hot water heater at no more than 120° F to avoid scalding.
- Disable appliances or items that are dangerous for the care recipient to use.

Social Groups

- Never leave the care recipient in the car unattended; an accident could happen.
- Arrange for a backup person to stay with the care recipient in case the caregiver is ill or must go out.
- Praise the care recipient for safe behaviors (e.g., watching where he or she is going, holding the handrail, paying attention).

Technical Supports

Physical Therapist

Indicators of the need for a physical therapist consultation include potential or actual problems related to poor balance, unsteadiness, debility, and low endurance; caregiver physical strain from helping the care receiver; and the occurrence of a safety-related event that triggers a catastrophic reaction. The physical therapist should

- Teach the caregiver to transfer the care recipient safely (e.g., bed to chair, chair to stand).
- Teach the caregiver back protection and back-strengthening techniques.
- Develop and monitor a program to improve the care recipient's mobility.
- Assess for and provide equipment to improve mobility.

Social Worker

During the consultation, the social worker should

- Help the caregiver obtain information about dementia and safety and suggest contacting the local library and Alzheimer's Association for materials about management of safety issues with people with dementia.
- Provide information about support groups and other community resource agencies that provide assistance, counseling, and respite.
- Provide information about the benefits of adult day care for respite from the daily pressures of providing personal assistance to a person with dementia. Give the caregiver specific information about adult day care in the area.
- Provide information about the benefits of partial respite gained by attending a senior citizen center with the care recipient. Give the caregiver specific information about senior citizen centers in the area.
- Help the caregiver obtain information from churches and religious organizations about volunteer or low-cost help for a range of services.

LEISURE AND INSTRUMENTAL ACTIVITIES OF DAILY LIVING

Object Layer

Use and Manipulation of Objects in Home

- Put out one interesting item, game, or activity where the care recipient will notice it. When interest decreases, replace with another item, game, or activity of similar interest and skill level.
- Ensure that objects used for work or leisure are simple to use and familiar.
- Simplify one area in the home, garage, or yard for the care recipient to roam and "putter" in freely.
- Set up an electronic monitor (such as those used to monitor infants) in the area where the care recipient is working or playing to make supervision easier.

Assistive Devices and Home Alterations

- Install window coverings to eliminate glare in areas throughout the house where the care recipient is engaged in a leisure activity.
- Because depth perception is likely to be impaired as a normal aspect of aging, consider the following techniques for stairways and passageways:
  - Paint a narrow strip at the edge of each step.
  - Paint the wall in the stairway a contrasting color from the steps to accentuate the stair rise.

- Add lighting to rooms or passageways where care recipient is engaged in leisure pursuits.
- Secure handrails, broken steps, and loose carpeting in key rooms, on stairs, and in passageways.
- Paint doors to key rooms a bright, eye-catching color.
- Order and install equipment to facilitate leisure or instrumental activities of daily living (e.g., games, long-handled reacher, remote control, environmental control unit).
- Create a safe area for leisure by installing
  - Safety gates where indicated (e.g., at the top of stairs),
  - Electronic monitors (such as those used to monitor infants) in key areas of the home,
  - Locks on key doors,
  - Locks on cabinet or appliance doors,
  - A shutoff switch on electric or gas lines, and
  - Bells or alarms on doors, cabinet doors, or drawers to alert the caregiver when the care recipient opens them.
- Purchase and install organizers for leisure materials.
- Install adequate lighting at the table, over countertops, and in work areas.
- Adjust the height of tables or chairs to position care recipient optimally.
- Install a screen or curtains to hide distracting items from view.

Task Layer

- Plan periods for work and leisure as a normal part of the daily routine.
- Relax the rules of the leisure activity and the standards of performance for work activities to provide a feeling of success. For example, if the bed is made incorrectly, praise the care recipient for his or her efforts and ignore the mistakes.
- Choose activities based on Levy's (1987) suggestions for pastimes. In general, choose activities that
  - Use gross motor skills,
  - Are highly familiar,
  - Are repetitive,
  - Have a predictable and notable effect on the environment,
  - Require one-step directions, or
  - Tap former interests or roles.
- Establish success experiences by, for example, allowing the care recipient to win a game, praising how he or she completed a task or the outcome, and commenting on how great it is to have the care recipient's help or companionship.

- On days when activities normally undertaken are impossible, reduce the challenge of the activity by simplifying it (e.g., reduce the number of objects or choices, give more verbal assistance, simplify the rules).
- Encourage exercise and activities that require no strenuous gross motor actions. Walking with another person is an excellent pastime for individuals with impairment as long as the route is safe. Choose a circular route for walking, because it is sometimes difficult to have the care recipient turn around and change directions. If this must be done, stop the care recipient, distract him or her by stopping to admire something, then casually start up again in the direction you want to go.
- Do not pull or push to get the care recipient to do what you want him or her to do. Move up behind and to one side, take the care recipient's elbow, and gently walk with him or her while calmly stating where the two of you are going. If the care recipient resists, do not force him or her to comply.
- Avoid competitive games or activities. Give preference to any leisure or work outlet that is cooperative.
- If traveling is an option, assess how well the care recipient handles small outings and changes in the daily routine. Irritability, catastrophic reactions, loss of appetite, and difficulty sleeping all indicate that the outing was too disruptive. However, if the care recipient accommodates these changes well, a trip away from home may be fairly well tolerated. Even when the care recipient tolerates travel well, however, the caregiver should expect the care recipient to be more confused and edgy than usual when traveling. The following are some considerations to accommodate the care recipient's and caregiver's needs when planning a trip:
  - Preserve the daily routine.
  - Plan times for rest (three rests plus meals are optimal).
  - Consider taking a third person along to help with the care recipient and to give the caregiver a rest. Traveling with a care recipient can be more work than simply staying at home.
  - Bring an "Occupied" sign to place on public restroom doors if the care recipient needs help to toilet. Alternately, look for family restrooms that allow caregivers to help care recipients in privacy.
  - Carry a recent photo of the care recipient in case he or she gets lost. Also, make note of the clothing worn each day by the care recipient, and make sure the person is carrying some form of identification. Place a card in the care recipient's pocket with the caregiver's name, the name of the hotel, an emergency number at home, and the name of the tour, if applicable.
  - Plan to provide extra help with dressing and bathing, because the surroundings will be unfamiliar and confusing.

- Keep travel plans flexible and arrival and departure dates open to accommodate the possibility that things do not proceed as anticipated.
- Be realistic. Vacations do not generally relax the care recipient, and he or she will not necessarily return "better off."
- If traveling by air, the caregiver should notify the airline that he or she is traveling with an individual who has an impairment.
- Keep a change of clothing and some premoistened towels handy.
- Bring a security object for the care recipient.

Social Groups

- Praise desirable behavior and ignore undesirable behavior. If undesirable behavior becomes intolerable, distract the care recipient.
- Convey the attitude that leisure outlets are valued and that work done by the care recipient contributes to the household.
- Keep contact with friends and family. Establish a regular routine that involves recreational visits by the same one or two people.
- Allow the care recipient to watch the activities of the neighborhood through the window or from the porch, as long as he or she is not disturbed by his or her observations. This vicarious involvement will expand the care recipient's social group.

Technical Supports

Social Worker
A social work consultation is indicated when community resources or home modifications are needed. During the consultation, the social worker should
- Help the caregiver obtain information about dementia and leisure and IADL and suggest contacting the local library and the Alzheimer's Association for materials about management of leisure and IADL for people with dementia.
- Provide information about support groups and other community resource agencies that provide assistance, counseling, and respite.
- Provide information about the benefits of adult day care for respite from the daily pressures of providing personal assistance to a person with dementia and as a leisure outlet. Give the caregiver specific information about adult day care in the area.
- Provide information about the benefits of partial respite gained by attending a senior citizen center with the care recipient. Give the caregiver specific information about senior citizen centers in the area.
- Help the caregiver obtain information from churches and religious organizations about volunteer or low-cost help for a range of services.

WANDERING

Wandering can manifest as trying to leave the home (elopement), aimless wandering or pacing inside the home, rummaging and looking for lost object, or collecting items throughout the home and hoarding them.

Object Layer

Use and Manipulation of Objects in Home

- For a care recipient who likes to rummage, provide objects that are interesting to touch and manipulate. People with dementia who rummage through drawers and closets may be seeking tactile stimulation. The objects may be left out for easy access or placed all together in places where the care recipient typically rummages.
- Place a large "Stop" or "Authorized Personnel Only" sign on doors that lead outside.
- Purchase an electronic monitor (such as those used to monitor infants) and supervise activities from another room.
- Place bells or alarms on key doors to alert the caregiver when the care recipient opens them. This strategy is especially useful in conjunction with a monitor.
- Use fabric or wallpaper to disguise the outside door. Fabric also can be used to cover the knob to camouflage it to prevent exiting behavior.
- Purchase a Medic Alert bracelet, or keep a card with the caregiver's name and address in the care recipient's pocket.
- Adjust the lighting to provide even illumination without shadows or pools of bright light. At night, use two or three dim sources of light in the bedroom. However, be careful not to overilluminate the bedroom and risk waking the care recipient.
- If the care recipient is looking for lost or misplaced items (e.g., keys, wallets), try purchasing duplicates and producing these items when necessary. In addition, replace important items with similar items that are not valuable. For instance, an old key can be used to replace the car keys, which are in turn kept out of sight.
- Eliminate as much clutter from the home as possible. A simple environment is less distracting and less likely to invite the care recipient to look for lost objects.
- If the care recipient hides objects and then looks for them, provide him or her with a special place where items can be kept safely.
- Install a high portable gate at the top of the stairs. Shop carefully to find one that is at least 3 feet high.

Assistive Devices and Home Alterations

- Install window coverings to eliminate glare in key rooms and in passageways throughout the house.
- Because depth perception is likely to be impaired as a normal aspect of aging, consider the following techniques for stairways and passageways to avoid accidents when the care recipient wanders:
  - Paint a narrow strip at the edge of each step.
  - Paint the wall in the stairway a contrasting color from the steps to accentuate the stair rise.
  - Add lighting to rooms or passageways where the care recipient wanders.
  - Secure handrails, broken steps, and loose carpeting in key rooms, on stairs, and in passageways.
  - Disguise doors to key rooms with a wall hanging or wallpaper.
- Install safety gates where indicated (e.g., at the top of stairs).
- Install an electronic monitor (such as those used to monitor infants) in key areas of the home.
- Install smoke and carbon monoxide detectors, and check the batteries regularly.
- Install or change the locks on key doors.
- Install locks on cabinet or appliance doors.
- Install a shutoff switch on electric or gas lines.
- Install a screen or curtains to hide distracting items from view.
- Install bells or alarms on doors, cabinet doors, or drawers to alert the caregiver to instances when the care recipient opens them.
- Provide exercise equipment.

Task Layer

- Provide acceptable outlets for wandering. Examples include visiting a museum, mall walking, and strolling around the neighborhood or yard.
- Increase the opportunities for exercise during the day.
- Distract the care recipient by providing some work or leisure outlet (see the section "Leisure and Instrumental Activities of Daily Living"). This strategy may be especially useful during times of the day when wandering typically happens, such as with sundowning (the state of increased agitation, activity, and negative behaviors that happen late in the day through the evening hours).
- Encourage the care recipient to use a platform rocker or chair when he or she feels restless.
- Take the care recipient into a room that is kept very simple to provide a low-stimulus rest if it appears that anxiety or too much stimulation is a factor in the wandering.

- Establish a routine before bed that prepares the care recipient for sleep, if patterns of sleep are reversed and the care recipient wanders during the night. Choose activities that are soothing and pleasant but not exciting.
- Avoid liquids for a couple of hours before bedtime to avoid the need to move around the house at night.

Social Groups

- Ask the physician or pharmacist about the possible side effects of medications.
- Consider using adult day care to provide supervised activity.
- Ask neighbors and police to watch for the care recipient and to alert the caregiver if the care recipient is seen unsupervised.
- Ask for or purchase help from a friend or neighbor to take the care recipient out for a walk every day.

Technical Supports

Social Worker

A social work consultation is indicated when additional or highly specialized community resources or home alterations are needed. During the consultation, the social worker should

- Help the caregiver obtain information about dementia and wandering and suggest contacting the local library and the Alzheimer's Association for materials about management of wandering in people with dementia.
- Provide information about support groups and other community resource agencies that provide assistance, counseling, and respite.
- Provide information about the benefits of adult day care for respite from the daily pressures of providing personal assistance to a person with dementia and as an outlet for urges related to wandering. Give the caregiver specific information about adult day care in the area.
- Provide information about the benefits of partial respite gained by attending a senior citizen center with the care recipient. Give the caregiver specific information about senior citizen centers in the area.
- Help the caregiver obtain information from churches and religious organizations about volunteer or low-cost help for a range of services.

CATASTROPHIC REACTIONS

Understanding and Avoiding Catastrophic Reactions

Catastrophic reactions are excessive emotional responses, such as crying, hitting, screaming, and pacing, in reaction to seemingly minor stresses (Corcoran &

Gitlin, 2001; Mace, 1987; Swanson, Maas, & Buckwalter, 1993). Catastrophic reactions are upsetting to both the caregiver and the care recipient and may occur without apparent provocation. Such emotional outbursts or fearful withdrawals are widely considered to be the care recipient's response to a perceived threat. The perceived threat may be external (e.g., excessive questioning by a caregiver or health professional, disturbing patterns of light) or internal (e.g., hallucinations, delusions, paranoia). Although it may be difficult to determine what stimulus the care recipient perceives as threatening, the caregiver should attempt to trace the catastrophic reaction to its source and, if possible, eliminate or modify the threatening stimulus to prevent further catastrophic reactions. The list of potential threatening stimuli is endless but can include

- Pain;
- Feelings of insecurity, anger, fear, or frustration;
- Arguments, contradictions, or scoldings;
- Caregiver impatience or irritation;
- Fatigue;
- Activities requiring close personal contact, such as toileting, bathing, or dressing;
- Rushed or hurried activities;
- Change in routine or location, including vacations or hospitalization;
- Noisy, confusing, or overly stimulating environments (including television viewing, which may be perceived as real);
- Strangers;
- Distortion of light, dark, time, space, or sleep cycles;
- Unmet needs, such as hunger, thirst, boredom, constipation, or full bladder; and
- Invasion of personal space or possessions.

An additional method for avoiding catastrophic reactions involves establishing a predictable routine that includes several periods in a low-stimulus environment. Many caregivers perceive that inactivity by their family member is to be avoided. However, Hall and Buckwalter (1987) reported a reduction in the frequency of catastrophic reactions when people with dementia were allowed to "shut down" for a short period several times a day. Hall and Buckwalter hypothesized that the confusion and uncertainty associated with dementia result in a greater number of stressors, largely because the care recipient is no longer able to make sense of the environment. In addition, dementia progressively reduces the care recipient's coping strategies and therefore his or her ability to deal with those added stressors.

During any given day, the stressors may stockpile until the care recipient's available coping strategies are completely overwhelmed and a catastrophic reaction ensues. This cycle may be quite short, resulting in frequent or almost constant catastrophic reactions. By periodically spending time in a low-stimulus environment, the care recipient may be able to reduce his or her stress level and renew his or her ability to use acceptable coping strategies.

A low-stimulus environment must be individually designed for each person but usually includes a quiet room with calming visual stimuli and a comfortable reclining or semireclining chair. Conversation should be avoided, although touch should be maintained (e.g., holding hands). Also, slow rhythmical stroking (neck, arms, or back) can be calming if the care recipient is not upset by touch.

Object Layer

- Install window coverings to eliminate glare in key rooms and in passageways throughout the house.
- Because depth perception is likely to be impaired as a normal aspect of aging, consider the following techniques for stairways and passageways:
  - Paint a narrow strip at the edge of each step.
  - Paint the wall in the stairway a contrasting color from the steps to accentuate the stair rise.
  - Add lighting to rooms or passageways where the care recipient must transfer or ambulate.
  - Secure handrails, broken steps, and loose carpeting in key rooms, on stairs, and in passageways.
  - Paint doors to key rooms a bright, eye-catching color.
  - Install a vertical strip of wallpaper or paint a vertical line as a visual cue to rise from a chair.
- Install equipment as needed for transfers (e.g., grab bars) and for safe mobility in key rooms and passageways (e.g., banisters, stair glides).
- Install equipment to eliminate the need to transfer or ambulate when these activities are unsafe (e.g., urinal, long-handled reacher, remote control, environmental control unit).
- Install safety gates where indicated (e.g., at the top of stairs).
- Install electronic monitors (such as those used to monitor infants) in key areas of the home.
- Modify doorways for accessibility (e.g., wider openings, lower thresholds).
- Install bells or alarms on doors, cabinet doors, or drawers to alert the caregiver when the care recipient opens them.
- Install adequate lighting in key areas.
- Install or change the locks on key doors.
- Install locks on cabinet or appliance doors.
- Install a shutoff switch on electric or gas lines.
- Adjust the height of tables or chairs to position care recipient optimally and comfortably.
- Install a screen or curtains to hide distracting items from view.

Task Layer

- Look for early-warning signs (e.g., wringing of hands, refusal to make eye contact, tense or upset expression, unusual voice pattern or pitch restlessness) and intervene immediately.
- Most importantly, the caregiver should protect himself or herself by staying out of the way if the care recipient directs his or her anger at the caregiver. The caregiver should not fight back, scream, or scold; he or she should just leave the room and tell the care recipient that he or she will come back when the care recipient feels better.
- Never turn your back on a person who is acting out.
- Avoid feeling rejected or guilty. If possible, ask another person to stay with the care recipient while you leave the room.
- Allay fears, offer reassurance, and let the care recipient know that everything is OK. Acknowledge feelings and use active listening (e.g., "You seem unhappy [or upset, or angry]").
- Avoid using humor or sarcasm.
- Use simple, clear, direct language.
- Use a gentle, firm touch if the care recipient allows it.
- Keep your hands in view.
- Avoid exaggerated or nervous gestures. Keep your actions minimal.
- Stand to one side, use "soft" eye contact that conveys empathy, and stay out of the care recipient's personal space (about 3 feet). Avoid standing over the care recipient.
- Appear nonconfrontational; avoid sounding angry, upset, or disappointed.
- Gently tell the care recipient what you want him or her to do, not what you want him or her to stop doing.
- Remove yourself from the situation; let the care recipient choose where he or she wishes to go in the home and where to sit, if desired.
- Do not restrain the care recipient from leaving; instead, go with him or her.
- Attempt to establish a quiet, soothing environment. Quietly indicate for others to leave the room.
- Distract the care recipient's attention.
- Allow the care recipient to express feelings, and listen to him or her without judgment. If the care recipient is aphasic, acknowledge the apparent emotions.

Technical Supports

Social Worker

A social work consultation is indicated when highly specialized or unusual community resources or home alterations are needed. During the consultation, the social worker should

- Help the caregiver obtain information about dementia and catastrophic reactions and contact the local library and Alzheimer's Association for materials about management of catastrophic reactions in people with dementia.
- Provide information about support groups and other community resource agencies that provide assistance, counseling, and respite.
- Provide information about the benefits of adult day care for respite from the daily pressures of providing personal assistance to a person with dementia and dealing with catastrophic reactions. Give the caregiver specific information about adult day care in the area.
- Provide information about the benefits of partial respite gained by attending a senior citizen center with the care recipient. Give the caregiver specific information about senior citizen centers in the area.
- Help the caregiver obtain information from churches and religious organizations about volunteer or low-cost help for a range of services.

CAREGIVER-CENTERED CONCERNS

Sources of caregiver-centered problems include
- Lack of information about dementia,
- Stress,
- Depression,
- Embarrassment,
- Fatigue or interrupted sleep,
- Boredom,
- Substance abuse,
- Poor health,
- Lack of social supports,
- Lack of formal resources,
- Fear for personal safety,
- Uncertainty about how to deal with catastrophic reactions, and
- Care recipient's resistance to care.

Object Layer

- Use a portable tape recorder with headphones to provide a small respite from repetitive questioning or other verbal perseveration.
- Supervision may be easier or allow more rest if an electronic monitor (such as those used to monitor infants) or gates in doorways are used.
- Contact the local library and Alzheimer's Association for materials about dementia management.
- Make a list of all the strategies that work well, and keep it handy.

- Keep available objects or activities to distract the care recipient if she or he is engaging in intolerable behavior.
- Getting others to help may be easier if the caregiver keeps an updated record of strategies that work and clues to communicating with the care recipient, including signals that he or she is upset.

Task Layer

- Practice, practice, practice energy conservation techniques.
- Interrupted sleep may be less of a problem if the caregiver can take a nap every day. An alternative may be to arrange for someone to spend the night once or twice a week so the caregiver can get a full night's sleep.
- The daily schedule can be planned to include exercise, even if it must be done with the care recipient (e.g., walking, stretching, running in place, stationary biking).
- Generous use of praise by the caregiver toward the care recipient has an interesting effect—the caregiver begins to focus on the care recipient's positive points. At first, the caregiver may have to give praise for very small and seemingly insignificant actions. It may even feel uncomfortable and stilted. Soon these feelings pass, and opportunities for praise are more apparent and meaningful.

Social Groups

- Contact the local Alzheimer's Association for information about support groups and other resource agencies that provide assistance, counseling, and respite resources.
- Make a schedule of daily helpers that indicates the focus of each helper's visit (e.g., leisure activities, self-care). The caregiver must clearly communicate the specifics of how to perform each task.
- Contact the local Area Agency on Aging to inquire about programs that may be beneficial (e.g., counseling, respite).
- Consider use of adult day care a few times a week. Call local adult day care providers for information (Appendix C lists some national organizations that may offer useful information).
- Attend a senior citizen center with the care recipient for partial respite and to get out of the house.
- Contact churches and religious organizations, which are good sources of volunteer or low-cost help for a range of services.
- Envision the best possible present and future for the household, and specify what that vision will look like and what needs to be done to make it reality.
- When asking for or arranging help, make sure the focus is on how the help will support the caregiver, who will in turn support the care recipient. For instance,

a neighbor, friend, or family member can be asked to watch television with the care recipient while the caregiver goes out or takes a nap.

- Spend some time thinking about which behaviors of the care recipient are intolerable and which are simply annoying. Ignore those behaviors that are annoying but systematically address intolerable behaviors as problems that are likely to benefit from an environmental approach.

- The caregiver may find it beneficial to ask himself or herself "Is this task really necessary? Can it be done later or by someone else?"

- Try to maintain a private area that the care recipient cannot easily enter to serve as a small refuge for short periods.

- The caregiver should plan to spend some time each day for himself or herself, even if it's just a couple of minutes to soak in a hot bath.

REFERENCES

Corcoran, M. A., & Gitlin, L. N. (2001). Family caregiver acceptance and use of environmental strategies provided in an occupational therapy intervention. *Physical and Occupational Therapy in Geriatrics, 19*, 1–20.

Eaton, M., Mitchell-Bonair, I. L., & Friedmann, E. (1986). The effect of touch on nutritional intake of chronic organic brain syndrome patients. *Journal of Gerontology, 41*, 611–616.

Hall, G. R., & Buckwalter, K. C. (1987). Progressively lowered stress threshold: A conceptual model for care of adults with Alzheimer's disease. *Archives of Psychiatric Nursing, 1*, 399–406.

Hoffman, B. F. (1990). Assessing the competence of people to consent to medical treatment: a balance between law and medicine. *Medicine & Law, 9*, 1122–30.

Hornbrook, M. C., Stevens, V. J., Wingfield, D. J., Hollis, J. F., Greenlick, M. R., & Ory M. G. (1994). Preventing falls among community-dwelling older persons: Results from a randomized trial. *The Gerontologist, 34*, 16–23.

Levy L. L. (1987, Winter). Psychosocial intervention and dementia: The cognitive disability perspective, part 2. *Occupational Therapy in Mental Health, 7*(4), 13–36.

Mace N. L. (1987, Spring). Principles of activities for persons with dementia. *Physical and Occupational Therapy in Geriatrics, 5*(3), 13–27.

Mattes, R. D. (1987). Sensory influences on food intake and utilization in humans. *Human Nutrition–Applied Nutrition, 41*, 77–95.

Shaw, F. E., Bond, J., Richardson, D. A., Dawson, P., Steen, I. N., McKeith, I. G., Kenny, R. A. (2003, Jan. 11). Multifactorial intervention after a fall in older people with cognitive impairment and dementia presenting to the accident and emergency department: Randomised controlled trial. *British Medical Journal, 326*(7380), 73–75.

Smith D., & Newman D. K. (1991, Aug.). Nursing management of urinary incontinence associated with Alzheimer's disease. *Journal of Home Health Care Practice, 3*(4), 25–32.

Swanson, E. A., Maas, M. L., & Buckwalter, K. C. (1993). Catastrophic reactions and other behaviors of Alzheimer's residents: Special unit compared with traditional units. *Archives of Psychiatric Nursing, 7*, 292–299.

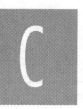

Resource List of Professional Organizations for Families and Health Professionals

Resource List of Professional Organizations for Families and Health Professionals

Organization	Web Site	Phone Number
Alzheimer's Association	www.alz.org	(800) 272-3900
Alzheimer's Disease Education & Referral Center	www.alzheimers.org	(800) 438-4380
Alzheimer's Store	www.alzstore.com	(800) 752-3238
Association for Frontotemporal Dementias	www.ftd-picks.org	
Caregivers Marketplace	www.caregiversmarketplace.com	(866) 327-8340
Children of Aging Parents	www.CAPS4caregivers.org	(800) 227-7294
Eldercare Locator	www.eldercare.gov	(800) 677-1116
Family Caregiver Alliance	www.caregiver.org	(800) 445-8106
National Association of Area Agencies on Aging	www.n4a.org	(202) 872-0888
National Family Caregivers Association	www.nfcacares.org	(800) 896-3650
National Parkinson Foundation	www.Parkinson.org	(800) 327-4545
National Resource Center on Supportive Housing and Home Modification	www.homemods.org	
National Stroke Association	www.stroke.org	(800) 787-6537
Well Spouse Foundation	www.wellspouse.org	(800) 838-0879

D

Home Environmental Skill-Building Program Road Map

Open the Contact

- Introduce yourself and your role.
- Provide road map for contact.
- Confirm that CG agrees and understands.

- Ask open-ended questions:
  - "Tell me about your day."
  - "How is it now vs. before?"
- Listen carefully without judgment.
- Summarize and reflect on what CG says.
- Express empathy, and validate when appropriate.

Negotiate the Agenda

- Identify problem areas using CAMP and open-ended questions.
- Offer options, and share how you view the situation.

- Elicit CG choice:
  - "What would you like to work on first?"
  - "What area is most upsetting, or what would you like to learn to handle better?"

Explore Cultural Values and Treatment Goals

- What would CG like to see happen?
- What is CG willing to change?
- What is CG's management style?
- What are CR's capabilities?
- What are the environmental supports and barriers?

Assess CG Readiness

1. Precontemplation
2. Contemplation
3. Preparation
4. Action and maintenance

Ask self:
- Why a 3, not a 2?
- What would need to be in place to move 1 to 2, 2 to 3, 3 to 4?

Tailor the Strategies

1 = Not ready
- Raise awareness.
- Make CG comfortable.
- Encourage and validate.

- Start with basic education about dementia.
- Ask, "How can I help you?"
- Ask, "What are you interested in learning or knowing more about?"
- Ask, "What would make your situation better?"

2 = Unsure
- Evaluate ambivalence.
- Determine if CG accepts role.
- Build readiness.

- Ask, "What is your immediate concern?"
- Ask, "What do you see as your next steps?"
- Ask, "What are you thinking about or feeling at this point?"
- Summarize as appropriate.

3–4 = Ready
- Strengthen understanding.
- Name and frame problem areas.
- Negotiate a plan.

- Problem solve characteristics of targeted problem.
- Identify treatment goal.
- Brainstorm potential strategies.
- Emphasize choice, and identify agreed on strategies.
- Instruct in strategy use.
- Role-play, practice new strategies, refine older strategies.

Close the Contact

- Review key contact activities and points.
- Express confidence in CG.

- Validate CG's capabilities.
- Specify homework (e.g., which strategies to practice and when).
- Arrange for next contact.

Note. CG = caregiver, CR = care recipient.

Articles by the Authors on or Related to Occupational Therapy and Family Caregiving

Corcoran, M. (2004). *Advanced occupational therapy for individuals with dementia* (Online Course). Bethesda, MD: American Occupational Therapy Association (with George Washington University).

Corcoran, M. (2004). *Fundamentals of occupational therapy for individuals with dementia* (Online Course). Bethesda, MD: American Occupational Therapy Association (with George Washington University).

Corcoran, M. (2004). *Occupational therapy for family, professional and paraprofessional caregivers.* (Online Course). Bethesda, MD: American Occupational Therapy Association (with George Washington University).

Corcoran, M., & Gitlin, L. N. (1997). The role of the physical environment in occupational performance. In C. H. Christiansen & M. C. Baum (Eds.), *Occupational therapy: Achieving human performance needs in daily living* (2nd ed., pp. 336–360). Thorofare, NJ: Slack.

Corcoran, M., & Gitlin, L. N. (2001). Family caregiver acceptance and use of environmental strategies in occupational therapy intervention. *Physical and Occupational Therapy in Geriatrics, 19*(1), 1–20.

Corcoran, M. A., Gitlin, L. N., Levy, L., Echkardt, S., Vause Earland, T., Shaw, G., et al. (2002). An occupational therapy home-based intervention to address dementia-related problems identified by family caregivers. *Alzheimer's Care Quarterly, 3,* 82–89.

Cornman-Levy, D., Gitlin, L. N., Corcoran, M., & Schinfeld, S. (2001). Caregiver aches and pains: The role of physical therapy in helping families provide daily care. *Alzheimer's Care Quarterly, 2,* 47–55.

Cotter, E. M., Burgio, L. D., Stevens, A. B., Roth, D. L., & Gitlin, L. N. (2001). Correspondence of the functional independence measure (FIM) self-care subscale with real-tine observations of dementia patients' ADL performance in the home. *Clinical Rehabilitation, 16,* 38–47.

Gitlin, L. N. (1998). Testing home modification interventions: Issues of theory, measurement, design, and implementation. In R. Schulz, M. P. Lawton, & G. Maddox (Eds.), *Annual review of gerontology and geriatrics. Intervention research with older adults* (pp. 190–246). New York: Springer.

Gitlin, L. N. (2000). Adjusting person-environment systems: Helping older people live the good life at home. In R. Rubenstein, M. Moss, & M. Kleban (Eds.), *The many faces of aging: Essays in honor of M.P. Lawton* (pp. 41–54). New York: Springer.

Gitlin, L. N., & Corcoran, M. (2000). Making homes safer: Environmental adaptations for people with dementia. *Alzheimer's Care Quarterly, 1,* 50–58.

Gitlin, L. N., Corcoran, M., Martindale-Adams, J., Malone, C., Stevens, A., & Winter, L. (2000). Identifying mechanisms of action: Why and how does intervention work? In R. Schulz (Ed.), *Handbook on dementia caregiving: Evidence-based interventions for family caregivers* (pp. 225–248). New York: Springer.

Gitlin L. N., Corcoran, M., Winter, L., Boyce, A., & Hauck, W. (2001). A randomized, controlled trial of a home environmental intervention: Effect on efficacy and upset in caregivers and on daily function of persons with dementia. *The Gerontologist, 41,* 4–14.

Gitlin, L. N., Corcoran, M., Winter, L., Boyce, A., & Marcus, S. (1999). Predicting participation and adherence to a home environmental intervention among family caregivers of dementia patients. *Family Relations, 48,* 363–372.

Gitlin, L. N., & Gywther, L. P. (2003). In-home interventions: Helping caregivers where they live. In D. Coon, D. Gallagher-Thompson, & L. Thompson (Eds.), *Innovative interventions to reduce caregiver distress: A clinical guide* (pp. 139–160). New York: Springer.

Gitlin, L. N., Hauck, W. W., Dennis, M. P., & Winter, L. (in press). Long-term effects of the Home Environmental Skill-Building Program for families caring for persons with Alzheimer's disease and related disorders. *Journal of Gerontology: Medical Sciences.*

Gitlin, L. N., Liebman, J., & Winter, L. (2003). Are environmental interventions effective in the management of Alzheimer's disease and related disorders? A synthesis of the evidence. *Alzheimer Care Quarterly, 4,* 85–107.

Gitlin, L. N., Schinfeld, S., Winter, L., Corcoran, M., & Hauck, W. (2002). Evaluating home environments of person with dementia: Interrater reliability and validity of the home environmental assessment protocol (HEAP). *Disability and Rehabilitation, 24,* 59–71.

Gitlin, L. N., Winter, L., Corcoran, M., Dennis, M., Schinfeld, S., & Hauck, W. (2003). Effects of the Home Environmental Skill-Building Program on the caregiver-care recipient dyad: Six-month outcomes from the Philadelphia REACH initiative. *The Gerontologist, 43,* 532–546.

Gitlin, L. N., Winter, L., Dennis, M., Corcoran, M., Schinfeld, S., & Hauck, W. (2002). Strategies used by families to simplify tasks for individuals with Alzheimer's disease and related disorders: Psychometric analysis of the task management strategy index (TMSI). *The Gerontologist, 42,* 61–69.

Shaw, G., Kearney, P. J., Vause Earland, T., & Eckhardt, S. M. (2003, March). Managing dementia-related behaviors. *Home and Community Health Special Interest Section Quarterly, 10,* 1–3.

Toth-Cohen, S., Gitlin, L. N., Corcoran, M., Eckhardt, S., Johns, P., & Lipsett, R. (2001). Providing services to family caregivers at home: Challenges and recommendations for health and human service professions. *Alzheimer's Care Quarterly, 2,* 23–32.

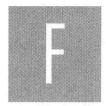

Key Equipment Considerations

Susan I. Klein, MA, Director, Housing Department and George Russell, Housing Program Manager, Philadelphia Corporation for Aging

Highlighted below are key considerations in recommending and/or ordering and installing the most common equipment offered in ESP to assist family caregivers, individuals with dementia, or members of the household.

A. GRAB BARS

1. Type of Grab Bar
- Knurled chrome grab bars are the standard. Grab bars should be a different color than the wall or tile in which it is placed and should be textured. Smooth grab bars will get slippery if a hand is wet and soapy.
- Grab bars come in a variety of sizes.
- Durable Medical Equipment (DME) providers can provide clamp-on grab bars for modern bathtubs.

2. Tub and Surrounding Area
- Ceramic tile may crack during wall-mounted grab bar installation. Make sure the homeowner, caregiver, or any interested party is aware of this. Consider a tub bench or tub seat with armrest instead of a clamp-on grab bar if this will be a problem.
- Fiberglass or other prefabricated tub surround walls probably *will* crack if drilled.

---

3. Installation

- Grab bars should be installed by professionals. They need to be solidly and securely installed into a stud or other backing. The installer needs to be aware of location of water pipes or other hazards. The purpose of grab bars is to prevent falls, and grab bars may have to tolerate significant pressure.

4. Size and Location

- Standard grab bar sizes are 18" and 24" lengths, but other sizes are available. There are some plastic pipe grab bars that can be used for custom sizes.
- Standard installation is a 24" grab bar on the inside tub wall (wall across from the opening—where the soap dish usually is located) and an 18" grab bar on the outside corner of the front wall (front wall is where the faucets are located).
- An occupational therapist should mark approximate locations with masking tape and instruct consumer or caregiver not to remove tape until bar is installed.
- Installation instructions should include
  - A. Size of grab bar
  - B. Location (which wall)
  - C. Direction (horizontal, diagonal, vertical)
  - D. Location measurements
- Example:
  Install 24" diagonal grab bar on inside tub wall, top 10" from front tub wall and 12" from top of tub, bottom 6" from top of tub. Marked with tape.
- Grab bars may also be placed next to toilets, doorjambs, or stairway elevators.

B. TUB SEATS, BOARDS, AND BENCHES

1. Type of Bathtub

- Old-fashioned tubs (cast iron, on claw feet) require different seats and boards than modern tubs.

2. Seats, Stools, and Benches

- Consider size and weight of the consumer.
- Does seat or bench need a back? (Stools don't have backs by definition.)
- Does the consumer need a padded seat or bench, or will molded plastic be sufficient?

- Does seat or bench need cutout?
- Does seat or bench need armrest?
- Does seat or bench need adjustable legs or extension legs?
- If ordering a transfer bench, discuss use of shower curtains and bench with caregiver to minimize wet floors. Caregiver can cut curtain around bench, which may reduce problem but will not solve it.
- Step stools with handles may help the consumer in/out of tub.

3. Tub Boards

- Tub boards rest on rim of tub.
- Will a clamp-on grab bar interfere with use of tub board?
- Is the consumer at risk for slipping and/or falling from tub board?
- Will tub board support consumer's weight and size?

C. HANDHELD SHOWERS AND SHOWER CURTAINS

- Handheld showers can be installed at existing overhead showers or from tub faucets. Overhead installation is appropriate if a caregiver will be helping the consumer to bathe. Faucet installation is appropriate if the consumer will be using a tub seat. Diverters are attached in either case.
- "Hook" for handheld showers attached to faucets is normally about 4" above the rim of the tub. If this is problematic, an occupational therapist can specify another location.
- Some handheld showers are installed on a rod so they can slide up and down depending on use.
- If a handheld shower is being installed, be sure there is a shower curtain rod and curtain(s) that can be used. Sometimes more than one curtain is needed. Be sure that water will not spill onto the bathroom floor.

D. RAISED TOILET SEATS, HANDICAP TOILETS, AND SAFETY FRAMES

- Consider who else will be using the toilet when ordering a raised toilet seat. Donut models are easier for others to remove, whereas types with clamps and armrests are sturdier for consumer.
- Consider replacing toilet with handicap-height toilet (16" high).
- Toilet safety frames mount to the toilet seat hinge and can be installed on regular or handicap-height toilets.
- Grab bars can be wall mounted next to toilets (horizontal, vertical, or diagonal) and "hinged" grab bars can be floor mounted. The "hinged" grab bars flip from horizontal to vertical positions.
- If bathroom floor is in disrepair, it may not be possible to replace a regular toilet with a handicap-height toilet without extensive plumbing work.

E. HOSPITAL BEDS AND RAILS

- Medicare may pay for hospital beds with one of the following conditions:
  1. Physician's approval
  2. Aspiration precaution
  3. Would decrease caregiver burden
- To assist the consumer getting out of bed, consider a bed assist and bed bars. There are two types: one is attached to plywood and slipped between the mattress and the box spring when the bed is supported with wood slats; the other is clamped on to the bed frame when the bed is supported with metal springs.

F. LIGHTING

- Consider motion detectors, three-way switches, and night-lights.

G. RAILINGS

- Indicate left or right ascending.
- Consider remaining space on the stairway. If railing takes up 5" of space, is remaining space sufficient for consumer and others using stairway?
- If railing extends beyond stairway, specify by length and location (top or bottom).
- If outside railing, is a separate railing needed for each flight or a continuous railing to include landings?
- If continuous outside railing, is a gate needed for access to lawn or alley?
- If outside, and the railing requested is on steps shared with neighbor, the railing can only be installed on consumer's side of steps. Railings cannot be installed in the middle of these stairways.
- If outside, and the railing requested is on steps leading to door, railing should be on "latch" side of door. (Railing on "hinge" side of door would be blocked when door opens.)
- Interior railings on masonry (concrete, brick, etc.) walls will be wrought iron. Railings on stud or plaster walls will be wood.

H. SEAT LIFT CHAIRS

- Seat lift chairs cost approximately $500.00.
- Lift chairs require a working receptacle (electrical outlet).
- Consider instructing the caregiver to place remote control in side pocket of chair so consumer doesn't play with it.

- Lift chairs assist consumer or caregiver in bringing consumer from sitting to standing position.
- Lift chairs are available in a variety of colors and in cloth or vinyl (for incontinence).

I. RAMPS

- For each inch of rise (height), a ramp must have one foot of run (length). A "landing area" is also needed at the top and bottom of the ramp, preferably 5'. Therefore, if a house has 3 cement steps (8" each) from the sidewalk to the front door, the ramp would have to be 24" in length with a 5' platform at the top and 5' of clear space at the bottom. In most homes in Philadelphia, ramping is not possible.
- Some properties might be accommodated if the house is set far back from the sidewalk and has few steps or if the property has a side exit or alley.
- Portable ramps tend to be too heavy for most caregivers. A 66" portable ramp weighs at least 42 pounds. When they are used because there isn't enough room for a regular ramp, they also tend to be too steep to be used easily.
- If there is a porch, the floor can be raised to meet the front door threshold. This allows the consumer to interact with people on the street, although it does not help the wheelchair user to leave the home.
- When installing a ramp, it is recommended that a lip is installed on both sides. A full railing in addition to the lip is preferred.

J. INTERCOMS

- Intercoms are effective for two-way communication. Baby monitors are more effective for monitoring.
- Intercoms can be installed with or without door releases (buzzers). Door releases usually decrease the security of the door since the consumer cannot use the deadbolt lock if he/she wants to be able to "buzz" someone in.
- Interior stations are usually wall mounted. They can be placed on a table (still wired), but this is only appropriate for very careful caregivers and consumers since spilling something on them or dropping them easily damages the unit.
- Intercoms require fine motor control to use. The buttons are small, close together, and must be pressed and held while talking. They are delicate mechanisms, and people forget how to use the different buttons despite written instructions.

K. STAIRWAY ELEVATORS

1. Consumer Qualifications
- Has severe difficulty ascending/descending stairs
- Often complains about discomfort associated with stairs
- Limits trips up/down steps to 4 or fewer times a day
- Has had a fall associated with ascending/descending stairs
- Needs to conserve energy
- Is not fearful and is receptive to use
- User weighs less than 250 pounds
- User has normal muscle tone and range of motion in major joints
- User willing to accept stairway elevator in his/her home
- User will be able to get on and off stairway elevator by themselves or with caregiver's assistance

2. Structural Qualifications
- Steps are in good condition.
- Steps are minimum of 30" wide.
- Top and bottom landings are large enough for stairway elevator to come to stop (30" x 30").
- There is a banister opposite the stairway elevator.
- Portion of stairway for stairway elevator is straight.
- A receptacle must be available within 6' of the top or bottom of steps.

3. Considerations
- Stairway elevators take up about 1/2 the width of the stairway. Non-riders must be able to use the stairway with the remaining space.
- Consumers who use wheelchairs need wheelchairs at top and bottom of the stairway.
- Stairway elevators have seatbelts.
- Stairway elevators are considered "attractive nuisances" to children. Consider this when ordering for a household with young children.
- Front-riding stairway elevators swivel at the top of the steps. User must be able to use hand on open side of stairway to operate swivel latch.

The information in this appendix is for general information purposes only. Qualified professionals should be consulted for advice concerning any specific circumstances and any building codes and other codes and other requirements applicable to a particular locality.

Index

Page number in *italics* refer to tables and figures; page numbers in **bold** refer to exhibits.

About the Contributors

Yeon Kyung Chee, PhD, research associate, Center for Applied Research on Aging and Health, Jefferson College of Health Professions, Thomas Jefferson University, Philadelphia

Mary A. Corcoran, PhD, OTR/L, FAOTA, research professor, Department of Health Care Sciences, George Washington University, Washington, DC; professor, Division of Occupational Therapy, Shenandoah University

Laura N. Gitlin, PhD, research sociologist; professor, Department of Occupational Therapy; director, Center for Applied Research on Aging and Health, Jefferson College of Health Professions, Thomas Jefferson University

Pamalyn Kearney, MS, OTR/L, assistant professor, Department of Occupational Therapy, University of the Sciences in Philadelphia; occupational therapy interventionist for ESP

Rosalyn S. Lipsitt, MHL, OTR/L, assistant professor, Department of Occupational Therapy, Temple University, Philadelphia; occupational therapy interventionist for ESP

Geri Shaw, OTR/L, independent contractor and home health care occupational therapist, Bensalem, PA; occupational therapy interventionist for ESP

Susan Toth-Cohen, PhD, OTR/L, associate professor, Department of Occupational Therapy, and research associate, Center for Applied Research on Aging and Health, Jefferson College of Health Professions, Thomas Jefferson University, Philadelphia

Tracey Vause Earland, MS, OTR/L, clinical coordinator, Center for Applied Research on Aging and Health, Thomas Jefferson University; occupational therapist, Genesis Health Ventures; instructor, Philadelphia University; occupational therapy interventionist for ESP